CYTOTOXIC ANTICANCER DRUGS: MODELS AND CONCEPTS FOR DRUG DISCOVERY AND DEVELOPMENT

DEVELOPMENTS IN ONCOLOGY

36. D.E. Peterson, G.E. Elias and S.T. Sonis, eds: Head and Neck Management of the Cancer Patient. 0–89838–747–7.
37. D.M. Green: Diagnosis and Management of Malignant Solid Tumors in Infants and Children. 0–89838–750–7.
38. K.A. Foon and A.C. Morgan, Jr., eds.: Monoclonal Antibody Therapy of Human Cancer. 0–89838–754–X.
39. J.G. McVie, W. Bakker, Sj.Sc. Wagenaar and D. Carney, eds.: Clinical and Experimental Pathology of Lung Cancer. 0–89838–764–7.
40. K.V. Honn, W.E. Powers and B.F. Sloane, eds.: Mechanisms of Cancer Metastasis. 0–89838–765–5.
41. K. Lapis, L.A. Liotta and A.S. Rabson, eds.: Biochemistry and Molecular Genetics of Cancer Metastasis. 0–89838–785–X.
42. A.J. Mastromarino, ed.: Biology and Treatment of Colorectal Cancer Metastasis. 0–89838–786–8.
43. M.A. Rich, J.C. Hager and J. Taylor-Papadimitriou, eds.: Breast Cancer: Origins, Detection and Treatment. 0–89838–792–2.
44. D.G. Poplack, L. Massimo and P. Cornaglia-Ferraris, eds.: The Role of Pharmacology in Pediatric Oncology. 0–89838–795–7.
45. A. Hagenbeek and B. Löwenberg, eds.: Minimal. Residual Disease in Acute Leukemia. 0–89838–799–X.
46. F.M. Muggia and M. Rozencweig, eds.: Clinical Evaluation of Antitumor Therapy. 0–89838–803–1.
47. F.A. Valeriote and L. Baker, eds.: Biochemical Modulation of Anticancer Agents: Experimental and Clinical Approaches. 0–89838–827–9.
48. B.A. Stoll, ed.: Pointers to Cancer Prognosis. 0–89838–841–4; Pb. 0–89838–876–7.
49. K.H. Hollmann and J.M. Verley, eds.: New Frontiers in Mammary Pathology. 0–89838–852–X.
50. D.J. Ruiter, G.J. Fleuren and S.O. Warnaar, eds.: Application of Monoclonal Antibodies in Tumor Pathology. 0–89838–853–8.
51. A.H.G. Paterson and A.W. Lees, eds.: Fundamental Problems in Breast Cancer. 0–89838–863–5.
52. M. Chatel, F. Darcel and J. Pecker, eds.: Brain Oncology, Biology, Diagnosis and Therapy. 0–89838–954–2.
53. M.P. Hacker, J.S. Lazo and T.R. Tritton, eds.: Organ Directed Toxicities of Anticancer Drugs. 0–89838–356–0.
54. M. Nicolini, ed.: Platinum and Other Metal Coordination Compounds in Cancer Chemotherapy. 0–89838–358–7.
55. J.R. Ryan and L.O. Baker, eds.: Recent Concepts in Sarcoma Treatment. 0–89838–376–5.
56. M.A. Rich, J.C. Hager and D.M. Lopez, eds.: Breast Cancer: Scientific and Clinical Progress. 0–89838–387–0.
57. B.A. Stoll, ed.: Women at High Risk to Breast Cancer. 0–89838–416–8.
58. M.A. Rich, J.C. Hager and I. Keydar, eds.: Breast Cancer. Progress in Biology, Clinical Management and Prevention. 0–7923–0507–8.
59. P.I. Reed, M. Carboni, B.J. Johnston and S. Guadagni, eds.: New Trends in Gastric Cancer. Background and Videosurgery. 0–7923–8917–4.
60. H.K. Awwad: Radiation Oncology: Radiobiological and Physiological Perspectives. The Boundary-Zone between Clinical Radiotherapy and Fundamental Radiobiology and Physiology. 0–7923–0783–6.
61. J.L. Evelhoch, W. Negendank, F.A. Valeriote and L.H. Baker, eds.: Magnetic Resonance in Experimental and Clinical Oncology. 0–7923–0935–9.
62. B.A. Stoll, ed.: Approaches to Breast Cancer Prevention. 0–7923–0995–2.
63. M.J. Hill and A. Giacosa, eds.: Causation and Prevention of Human Cancer. 0–7923–1084–5.
64. J.R.W. Masters, ed.: Human Cancer in Primary Culture. A Handbook. 0–7923–1088–8.
65. N. Kobayashi, T. Akera and S. Mizutani, eds.: Childhood Leukemia. Present Problems and Future Prospects. 0–7923–1138–8.
66. P. Padetti, K. Takakura, M.D. Walker, G. Butti and S. Pezzota, eds.: Neuro-Oncology. 0–7923–1215–5.

CYTOTOXIC ANTICANCER DRUGS: MODELS AND CONCEPTS FOR DRUG DISCOVERY AND DEVELOPMENT

Proceedings of the
Twenty-Second Annual Cancer Symposium
Detroit, Michigan, USA - April 26–28, 1990

edited by

Frederick A. Valeriote
Thomas H. Corbett
Laurence H. Baker

Wayne State University School of Medicine
Detroit, Michigan

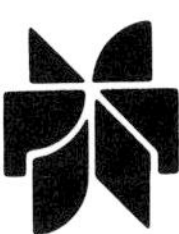

Kluwer Academic Publishers
Boston / Dordrecht / London

Distributors for North America:
Kluwer Academic Publishers
101 Philip Drive
Assinippi Park
Norwell, Massachusetts 02061 USA

Distributors for all other countries:
Kluwer Academic Publishers Group
Distribution Centre
Post Office Box 322
3300 AH Dordrecht, THE NETHERLANDS

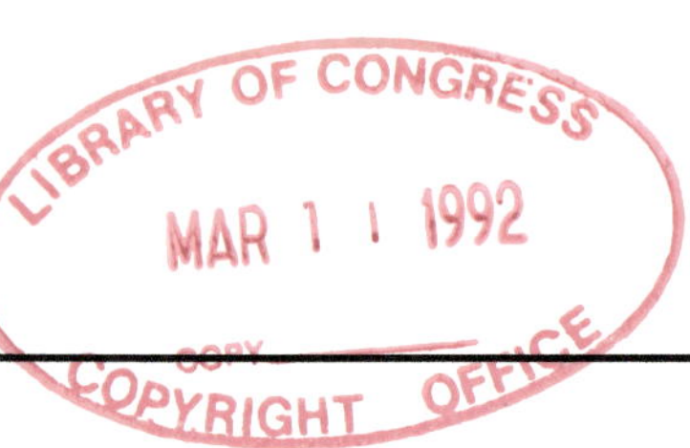

Library of Congress Cataloging-in-Publication Data

Detroit Cancer Symposium (22nd : 1990)
    Cytotoxic anticancer drugs : models and concepts for drug
discovery and development : proceedings of the Twenty-Second Annual
Detroit Cancer Symposium, Detroit, Michigan, USA., April 26–28, 1990
/ edited by Frederick A. Valeriote, Thomas H. Corbett, Laurence H.
Baker.
        p.   cm. — (Developments in oncology : 68)
    Includes bibliographical references.
    ISBN 0–7923–1629–0
    1. Antineoplastic agents—Congresses.   I. Valeriote, Frederick.
II. Corbett, Thomas H.   III. Baker, Laurence H.   IV. Title.
V. Series.
    [DNLM: 1. Antineoplastic Agents—congresses.   2. Drug Design-
-congresses.   3. Pharmacology, Clinical—congresses.   4. Technology,
Pharmaceutical—congresses.   W1 DE998N v. 68]
    RC271.C5D49   1990
    616.99'4061—dc20
    DNLM/DLC
    for Library of Congress   92-3035
                                                                                      CIP

CONTENTS

David S. Alberts, M.D.
Section of Hematology-Oncology
Department of Medicine
Medical College
University of Arizona
Tucson, AZ 85724

Kenneth Bair, Ph.D.
Burroughs-Wellcome
Div. of Organic Chemistry
3030 Cornwallis Road
Research Triangle Park, NC 27709

Laurence Baker, D.O.
Div. Hematology and Oncology
Wayne State University
5 Hudson, Harper Hospital
P.O. Box 02188
Detroit, MI 48201

Andy Barker, Ph.D.
ICI Pharmaceuticals
Mereside Alderley Park
Macclesfield, Cheshire
UK 104TGG

Bijoy K. Bhuyan, Ph.D.
Cancer Research
The Upjohn Company
Kalamazoo, MI 49001

Marie-Christine Bissery, Ph.D.
Anticancer Research Programme
Rhone-Poulenc
Centre de Recherches de Vitry
13 quai Jules Guesde
B.P. 14 - 94403 Vitry Sur Seine
Cedex, FRANCE

Michael Boyd, M.D., Ph.D.
Developmental Therapeutics
Executive Plaza North, Room 843
Division of Cancer Treatment
National Cancer Institute
Bethesda, MD 20892

Paul Cavanaugh, Jr., Ph.D.
Eastman Pharmaceuticals
Division of Eastman Kodak Company
9 Great Valley Parkway
Great Valley Corporate Center
Great Valley, PA 19355

Thomas Corbett, Ph.D.
Div. Hematology and Oncology
Wayne State University
418 Hudson, Harper Hospital
P.O. Box 02188
Detroit, MI 48201

Daniel Dexter, Ph.D.
Medical Products
E.I. Dupont de Nemours & Co.
Glenolden Laboratory
500 South Ridgeway Avenue
Glenolden, PA 19036

Dr. Terrence Doyle
Pharmaceutical Research
    and Development
Bristol-Myers Company
536 Research Parkway
Wallingford, CT 06492

Paul Fischer, Ph.D.
Pfizer Inc.
Pfizer Central Research
Eastern Point Road
Groton, CT 06340

Michael Friedman, M.D.
Cancer Therapy Evaluation Program
Division of Cancer Treatment
National Cancer Institute
National Institutes of Health
Executive Plaza North, Room #742
Bethesda, MD 20892

Charles Grieshaber, Ph.D.
Toxicology Branch
Developmental Therapeutics Program
Division of Cancer Treatment, NCI
843 Executive Plaza North
Bethesda, MD 20892

Fred Hausheer, M.D.
Cancer Therapy and Research Center
4450 Medical Drive
San Antonio, Texas 78229

George Johnson, Ph.D.
Grants & Contracts Operations Branch
Executive Plaza North, Room 830B
Developmental Therapeutics Program
Division of Cancer Treatment
National Cancer Institute
Bethesda, MD 20892

Dick Leopold, Ph.D.
Tumor Biology Section
Pharmaceutical Research Division
Warner Lambert/Parke Davis
2800 Plymouth Road
Ann Arbor, MI 48105

Jacob J. Lokich, M.D.
The Cancer Center
125 Parker Hill Avenue
Boston, MA 02120

John Murphy, Ph.D.
Dept. of Biomolecular Medicine
Boston University
University Hospital
Evans Building, Suite 613
88 East Newton Street
Boston, MA 02118

Dr. Kenneth Paull
National Institutes of Health
Executive Plaza North
Room 811
6130 Executive Blvd.
Bethesda, MD 20892

Carl Porter, Ph.D.
Dept. of Experimental Therapeutics
Grace Cancer Drug Center
Roswell Park Memorial Institute
666 Elm Street
Buffalo, NY 14263

Lawrence Rubinstein, Ph.D.
National Institutes of Health
Executive Plaza North
Room 739
6130 Executive Blvd.
Bethesda, MD 20892

Matthew Suffness, Ph.D.
Executive Plaza North, Room #832
Developmental Therapeutics Program
Division of Cancer Treatment
National Cancer Institute
Bethesda, MD 20892

Raymond Taetle, M.D.
Department of Pathology
Univ. of California, San Diego
Medical Center
225 Dickinson Street
San Diego, CA 92103

Manuel Valdivieso, M.D.
Div. Hematology and Oncology
Wayne State University
5-Hudson, Harper Hospital
P.O. Box 02188
Detroit, MI 48201

Frederick Valeriote, Ph.D.
Div. Hematology and Oncology
Wayne State University
418 Hudson, Harper Hospital
P.O. Box 02188
Detroit, MI 48201

Daniel D. Von Hoff, M.D.
Department of Medicine
Division of Oncology
University of Texas Health
    Science Center
7703 Floyd Curl Drive
San Antonio, TX 78284

Wendell Wierenga, Ph.D.
The Upjohn Company
7000 Portage Road
Kalamazoo, MI 49001

ACKNOWLEDGMENTS

Major funding for this Symposium was obtained from:

- The Public Health Service under grant # 1R13 CA-52454
  from the National Cancer Institute, DHHS.
- Harper-Grace Hospitals
- Wayne State University Ben Kasle Trust for Cancer
  Research
- Meyer L. Prentis Comprehensive Cancer Center of Metro-
  politan Detroit

Generous support from the following donors were critical to
the success of this Symposium:

- Glaxo Pharmaceuticals (Division of Glaxo, Inc.)
- MeadJohnson Oncology Products (Division of Bristol-Myers)
- Schering Laboratories
- Sterling Drug, Inc. (Subsidiary of Eastman Kodak Company)
- Upjohn Company

Editorial assistance and typing was provided by Ms. Linda
Leino, Ms. Loretta Lisow, Ms. Sandy Essenmacher and Mr. Darren
Lisow.

CYTOTOXIC ANTICANCER DRUGS: MODELS AND CONCEPTS FOR DRUG DISCOVERY AND DEVELOPMENT

1

DRUG DISCOVERY - 1990

Frederick Valeriote, Thomas Corbett and Laurence Baker

This is the first of what we hope will become a regular meeting held on the alternate years of the EORTC-NCI joint European (Amsterdam) meeting. Our focus is on the presentation and discussion of cytotoxic agents, with a significant portion of the Symposium to include the exciting frontiers of drug discovery being explored by the National Cooperative Drug Discovery Groups (NCDDG) Program. Like most areas of cancer research, cytotoxic research has gone through its ups and downs. A few years ago, with the lack of active agents coming through the pipeline, together with the excitement concerning new modalities and new approaches such as biological response modifiers, immuno-conjugates, hyperthermia, radiation sensitizers, biochemical modulation and antisense therapy, both expectation about finding new cytotoxics, and subsequently funding, waned and the number of new cytotoxics declined significantly. We are now observing a redressing of this problem and a more balanced national approach. Of significance this year has been the initiation of renewed efforts in the area of natural product drug discovery. While the entire field of Developmental Therapeutics (including both Exper-imental and Clinical Therapeutics) has many potentials for dis-covery of curative therapy, the area of discovery of new cyto-toxics is particularly promising at present.

There have been a number of major changes during the past decade in research on drug discovery of cytotoxic agents. For over 30 years, from the inception of an organized drug discovery program, murine leukemia cells (specifically P388 and L1210 lymphocytic leukemias) _in vivo_ or KB cells _in vitro_ were the foci and funnel of cytotoxic research programs which not only discovered new active agents but also defined the direction of analog synthesis. Increased therapeutic efficacy was defined in terms of greater increase in lifespan of the leukemia-bearing mice at the drug's maximal tolerated dosage. The success of this program can be assessed by the discovery of a host of agents active against lymphocytic leukemia and lymphoma. By the standard of the murine leukemia models finding drugs effective against the human tumor counterparts, the program was successful. The frustration and subsequent decline in funding of the program resulted not from having cured human leukemias but from its inability to discover major leads against human solid tumors. Cure rates for cancers of the lung, breast, colon and pancreas did not seem to budge following treatment with the alphabet soup of drugs which became available from this leukemia-based drug discovery program.

The poor record of discovery of new structural leads during the 1970's, and especially the dearth of agents active against solid tumors, led to a re-thinking of the underlying screen. As evidenced by the first two presentations in this Symposium, a radical break with the past occurred in the early 1980's and emphasizes the present screening philosophy: "You get what you fish for!" As shown in Figure 1A, if you use leukemia cells as your screening "bait", you will pull out antileukemic agents. Figure 1B, by analogy indicates that if you use solid tumors you will find agents active against solid tumors. Further, and most important, it seems that there may be little overlap between the specific compounds most effective against either tumor type.

Some investigators believed that since we are searching for agents active against human solid tumors, then the human tumors must be the bait on the hook. Use of human tumors directly from the patient has been attempted but is technically difficult and expensive for a primary screen. Also, there is a problem of reproducibility since each specimen is consumed quickly so that there is no "standard" from one run to the next. As discussed in this Symposium, their use in a Phase 2 setting is profitable. A

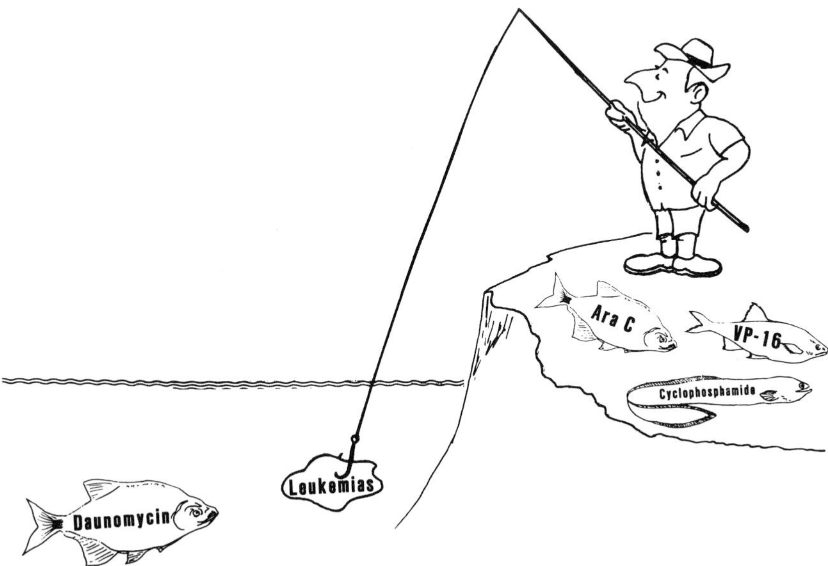

Figure 1A. Cartoon of present anticancer screening philosophy for antileukemic agents.

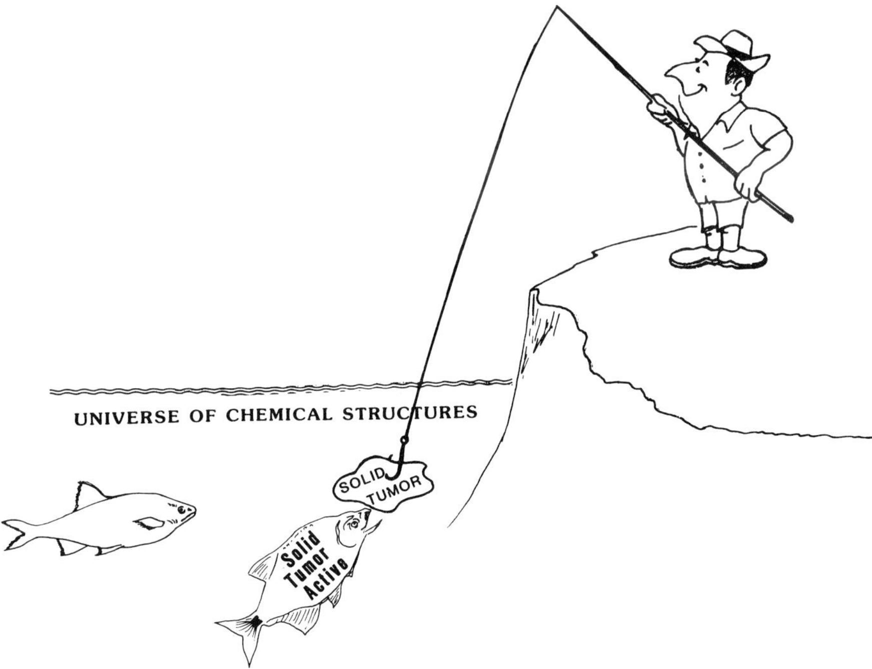

Figure 1B. Cartoon of present anticancer screening philosophy for solid tumor selective agents.

way around the primary screen problem for human tumors has been to use human solid tumor cell lines. Not only can a "standard" be maintained, but a variety of pathological types can be assessed so as to represent the heterogeneity of human tumors. However, a major problem here is that after many passages _in vitro_, the cell line may not represent the sensitivity of the original (or any) human tumor in situ. The advantages outweigh the disadvantages at the present time and NCI as well as many others have implemented the use of various sets of human tumor cell lines as the primary screen for new agents.

Subsequent testing of human cells _in vivo_ has been made possible through the development of immune-deficient mice (such as nude mice) in which the human tumor lines could grow as solid tumors. This _in vivo_ intermediary between the _in vitro_ screen and the clinical trial, whether xenografts in nude mice or, probably as important, standard murine solid tumors, is essential in experimental therapeutics. The critical factor of activity _in vivo_ which reflects a variety of components including drug passage across various physiological barriers, and the metabolism and toxicity of the agent must all be assessed with an aim of defining therapeutic effectiveness before being introduced into the clinic.

Besides using human solid tumor cell lines in the initial screen, another fruitful approach is to use standard murine solid tumor cells directly from mice. The advantage of this is that the _in vivo_ response is maintained, the standard tumors are very resistant to most known anticancer agents, and their biology and therapeutic response often parallel that of the corresponding human tumors.

In terms of the chemical structures themselves, there are two basic approaches to the search for agents: random screening and rational synthesis. In the case of random screening, there is little if any decisions made about the specific structures (or organisms) to be examined but rather any agent or extract in the universe of chemical compounds and organisms is a candidate for the screen. While this can be inefficient, its advantage is that it is the only effective way at the present time to obtain new and unique classes of agents in terms of mechanism of action.

Our Detroit experience to date with various chemical inventories is that with our _in vitro_ assay about 1% of randomly selected agents demonstrate sufficient solid tumor selectivity to proceed to _in vivo_ testing. Subsequently, about 1 in 20 of the _in vivo_ tests show significant antitumor activity. Of these, only a small fraction are considered potential clinical candidates; most represent leads for further analog searches and analog synthesis programs. Unfortunately, we don't yet know how many of such agents will have significant human tumor activity. If it is 1 in 5, then we can predict that each inventory of 20,000 different chemical structures, regardless of structural type, would contain an agent clinically active against some human solid tumor(s).

The second basic approach is rational synthesis in which case numerous structural analogs are synthesized around the lead or parent compound. This is a standard approach that has been made for nearly all compounds which appear to be going towards the clinic or demonstrate activity in the clinic. Large programs in the past which aim at synthesizing more effective analogs are typified by the nitrogen mustard series in which thousands of structural modifications were made but keeping the active moiety-the bis chlorethyl group. Also, the search for a better anthracycline has occupied the talents of a multitude of investigators synthesizing and testing thousands of compounds. Similar enterprises existed for the antifolates with aminopterin as the parent, the nucleoside analogs, and a number of other clinically active compounds.

Irrespective of the manner in which the chemical structure is presented to the laboratory for screening of activity, the screen itself must provide a target or vulnerability which will detect the desired biological activity. This "target-oriented" approach could be a cellular target (solid tumors) as defined by the Corbett and NCI models; or, it could be a biochemical or molecular

target. The latter are exemplified by an enzyme such as ribonucleotide reductase or topoisomerase I, or a structural protein
such as tubulin or laminin, or even a broad function such as DNA
repair, protein kinases, or specific gene shutoff with antisense
probes.

The problem with the cellular approach is that it is viewed
by many as very broad and not sufficiently selective (or rational). The problem with the specific target approach is that it is
very narrow in focus and is extremely inefficient in a broad-based
random screen. The problem with the functional approach is that
it is neither known nor often expected that inhibition of these
broad functions would lead to preferrential killing of tumor
cells.

For the non-cellular, specific-target approach, one often
begins with an active parent compound, and then institutes a large
analog synthesis program with appropriate structure-activity
relationships to obtain the best compound for eventual clinical
trial. Many of the presentations in this Symposium have taken
this molecular target-oriented approach with promising results.

In some cases, random screening is the only way to proceed,
for example with natural products. Here, one is not dealing with
inventories of known chemical products but rather with inventories
of organisms (from bacteria to plants) which contain storehouses
of many different structural classes. The screening assay is
critical in identifying an extract which might harbor an anticancer agent. A major problem with analysis of such extracts is
that they may contain more than one toxic substance which can
obfuscate the assay or even lead to a false negative classifica-
tion. The advantages of analyzing natural products is that the
structures that exist in a given bacteria, alga, marine organism
or plant are usually unknown, and are often difficult or impossible to synthesize and thus would never show up in the
chemist's test tube.

One note of caution about the bandwagon that many of us have
jumped on; the search for solid tumor active agents. This empha-

sis has had a negative impact on the search for new antileukemic agents. As with the bait for solid tumor actives, we can also examine a change of the lymphocytic leukemia bait for that of myelogenous leukemia or myeloma to try to fish out compounds active against these human diseases which have very high failure rates. The antileukemics certainly should not be overlooked especially since some of the new screening models are capable of identifying such leads as well.

There must be some concern for past inventories which have been screened for anticancer agents. If we are correct in our fishing hook concept then these inventories represent fertile ground for harvesting the solid tumor active agents. Also, there are large inventories in chemical and pharmaceutical companies which have yet to be systematically searched and likely contain active compounds as leads against many of the presently resistant cancers.

One major problem with large inventories is whether they can be pared down to a size sufficient for rapid testing. For example, with a chemical inventory of 100,000 compounds, testing 5,000 each year represents a 20-year project. The chemist's approach to this is to break the compounds into specific classes and screen only a "representative" number. However, it is our experience that we do not have sufficient knowledge to define what fraction of an inventory is sufficient to be representative of the entire inventory. If we examine 2,000 random compounds from an inventory, we predict that we will find an _in vivo_ murine solid tumor active agent. Certainly, if we examine analogs of that structure, then the fraction of _in vivo_ actives increases by at least an order of magnitude. However, if we take _any other_ set of 2,000 compounds from the inventory, we will, in an unpredictable manner, come up with another _in vivo_ active.

Thus, there probably is no way in which, even if 99% of an inventory is searched that we are assured that the remaining 1% does not contain a very active lead. One can use the concept of a gold mine as shown in Figure 2. While once you hit gold, analog synthesis will allow you to move up the seam with lots of actives, if you head off in a random direction you may eventually hit another vein or even the mother lode. The conclusion must be that at the present time, the vast majority, if not all, of an inventory needs to be tested to ensure that important leads are not excluded.

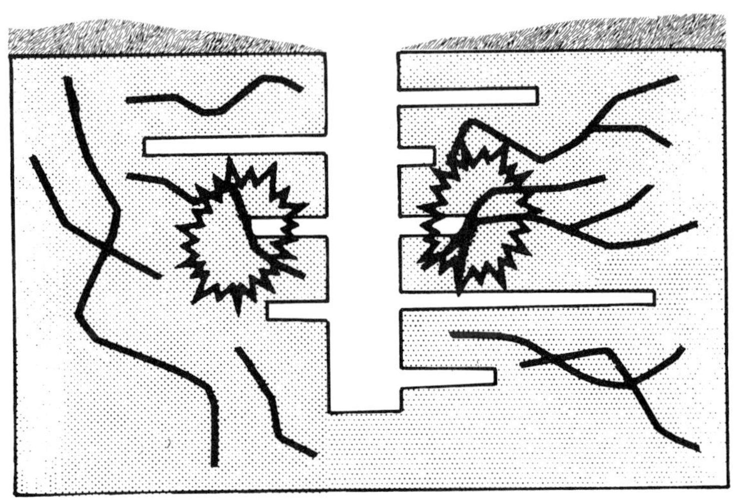

Figure 2. Gold mine analogy to inventory screening.

    A recent development which is to be much applauded and which portends to great discoveries is the new relationship formed between Government, University and Industry (Figure 3). The NCDDG mechanism which stimulates this interaction is an inexpensive manner to greatly magnify the drug discovery and development effort nationally.

    The years ahead promise to be exciting times for the search for new active solid tumor cytotoxics and it is our hope that this forum will become the major mode for bringing together the 3 different components in the equation to regularly discuss their results and ideas.

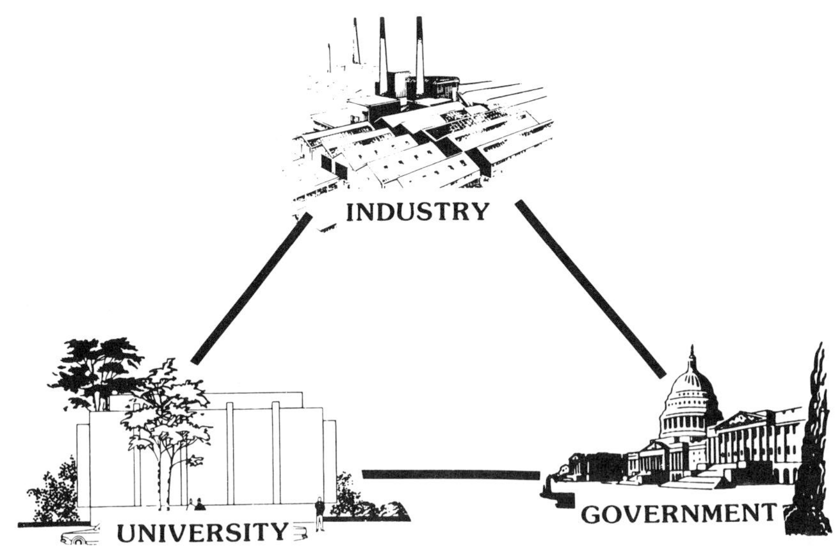

Figure 3. The National Cooperative Drug Discovery Group concept which brings together NCI, Industry and Universities (or other research institutions).

2

DATA DISPLAY AND ANALYSIS STRATEGIES FOR THE NCI DISEASE-ORIENTED IN VITRO ANTITUMOR DRUG SCREEN

M.R. Boyd, K.D. Paull and L.R. Rubinstein

INTRODUCTION

For the past five years, NCI staff and collaborators have been pursuing the development and implementation of an unprecedented new investigational antitumor drug discovery screen. These efforts have not only been controversial, but have also been undertaken during an era of diminishing resources for antitumor drug screening and drug development at NCI. Moreover, numerous unanticipated obstacles, not only in the scientific and technical aspects, but also with respect to issues of management, organization, budget, personnel, laboratory facilities and space, have repeatedly threatened the viability of the project. There has also been immense pressure created by the reliance of many investigators worldwide for antitumor drug screening heretofore provided by NCI, and the fact that NCI has been essentially unable to provide any kind of routine screening support during most of the time the new screen has been under development. During 1986-87, the P-388 screen and other elements of the prior screening program were phased out entirely to free up necessary resources for research and development of the new screen.

Periodic reviews of all of the various developmental aspects of the new screen have been conducted by several external groups, including an Ad Hoc Expert Advisory Committee, the Division of Cancer Treatment's Board of Scientific Counselors and the National Cancer Advisory Board (1-10). The most recent reviews, during November and December of 1989, resulted in consensus recommendations by these groups that the screen had reached a sufficient level of refinement that it should be placed immediately into operational status, and that further developmental efforts could proceed in parallel (4). As the result of these reviews and recommendations, some additional refinements of the cell line panel and the screening laboratory procedures were made, a standardized screening data report portfolio was completed, and full-scale (300-400 compounds per week) screening operations were formally initiated in March, 1990.

The new screen is "disease-oriented", in the sense that multiple, "disease-specific" tumor models are used for the initial (primary) screen. This is in contrast to previous screens used by NCI, such as the P-388 _in vivo_ screen, wherein the initial testing and selection of leads for follow-up were based principally upon a single disease-specific (e.g., leukemia) tumor model. The rationale, background, technical aspects of development, and the current status of the new screen have been reviewed elsewhere (11-14). Briefly, as depicted in Figure 1, the first stage of the screen consists of a diverse assortment of human tumor lines organized in "disease-specific" subpanels (i.e. grouped by histologic types). Initially, each compound is tested, over a wide range of concentrations, against each cell line in the panel.

In the second stage _in vivo_ component of the screen (Figure 1), compounds of interest are tested against a selected subset of the same cell lines found sensitive to the respective compounds in the initial _in vitro_ testing. All _in vivo_ evaluations use the athymic nude mouse xenograft model. Although the _in vivo_ component is an integral part of the overall new screening strategy, it is the _in vitro_ screen that has thus far posed the greatest challenge to implementation of the program. The _in vitro_ screen has also posed unprecedented requirements for data processing, display, analysis, optimal use and exploitation of the wealth of information that is produced.

The development of a variety of alternative approaches for display and analysis of the _in vitro_ screening data is an evolving and intensive effort within the NCI program. Nevertheless, some new methodologies have already been developed which appear quite

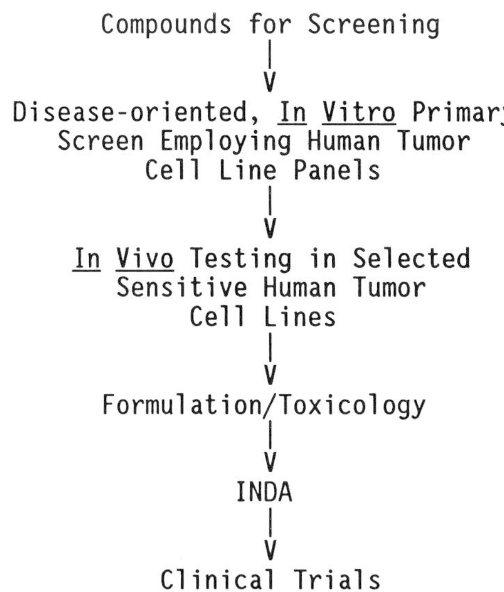

Figure 1. New investigational disease-oriented preclinical drug development strategy.

useful and which will be provided to suppliers of compounds for screening in the NCI program.

In the following, we briefly review some points of interest with respect to the current screening protocol and laboratory operations. Thereafter, we describe the various components that comprise the present version of the screening data report package. We do this in anticipation of the impending release of screening data accrued on several thousand compounds evaluated in pilot-screening operations during the previous year and hereafter on new compounds submitted for testing in the current operational version of the NCI in vitro screen. We welcome the critique and other input from users of the NCI screen and others who receive NCI screening data. The screening data report package will be subject to any modifications which would enhance its utility to the user community.

SCREENING ASSAY AND LABORATORY OPERATIONS

Key aspects of research, development and evaluation of various components of the screen are elsewhere in a series of more detailed reports (15-25). Those reports also contain detailed descriptions of the screening assay parameters and methodologies, and the basis for their selection or development. Tables 1 and 2

Table 1

Assay Protocol and Parameters for the NCI Disease-Oriented In Vitro Antitumor Screen

CELL LINE PANEL

- 60 lines total
- 8 subpanels (non-small cell lung, small cell lung, colon, renal, ovary, melanoma, brain, leukemia)
- lines used at $\leq$ 20 passages from master stock

CULTURE MEDIUM

- RPMI 1640
- 5% serum

CELL INOCULATION DENSITIES

- 5,000-40,000 cells per well (95-well microtitre plate)

PRE-INCUBATION: 24 hrs (no drug)

DRUG DILUTIONS

- Routinely 10^{-4}, 10^{-5}, 10^{-6}, 10^{-7}, and 10^{-8}; or, range as desired

- Duplicates performed at all concentrations

- T_{zero} and "no-drug" controls included

- Minimal sample requirement (grams) for 1 routine test: M.W. of compound x 10^{-4} x 0.04

DRUG INCUBATION: 48 hrs

END-POINT ASSAY: Sulforhodamine B protein stain

Table 2

Screening Laboratory Operations and Logistics

LABORATORY:
- 8,051 ft^2 total space
- 2 floors
- 4 general support modules
- 20 screening modules
- 50 laminar-flow hoods

STAFFING:
- 44 technicians
- 2 senior supervisors (Ph.D.)

CELL INOCULATIONS/DRUG ADDITIONS
- 6 lines assigned per technician
- 3 lines/2 compounds per 96-well plate

COLORIMETRIC END-POINT DETERMINATIONS
- 10 plates/compound
- 4,000 plates/week
- 12 automated plate readers

QUALITY CONTROL
- Manual
- Automated

COMPUTER SUPPORT
- 20 microcomputers (Compaq 386's)
- Central computer (VAX 8820)

CALIBRATION/STANDARDIZATION OF SCREEN
- Daily standards
- Monthly standards
- Standard agent database

briefly summarize some selected aspects of the screen which are pertinent for the present discussion or which otherwise may be of interest to submitters of compounds and users of screening data derived therefrom.

Presently, the cell line panel consists of 60 lines, organized into eight, disease-related subpanels including leukemia, non-small cell lung, small cell lung, colon, renal, ovary, melanoma, and brain cancers. Cryopreserved master stocks of all of the lines are maintained, and cultures used for screening are replaced from the master stock after no more than twenty passages in the screening laboratory. The culture medium presently used is RPMI 1640, containing 5% fetal calf serum. A new CO_2-independent cell culture medium has been developed (20), and is undergoing feasibility studies as a possible future replacement for the RPMI medium.

The screening assay is performed on 96-well microtitre plates. Relatively high initial inoculation densities are used, in order to permit measurement of "time-zero" values (see further discussion below) and to enhance the screen's ability to detect and provide some differentiation between antiproliferative and cytotoxic response parameters. The specific inoculation densities (which range from 5,000 to 40,000 cells/well) used for each cell line are those which, for the respective line, were determined to give an optical density signal for both the "time-zero" value (at 24 hrs) and the "no-drug" control (at 72 hrs) above the noise level and within the linear range of the end-point assay (which measures cellular protein). The inoculated microtitre plates are pre-incubated for 24 hrs at 37^0 prior to drug additions.

The five drug dilutions tested routinely range from 10^{-4} to 10^{-8} molar. Higher or lower concentration ranges may be selected on a nonroutine basis if appropriate solubility and/or prior biological information or other screening data so dictate. Duplicate wells are prepared for all concentrations; "time-zero" and "nodrug" controls are also provided for each test. The minimum amount of compound required for a 1-time evaluation in the routine screen can be calculated from the knowledge that each test requires a total of approximately 40 ml (0.04 liter) of cell culture medium containing the highest desired drug concentration. Thus, the amount (grams) of sample required (assuming an upper test concentration limit of 10^{-4} M) is: molecular weight of compound x 10^{-4} x 0.04.

After a 48 hour incubation (37^0) with the test compound, the cells are fixed _in situ_ to the bottoms of the microtitre wells by addition of 50 ul of either 50% trichloroacetic acid (for adherent cell lines) or 80% trichloroacetic acid (for settled cell suspension lines), followed by incubation for 60 minutes at 4^0.

The cellular protein in each well is assayed using a new sulforhodamine B (SRB) stain procedure described in detail elsewhere (21).
Briefly, after discarding the supernatants, the microtitre plates
are washed 5 times with deionized water and air-dried. One hundred microliters of SRB solution (0.4% w/v in 1% acetic acid) is
added to each microtitre well and incubated for 10 minutes at room
temperature. Unbound SRB is removed by washing 5 times with 1%
acetic acid. The plates are air-dried, the bound stain is solu-
bilized with Tris buffer, and the optical densities read at 515
nm. SRB is a bright pink anionic dye which, in dilute acetic
acid, binds electrostatically to the basic amino acids of TCA-
fixed cells (21).

While the above-described procedure is very simple to perform
on a small laboratory research scale, its application in a high-
flux screening laboratory environment offers yet a different perspective, as illustrated in Table 2. Currently the NCI _in vitro_
screening laboratory is comprised of a total of 8,051 square feet
of laboratory space subdivided onto two floors containing a total
of 4 general lab support modules and 20 screening modules. The
laboratory contains a total of 50 laminar flow cell culture hoods,
and the staff includes 44 technicians and 2 Ph.D.-level supervisors. Each technician regularly works with 6 assigned cell
lines. Each microtitre plate is prepared such that it contains 3
cell lines and 5 concentrations of each of 2 different compounds.
The testing of one compound requires a total of 10 microtitre
plates; one week of screening thus consumes about 4,000 microtitre
plates. The plates are read on one of the 12 automated plate readers in the laboratory. Quality control measures are applied both
manually (e.g., by technicians who may have reason to flag suspect
data), as well as by an extensive in-lab, computer-automated procedure. Computer support for screening laboratory management,
quality control, data acquisition, transmission, storage and analysis is provided by a network of 20 in-lab microcomputers (Compaq
386's) interfaced to a dedicated central computer (VAX 8820).
Calibration and standardization of the screen is performed routinely by monitoring the performance of the screen with one or two

standard agents tested daily and 40 standard agents tested monthly, with respect to a standard agent database. The standard agent
database was constructed by the repetitive (10-20 times each) screening of approximately 180 selected compounds (including all commercial anticancer drugs, all drugs receiving investigational new
drug [IND] approval status since 1970, and all other drugs that
have been in some phase of preclinical development by NCI during
the last decade).

DATA DISPLAY AND ANALYSIS; THE SCREENING DATA REPORT PACKAGE

Presently, the screening data report package consists of five
separate but interrelated components (Table 3). These include:
the data sheet, which contains the experimental optical density
(OD) values and certain calculated parameters used for construct-
ing the other display components; dose-response curves; mean
graphs for each of three different response parameters; a dose response matrix; and, a series of calculated measures of subpanel
selectivity. The derivation, use and interpretation of each of
the components is described in further detail below.

Table 3

Screening Data Report Components

- The data sheet
- Dose-response curves
- Mean graphs for GI_{50}, TGI & LC_{50}
- Dose-response matrix
- Selectivity analyses

<u>The Data Sheet</u>

The first page of the screening data report package (see
example, Figure 2) presents the experimental data collected
against each cell line. The measured effect, which we will term
percentage growth (PG), of the compound on a cell line is

<table>
<tr><td colspan="16">National Cancer Institute Developmental Therapeutics Program
In-Vitro Testing Results</td></tr>
<tr><td colspan="7">NSC:</td><td colspan="5">Experiment ID: 8909MD21</td><td colspan="2">Test Type: 8</td><td colspan="2">Units: Molar</td></tr>
<tr><td colspan="7">Report Date: March 18, 1991</td><td colspan="5">Test Date: September 19, 1989</td><td colspan="2">QNS:</td><td colspan="2">MC:</td></tr>
<tr><td colspan="7">COMI:</td><td colspan="5">Stain Reagent: PRO</td><td colspan="2">SSPL:</td><td colspan="2"></td></tr>
</table>

Panel/Cell Line	Time Zero	Ctrl	Mean Optical Densities −8.0	−7.0	−6.0	−5.0	−4.0	Percent Growth −8.0	−7.0	−6.0	−5.0	−4.0	GI50	TGI	LC50
Leukemia															
CCRF-CEM	0.340	1.116	1.148	1.187	0.981	0.565	0.313	104	109	83	29	−8	4.05E-06	6.09E-05	>1.00E-04
HL-60(TB)	0.396	1.205	1.318	1.363	1.485	1.164	0.439	114	120	135	95	5	3.17E-05	>1.00E-04	>1.00E-04
K-562	0.134	0.773	0.856	0.810	0.745	0.303	0.144	113	106	96	26	1	4.56E-06	>1.00E-04	>1.00E-04
MOLT-4	0.358	1.577	1.589	1.483	1.108	0.621	0.438	101	92	61	22	7	1.94E-06	>1.00E-04	>1.00E-04
RPMI-8226	0.833	2.157	2.116	2.065	1.712	1.497	0.905	97	93	.	50	5	1.01E-05	>1.00E-04	>1.00E-04
Non-Small Cell Lung Cancer															
A549/ATCC	0.217	0.966	0.914	0.799	0.385	0.242	0.181	93	78	22	3	−17	3.17E-07	1.47E-05	>1.00E-04
HOP-18	0.337	0.676	0.657	0.642	0.604	0.529	0.298	94	90	79	57	−12	1.25E-05	6.77E-05	>1.00E-04
HOP-62	0.540	1.022	1.033	1.026	0.744	0.481	0.408	102	101	42	−11	−24	7.38E-07	6.21E-06	>1.00E-04
HOP-92	0.436	0.776	0.767	0.816	0.796	0.596	0.361	97	112	106	47	−17	8.86E-06	5.39E-05	>1.00E-04
NCI-H226	0.462	1.071	1.037	0.995	0.741	0.425	0.118	94	87	46	−8	−75	7.89E-07	7.07E-06	4.27E-05
NCI-H23	0.459	0.948	1.010	1.023	0.776	0.348	0.149	113	115	65	−24	−68	1.46E-06	5.33E-06	3.93E-05
NCI-H322M	0.433	1.303	1.271	1.204	0.878	0.526	0.300	96	89	51	11	−31	1.07E-06	1.81E-05	>1.00E-04
NCI-H460	0.138	0.837	0.844	0.785	0.630	0.182	0.028	101	92	70	6	−80	2.07E-06	1.18E-05	4.51E-05
NCI-H522	0.486	0.964	1.039	0.978	0.672	0.273	0.094	116	103	39	−44	−81	6.72E-07	2.96E-06	1.48E-05
Small Cell Lung Cancer															
DMS 114	0.184	0.605	0.561	0.524	0.272	0.122	0.100	89	81	21	−34	−46	3.27E-07	2.42E-06	>1.00E-04
DMS 273	0.659	2.012	2.054	2.039	1.509	0.736	0.231	103	102	63	6	−65	1.68E-06	1.20E-05	6.13E-05
Colon Cancer															
COLO 205	.	.	.	.	.	.	.	.	.	.	.	.	.	.	.
DLD-1	0.316	0.910	0.859	0.879	0.677	0.427	0.361	91	95	61	19	8	1.80E-06	>1.00E-04	>1.00E-04
HCC-2998	0.252	1.292	1.186	1.139	1.097	1.131	0.994	90	85	81	85	71	>1.00E-04	>1.00E-04	>1.00E-04
HCT-116	0.306	1.748	1.789	1.772	1.634	0.785	0.307	103	102	92	33	0	5.18E-06	>1.00E-04	>1.00E-04
HCT-15	0.222	1.037	1.057	1.086	0.990	0.835	0.685	102	106	94	75	57	>1.00E-04	>1.00E-04	>1.00E-04
HT29	0.128	0.907	0.987	0.920	0.947	0.435	0.183	110	102	105	39	7	6.90E-06	>1.00E-04	>1.00E-04
KM12	0.205	0.899	0.882	0.806	0.431	0.243	0.186	98	87	33	5	−9	4.76E-07	2.35E-05	>1.00E-04
SW-620	.	.	.	.	.	.	.	.	.	.	.	.	.	.	.
CNS Cancer															
SF-268	0.409	0.934	0.900	0.805	0.394	0.129	0.067	94	75	−4	−68	−84	2.10E-07	9.02E-07	5.20E-06
SF-295	0.246	0.717	0.753	0.672	0.321	0.179	0.114	108	91	16	−27	−54	3.49E-07	2.33E-06	7.16E-05
SF-539	0.758	1.542	1.578	1.503	0.991	0.484	0.159	105	95	30	−36	.	4.89E-07	2.83E-06	>1.00E-05
SNB-19	0.349	1.069	1.026	0.979	0.502	0.274	0.279	94	88	21	−21	−20	3.68E-07	3.14E-06	>1.00E-04
SNB-75	0.348	0.661	0.641	0.554	0.284	0.171	0.104	94	66	−19	−51	−70	1.54E-07	6.03E-07	9.40E-06
SNB-78	0.331	0.737	0.725	0.706	0.528	0.412	0.314	97	92	49	20	−5	9.28E-07	6.18E-05	>1.00E-04
U251	0.386	1.355	1.338	1.285	0.535	0.197	0.120	98	93	15	−49	−69	3.57E-07	1.73E-06	1.11E-05
XF 498	0.405	0.693	0.691	0.715	0.646	0.400	0.290	99	107	84	−1	−29	2.49E-06	9.67E-06	>1.00E-04
Melanoma															
LOX IMVI	0.154	0.768	0.831	0.873	0.815	0.581	0.152	110	117	108	70	−2	1.88E-05	9.49E-05	>1.00E-04
MALME-3M	0.639	1.171	1.168	1.156	0.996	0.489	0.386	99	97	67	−24	−40	1.55E-06	5.50E-06	>1.00E-04
M19-MEL	1.042	2.017	1.990	1.981	1.940	1.960	1.972	97	96	92	94	95	>1.00E-04	>1.00E-04	>1.00E-04
SK-MEL-28	0.154	0.454	0.446	0.469	0.408	0.225	0.040	97	105	85	24	−74	3.72E-06	1.75E-05	5.68E-05
SK-MEL-5	0.320	1.135	1.088	1.066	0.863	0.332	0.119	94	92	67	1	−63	1.80E-06	1.05E-05	6.32E-05
UACC-257	0.303	0.708	0.737	0.720	0.676	0.442	0.242	107	103	92	34	−20	5.35E-06	4.26E-05	>1.00E-04
Ovarian Cancer															
IGROV1	0.400	1.076	0.981	1.020	0.957	0.655	0.439	86	92	82	38	6	5.33E-06	>1.00E-04	>1.00E-04
OVCAR-3	0.275	0.784	0.775	0.725	0.688	0.402	0.186	98	89	81	25	−32	3.58E-06	2.72E-05	>1.00E-04
OVCAR-4	.	.	.	.	.	.	.	.	.	.	.	.	.	.	.
OVCAR-5	0.367	0.926	0.930	0.956	0.943	0.738	0.615	101	105	103	66	44	5.53E-05	>1.00E-04	>1.00E-04
OVCAR-8	0.373	1.360	1.315	1.200	0.756	0.497	0.372	95	84	39	13	0	5.63E-07	9.53E-05	>1.00E-04
SK-OV-3	0.337	0.817	0.757	0.804	0.708	0.580	0.470	87	97	77	51	28	1.05E-05	>1.00E-04	>1.00E-04
Renal Cancer															
A498	0.699	1.148	1.179	1.202	1.068	0.967	0.860	107	112	82	60	36	2.59E-05	>1.00E-04	>1.00E-04
CAKI-1	.	.	.	.	.	.	.	.	.	.	.	.	.	.	.
RXF-393	0.297	0.659	0.673	0.682	0.495	0.350	0.295	104	106	55	14	−1	1.31E-06	9.03E-05	>1.00E-04
SN12C	0.298	1.109	1.046	0.912	0.412	0.209	0.126	92	76	14	−30	−58	2.61E-07	2.08E-06	5.21E-05
SN12K1	0.293	1.541	1.501	1.373	0.802	0.340	0.112	97	87	41	4	−62	6.28E-07	1.14E-05	6.61E-05
UO-31	0.684	1.386	1.413	1.414	1.370	1.424	1.465	104	104	98	105	111	>1.00E-04	>1.00E-04	>1.00E-04
Miscellaneous															
MCF7	0.092	0.402	0.398	0.372	0.316	0.117	0.065	99	90	72	8	−30	2.22E-06	1.64E-05	>1.00E-04
MCF7/ADR-RES	0.474	1.331	1.364	1.313	1.118	1.061	0.932	104	98	75	69	53	>1.00E-04	>1.00E-04	>1.00E-04
P388	0.073	0.646	0.605	0.683	0.375	0.100	0.055	93	106	53	5	−25	1.14E-06	1.44E-05	>1.00E-04
P388/ADR	0.082	0.689	0.697	0.712	0.727	0.729	0.481	101	104	106	107	66	>1.00E-04	>1.00E-04	>1.00E-04

Figure 2. An example of the "data sheet" component of the screening data report package.

currently calculated according to one or the other of the following two expressions:

If (Mean OD_{test} − Mean OD_{tzero}) ≥ 0, then

$$PG = 100 \times (\text{Mean } OD_{test} - \text{Mean } OD_{tzero})/(\text{Mean } OD_{ctrl} - \text{Mean } OD_{tzero})$$

If (Mean OD_{test} − Mean OD_{tzero}) < 0, then

$$PG = 100 \times (\text{Mean } OD_{test} - \text{Mean } OD_{tzero})/\text{Mean } OD_{tzero}$$

Where:

Mean OD_{tzero} =   The average of 24 optical density measurements of SRB-derived color at the time just before exposure of cells to the test compound (denoted tzero).

Mean OD_{test} =   The average of the 2 optical density measurements of SRB-derived color after 48 hr exposure of cells to the test compound.

Mean OD_{ctrl} =   The average of 4 optical density measurements of SRB derived color after 48 hr with no exposure to the test compound.

On the first two columns of the data sheet page the subpanels (e.g., leukemia) and cell lines (e.g., CCRF-CEM) are identified. The next two columns list the Mean OD_{tzero} and Mean OD_{ctrl}. The following five columns list the Mean OD_{test} for each of five different concentrations. Each concentration is expressed by its $\log_{10}$ (molar or ug/ml). The individual optical density measurements, which contribute to the means in these seven columns, are accurate to at least 4 significant digits. The Mean OD_{tzero} and Mean OD_{ctrl} values (averages of 24 and 4 individual values, respectively) are justifiably reported to 4 significant digits. The Mean OD_{test} values (averages of 2 individual values) are reported to 3 significant digits. The next five columns list the calculated PG's for each concentration. The response parameters GI50, TGI, and LC50 are interpolated values representing the concentrations at which the PG is +50, 0, and -50, respectively:

GI50 is the concentration for which the PG=+50. At this value, the increase from time t_{zero} in the number or mass of cells in the test well is only 50% as much as the corresponding increase in the control well during this period of the experiment. A drug effect of this intensity is interpreted as primary growth inhibition.

TGI is the concentration for which the PG=0. At this value, the number or mass of cells in the test well at the end of the experiment equals the number or mass of cells in the well at time tzero. A drug effect of this intensity is regarded as cytostasis.

<u>LC50</u> is the concentration for which the PG=-50. At this value, the number or mass of cells in the test well at the end of the experiment is half that at time t_{zero}. This is inter- preted as cytotoxicity.

The above response parameters cannot always be obtained by interpo- lation. If, for instance, all of the PG's on a given row exceed +50, then none of the three parameters can be obtained by interpo- lation. In such a case, the value given for each response para- meter is the highest concentration tested and is preceded by ">" sign. This practice is extended analogously to the other possible situations where a response parameter cannot be obtained by inter- polation.

Dose-Response Curves

The second page of the screening data report package (see example, Figure 3) is created by plotting the PG's against the

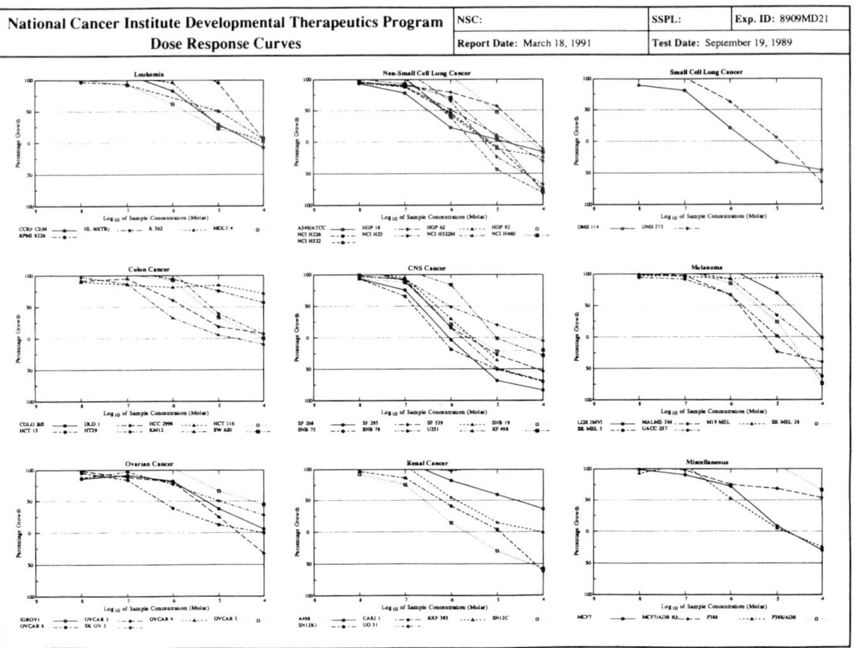

Figure 3. An example of the "dose-response curves" component of the screening data report package.

$\log_{10}$ values of the corresponding concentrations for every cell line. The individual curves for each cell line are grouped by sub-panel. Horizontal lines are provided at the PG values of +50, 0 and -50. The concentrations corresponding to points where the curves cross these lines are the respective GI50, TGI, and LC50 values. These curves provide a means of visualization of the drug effect at each concentration and also give an overall indication of the quality of the screening experiment (e.g., consistency, appropriateness of dose-range, etc.). This is in contrast to the mean graphs (below) which depict the relative dose, per cell line, required to achieve a specified level of drug effect.

The Mean Graphs

The third page of the screening data report package (see example, Figure 4) is a composite of three mean graphs, one for each

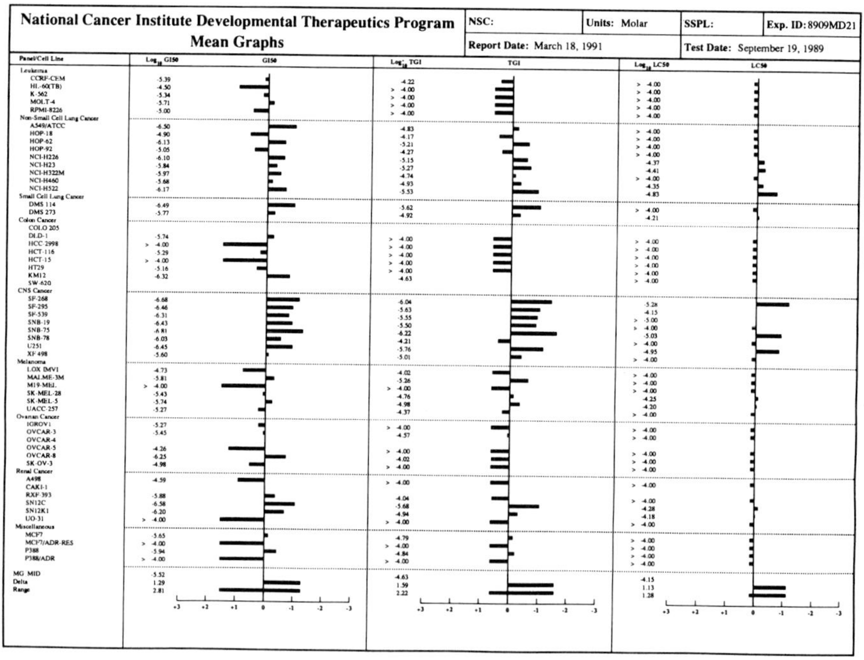

National Cancer Institute Developmental Therapeutics Program — Mean Graphs			
NSC:	Units: Molar	SSPL:	Exp. ID: 8909MD21
Report Date: March 18, 1991		Test Date: September 19, 1989	

Panel/Cell Line	$\log_{10}$ GI50	$\log_{10}$ TGI	$\log_{10}$ LC50
Leukemia			
CCRF-CEM	-5.39	-4.22	> -4.00
HL-60(TB)	-4.50	> -4.00	> -4.00
K-562	-5.34	> -4.00	> -4.00
MOLT-4	-5.71	> -4.00	> -4.00
RPMI-8226	-5.00	> -4.00	> -4.00
Non-Small Cell Lung Cancer			
A549/ATCC	-6.50	-4.83	> -4.00
HOP-18	-4.90	-4.17	> -4.00
HOP-62	-6.13	-5.21	> -4.00
HOP-92	-5.05	-4.27	> -4.00
NCI-H226	-6.10	-5.15	-4.37
NCI-H23	-5.84	-5.27	-4.41
NCI-H322M	-5.97	-4.74	> -4.00
NCI-H460	-5.68	-4.93	-4.35
NCI-H522	-6.17	-5.53	-4.83
Small Cell Lung Cancer			
DMS 114	-6.49	-5.62	> -4.00
DMS 273	-5.77	-4.92	-4.21
Colon Cancer			
COLO 205			
DLD-1	-5.74	> -4.00	> -4.00
HCC-2998	> -4.00	> -4.00	> -4.00
HCT-116	-5.29	> -4.00	> -4.00
HCT-15	> -4.00	> -4.00	> -4.00
HT29	-5.16	> -4.00	> -4.00
KM12	-6.32	-4.63	> -4.00
SW-620			
CNS Cancer			
SF-268	-6.68	-6.04	-5.28
SF-295	-6.46	-5.63	-4.15
SF-539	-6.31	-5.55	> -5.00
SNB-19	-6.43	-5.50	> -4.00
SNB-75	-6.81	-6.22	-5.03
SNB-78	-6.03	-4.21	> -4.00
U251	-6.45	-5.76	-4.95
XF 498	-5.60	-5.01	> -4.00
Melanoma			
LOX IMVI	-4.73	-4.02	> -4.00
MALME-3M	-5.81	-5.26	> -4.00
M19-MEL	> -4.00	> -4.00	> -4.00
SK-MEL-28	-5.43	-4.76	-4.25
SK-MEL-5	-5.74	-4.98	-4.20
UACC-257	-5.27	-4.37	> -4.00
Ovarian Cancer			
IGROV1	-5.27	> -4.00	> -4.00
OVCAR-3	-5.45	-4.57	> -4.00
OVCAR-4			
OVCAR-5	-4.26	> -4.00	> -4.00
OVCAR-8	-6.25	-4.02	> -4.00
SK-OV-3	-4.98	> -4.00	> -4.00
Renal Cancer			
A498	-4.59	> -4.00	> -4.00
CAKI-1			
RXF-393	-5.88	-4.04	> -4.00
SN12C	-6.58	-5.68	-4.28
SN12K1	-6.20	-4.94	-4.18
UO-31	> -4.00	> -4.00	> -4.00
Miscellaneous			
MCF7	-5.65	-4.79	> -4.00
MCF7/ADR-RES	> -4.00	> -4.00	> -4.00
P388	-5.94	-4.84	-5.00
P388/ADR	> -4.00	> -4.00	> -4.00
MG MID	-5.52	-4.63	-4.15
Delta	1.29	1.59	1.13
Range	2.81	2.22	1.28

Figure 4. An example of the "mean graphs" component of the screening data report package.

of the selected response parameters, GI50, TGI and LC50. A detailed description of the derivation and characteristics of the mean
graph display format has been published elsewhere (24). Simplis-
tically, mean graphs facilitate visual scanning of data for patterns of selectivity for particular cell lines or for particular
subpanels with respect to a selected response parameter. Bars
extending to the right represent sensitivity of the cell line to
the test agent in excess of the average sensitivity of all tested
cell lines. Since the bar scale is logarithmic, a bar 2 units to
the right indicates the compound achieved the response parameter
(e.g., GI50) for the cell line at a concentration one hundredth
the geometric mean concentration required over all cell lines;
thus the cell line is unusually sensitive to that compound. Bars
extending to the left correspondingly indicate sensitivity less
than the mean. If, for a particular drug cell line, it was not
possible to determine the desired response parameter by interpola-
tion, the bar length shown corresponds to the highest concentration tested (and the listed $\log_{10}$ of the response parameter will
be preceded by a ">"). Differences in apparent selectivity patterns in the mean graphs may occur for the same compound against
the same cell lines with respect to the different response parameters (e.g., see examples in Figure 4).

The mean graph patterns are conveniently amenable to further
analyses by computer, using a pattern-recognition algorithm called
COMPARE, which has also been described in detail elsewhere (24).
Although this technique is not applied routinely to screening
data, and is not a regular part of the data report package, there
are a number of specialized applications that merit mention. For
example, COMPARE provides a means for monitoring the reproducibility of the overall cellular response profiles for standard compounds tested periodically against the cell line panel (e.g., by
matching/comparisons of the characteristic mean graph "fingerprints"). Also, COMPARE-based sorting of mean graphs contained in
the screening database is useful to group compounds with similar
mean graph fingerprints. Interestingly, such grouped compounds
often have very similar structures and/or mechanisms of action.

24

For example, alkylating agents tend to show highly related mean graph fingerprints; likewise, certain classes of DNAbinders group closely; and so on. The COMPARE method should, therefore, be useful not only for applications such as the monitoring of performance of standard agents in the screen, but also for support of analog development and lead optimization. Likewise, COMPARE analysis may assist in the identification of agents giving cellular response profiles quite unlike those of the "standard agents" or other known compounds. Compare analyses may therefore assist in the search for novel agents acting by mechanisms for which there are few, if any, known prototypes.

The Dose-Response Matrix

While clearly the mean graph provides a useful visual representation of potential subpanel selectivity, it is tied to the particular mean level of effect (GI50, TGI or LC50) to which it relates. Also, the mean graph reflects differences (across cell lines) in required dose to achieve a given level of effect; it does not directly reflect differences in the effect (across cell lines) at a fixed dose level.

The fourth page of the screening data report package includes a dose-response matrix (an example of which is shown in Figure 5). This display complements the 3 mean graphs by providing a visualization of potential subpanel selectivity that is not tied to a particular level of effect, and which directly reflects differences in effect (across cell lines) at the 5 dose levels used in testing. The matrix is created as follows: The rows correspond to the cell lines, arranged by subpanel. The columns correspond to the 5 dose levels. Each element (square) in the matrix is color-coded according to the level of effect achieved by the compound against the given cell-line at the given dose level:

White:	Percentage growth > 50 (GI50 not achieved)
Light gray:	Percentage growth ≤ 50 (GI50 achieved)
Dark gray:	Percentage growth ≤ 0 (TGI achieved)
Black:	Percentage growth ≤ -50 (LC50 achieved)

25

NCI Developmental Therapeutics Program	NSC: ______	Exp. ID: 8909MD21
Dose Response Matrix	Test Date: September 19, 1989	Stain: PROTEIN-51
	Report Date: March 18, 1991	SSPL:

Log$_{10}$ Concentration (Molar): PG (-5.0) -4.0 -5.0 -6.0 -7.0 -8.0

PG	Panel/Cell Line	Log$_{10}$ TGI
	Leukemia	
29	CCRF-CEM	-4.22
95	HL-60(TB)	> -4.00
26	K-562	> -4.00
22	MOLT-4	> -4.00
50	RPMI-8226	> -4.00
	Non-Small Cell Lung Cancer	
3	A549/ATCC	-4.83
57	HOP-18	-4.17
-11	HOP-62	-5.21
47	HOP-92	-4.27
-8	NCI-H226	-5.15
-24	NCI-H23	-5.27
11	NCI-H322M	-4.74
6	NCI-H460	-4.93
-44	NCI-H522	-5.53
	Small Cell Lung Cancer	
-34	DMS 114	-5.62
6	DMS 273	-4.92
	Colon Cancer	
	COLO 205	
19	DLD-1	> -4.00
85	HCC-2998	> -4.00
33	HCT-116	> -4.00
75	HCT-15	> -4.00
39	HT29	> -4.00
5	KM12	-4.63
	SW-620	
	CNS Cancer	
-68	SF-268	-6.04
-27	SF-295	-5.63
-36	SF-539	-5.55
-21	SNB-19	-5.50
-51	SNB-75	-6.22
20	SNB-78	-4.21
-49	U251	-5.76
-1	XF 498	-5.01
	Melanoma	
70	LOX IMVI	-4.02
-24	MALME-3M	-5.26
94	M19-MEL	> -4.00
24	SK-MEL-28	-4.76
1	SK-MEL-5	-4.98
34	UACC-257	-4.37
	Ovarian Cancer	
38	IGROV1	> -4.00
25	OVCAR-3	-4.57
	OVCAR-4	
66	OVCAR-5	> -4.00
13	OVCAR-8	-4.02
51	SK-OV-3	> -4.00
	Renal Cancer	
60	A498	> -4.00
	CAKI-1	
14	RXF-393	-4.04
-30	SN12C	-5.68
4	SN12K1	-4.94
105	UO-31	> -4.00
	Miscellaneous	
8	MCF7	-4.79
69	MCF7/ADR-RES	> -4.00
5	P388	-4.84
107	P388/ADR	> -4.00

TGI scale: +4 +3 +2 +1 0 -1 -2 -3 -4

Legend	D values	Statistics
PG > GI50	D$_{GI50}$ = 66.0 (-6.0)	MG MID TGI = -4.63
PG ≤ GI50	D$_{TGI}$ = 71.0 (-5.0)	Delta = 1.59
PG ≤ TGI	D$_{LC50}$ = 37.0 (-4.0)	Range = 2.22
PG ≤ LC50	D$_H$ = 79.17 (-5.0)	MGD$_H$ = 80.50

Figure 5. An example of the "dose-response matrix component of the screening data report package.

The example in Figure 5 shows the result from testing of an
actual compound against 50 cell lines. The pattern of coloring
shows the brain tumor (CNS) subpanel to be the most sensitive,
with the small-cell lung and non-small-cell lung subpanels also
demonstrating sensitivity. The rows of the dose-response matrix
can be viewed as a condensation of the data presented in the dose-
response curves. For example, the coloring pattern of the boxes
forms bars associated with the cell lines; these bars correspond
roughly with the respective bars of one or more of the mean
graphs. In this instance (Figure 5), the bars formed by the black
and dark gray boxes are correlated most directly with the bars of
the TGI mean graph, which is automatically reprinted alongside the
dose-response matrix on page 4 of the screening data report pack-

age. If the light gray boxes were also included, there would be corresponding correlations with the GI50 mean graph. The rows of dose-response matrix can also be viewed as a condensation of the data presented in the dose-response curves. The dose-response matrix can also be viewed column by column, to ascertain possible selectivity at each separate dose level. The boxes with dots indicate data which are missing due to violations of quality control criteria.

<u>Scoring the Mean Graphs and the Dose-Response Matrix for Subpanel Selectivity</u>

One important goal of the new screen is to facilitate the discovery of new agents, or the "rediscovery" of "old" agents, which may have heretofore escaped detection and which produce growth inhibitory and/or cytotoxic activity preferentially against certain histologic types of cancer. For example, in the new screening strategy, the detection of a "disease-specific" antitumor agent (e.g., active against the non-small cell lung cancer cell line subpanel and/or the colon cancer subpanel and/or the new brain tumor subpanel, etc.) would be followed by the testing of the respective compound against a selection of the appropriate cell lines implanted in nude mice. Conceivably, the information provided by this preclinical screening strategy could help obviate the subsequent need for broad ("disease-oriented") clinical evaluation of a new investigational drug having shown a pattern of disease-specific activity and focus the early emphasis upon a more limited subset of cancer patients.

We have developed a way of objectively scoring the degree of subpanel selectivity shown in the mean graph for a screened compound. Visually, a mean graph shows subpanel selectivity when the sensitive cell lines, represented by bars extending to the right, are concentrated in one or more histologic subpanels, rather than being dispersed throughout the panel. We score this phenomenon numerically in the following manner:

We first rank the cell lines from 1 to N (where N is the total number of cell lines for which data passed the quality control requirements) in order of increasing sensitivity, as measured by positive (rightward) or negative (leftward) extension of the mean graph bars. Tied values are assigned the mean rank of the ties. We then calculate the mean rank within each subpanel and order the subpanels by increasing mean rank (increasing sensitivity). We then compute 3 separate differences:

1. The difference between the highest subpanel mean rank (R_1) and the mean of the remaining ranks (R_1').
2. The difference between the mean rank of the 2 highest subpanels taken together (R_2) and the mean of the remaining ranks (R_2').
3. The differences between the mean rank of the 3 highest subpanels taken together (R_3) and the mean of the remaining ranks (R_3).

We then rescale the maximum of the above 3 differences ($Max[R_I-R_I']$; $I = 1,2,3$), so that it varies between 1 and 100. Without rescaling, the maximum of the above 3 differences will have an upper limit of N/2, which will be achieved if the cell lines in the most sensitive 1, 2 or 3 subpanels have ranks uniformly higher than the ranks of the remaining lines. For instance, if N = 50 cell lines that have been successfully tested against a compound, and the 2 most sensitive subpanels include 12 lines, ranked 39-50, then their mean rank is 44.5, while the mean of the remaining ranks (1-38) is 19.5, yield a difference of 25 (which is N/2). Rather than allowing the range of our score to be determined in this way by the varying number of cell lines successfully tested against a compound, we rescale the score to a range of 1-100 by multiplying by 200/N.

An example, using the TGI mean graph in Figure 5, will further elucidate this method of scoring. We use the log_{10} dose values to rank the cell lines (from 1-50) in order of increasing sensitivity and also to order the subpanels by mean rank. We calculate that the CNS, small cell lung, and non-small cell lung panels are the 3 most sensitive, with mean ranks of 42.25, 39, and 33.22, respectively, as shown in Table 4. The greatest mean rank difference is obtained by calculating the mean rank of the CNS and

28

small cell lung subpanels taken together (R_2=41.6), and subtracting the mean rank of the remaining cell lines (R_2'=21.475). The difference (20.125) is rescaled by a factor of 200/N (N=50), to equal 80.5. The score is denoted MGD_H (<u>M</u>ean <u>G</u>raph <u>D</u>ifference relating to <u>H</u>istology), and, if appropriate, this value may be provided on page 3 or 4 of the screening data report package (e.g., Figure 5). The subpanels indicated as sensitive by MGD_H are marked with dots placed to the right of their names.

Table 4

Scoring Selectivity for Compound X with Mean Graph: An Example

<u>Subpanel</u>	<u>Ranks</u>	<u>Mean Rank</u>	$\underline{R}_I$	$\underline{R}_I$-$\underline{R}_I{}'$
CNS	22,37,42,44, 46,48,49,50	42.25	42.25	19.94
SCLC	33,45	39.00	41.60	20.125
NSCLC	21,24,28,31,34, 38,39,41,43	33.22	37.63	19.57

$MGD_H = (200/50) \times 20.125 = 80.5$

The primary purpose of the MGD_H score is to allow us to assign objective relative rankings to the degrees of subpanel selectivity demonstrated by the mean graphs associated with the compounds tested. Therefore, score levels that will be used as cutoff criteria, to determine which compounds get further attention, will be set empirically. However, computer simulations involving the null-hypothesis case of no subpanel selectivity indicate that an MGD_H score of at least 75 is statistically significant at the 0.01 level.

The MGD_H score is closely related to the commonly used non-parametric 2-sample Wilcoxon rank-sum test. We have altered this test so that our test is sensitive to the particular case of interest, namely where 1, 2 or 3 subpanels demonstrate sensitivity markedly greater than the remainder of the panel. Like the Wilcoxon statistic, the MGD_H score is based on the ranks of the cell lines (determined by the dose levels represented by the mean graph). Alternatively, one could calculate the analogous score based on the dose level values, themselves, or based on the $\log_{10}$ values of those dose levels, or even based on some other mathematical transformation of the dose level. However, the choice of the proper scale would be arbitrary. Basing the score on the ranks lets the distribution of the dose levels determine the scale, since the scale of the ranks is the percentiles associated with the distribution of the dose levels.

Scoring the Dose-Response Matrix for Subpanel Selectivity

We have also developed an objective method of scoring the degree of subpanel selectivity represented by the dose-response matrix. We first score the selectivity at each dose level separately. The score is computed in a manner identical to that used in scoring the mean graph, except that the cell lines are ranked from least to most sensitive according to PG value (percentage growth) at the given level. The maximum of the five separate computed scores is denoted as the overall score.

The example in Figure 5 again provides further elucidation. The score is first calculated for each dose, but the $\log_{10}$ (molar) concentration of -5 yields the highest score. The PG values of the cell lines for this dose are given on the left-most column of Figure 5. Using these values to rank the cell lines, we find that the 3 most sensitive subpanels are again CNS, small cell lung, and non-small cell lung, with mean ranks 42, 37.25, and 31.2, respectively, as shown in Table 5. The greatest mean rank difference (19.6) is obtained by subtracting from the CNS mean rank (R_1=42) the mean of the remaining ranks (R_1'=22.4). This score is rescaled by a factor of 200/N (N=50) to equal 78.6. This score is denoted as D_H (at the bottom of the middle column of Figure 5). The subpanel(s) indicated as most sensitive by D_H are marked by a dot to the left of the respective subpanel name(s). We see that D_H, in this example, is in good agreement with MGD_H, even though they are two different statistics. As for MGD_H, a D_H score of at least 75

75 has been determined by null-hypothesis simulations to be statistically significant. However, actual cut-off criteria will be determined empirically.

Table 5

Scoring Selectivity for Compound X with the Dose-Response Matrix = An Example (Most Selective Dose = 10^{-5})

Subpanel	Ranks	Mean Rank	$\underline{R}_I$	$\underline{R}_I - \underline{R}_{I'}$
CNS	23,37,40,43, 46,48,49,50	42.00	42.00	19.64
SCLC	29.5,45	37.25	41.05	19.44
NSCLC	11,13,27,29.5, 35,38,39,41.5,47	31.22	36.39	17.57

$D_H = (200/50) \times 19.64 = 78.57$

We have developed 3 additional scores, based on the dose-response matrix, which relate specifically to achievement of GI50, TGI, and LC50, respectively. These 3 scores are analogous, so we will only describe how we calculate the one relating to achievement of GI50. We score each dose level separately, as follows. We first calculate for each subpanel the percentage of cell lines for which $PG \leq 50$ (GI50 is achieved), and thereby rank the subpanels in order of increasing sensitivity. We then compute 3 differences: the difference between the percentage achieving GI50 and in the I most sensitive subpanels (P_I) and the percentage achieving GI50 among the remaining cell lines (P_I') <u>where</u> I = 1, 2, or 3. The score for the given dose level is the maximum of the above 3 differences ($Max[P_I - P_I']$; I=1,2,3), and the overall score is the maximum over is the maximum over the 5 dose levels, and is denoted D_{GI50}. The analogous scores relating to TGI and LC50 are denoted D_{TGI} and D_{LC50}.

We again use the example in Figure 5 for elucidation. In this example D_{TGI} is greater than D_{GI50} and D_{LC50}, and it is calcu-

lated as follows. The dose that maximizes this score is -5. At
this dose, 87.5% of the cell lines in the CNS subpanel achieve
TGI, as do 50% and 44% of the small cell lung and non-small cell
lung subpanels, respectively, as shown in Table 6. The greatest

Table 6

Scoring Selectivity Related to Achievement of
TGI for Compound X: (Most Selective Dose = 10^{-5})

Subpanel	% Achieving TGI	P_I	$P_I\text{-}P_I{}'$
CNS	87.5	87.50	70.83
SCLC	50	80.00	65.00
NSCLC	44	63.16	56.71
Renal	20		
Melanoma	16		
Others	0		

$D_{TGI} = 70.8\ (-5)$

percentage difference (70.8%) is obtained by subtracting from the
CNS TGI percentage (P_1=87.5%), the percentage of the remaining
lines achieving TGI ($P_1{}'$=16.7%).

The scores D_{GI50}, D_{TGI} and D_{LC50} can be viewed as measures
of difference in "percentage of responders" between the most and
least sensitive subpanels. Taking D_{GI50}, in particular, we
start by equating "response" with _in vitro_ achievement of GI50.
Thus, D_{GI50} is the difference in percentage of response between
the most and least sensitive subpanels, where we maximize over the
5 doses and over the choice of the top 1, 2, or 3 subpanels to be
grouped together. Viewed in this way, the scores take on intui-
tive meaning. We use these scores primarily as objective relative
measures of selectivity, so that the cut-off criteria, used to
decide which compounds deserve further attention, will be determined empirically. However, computer simulations involving the
null hypothesis case of no subpanel selectivity indicate that,
roughly speaking, a score of at least 50 is statistically significant.

32

We see, in the example of Figure 5, that D_{GI50} is maximized
at $\log_{10}$ concentration equal to -6, while D_{TGI} and D_{LC50} are maximized at $\log_{10}$ concentrations equal to -5 and -4, respectively.
The maximum of these three scores determines which of the 3 corresponding mean graphs is displayed with the dose-response matrix
analysis; in this case D_{TGI} is the maximum. It is interesting
to note that in this case the dose that maximizes D_{TGI} also maximizes the overall score D_H. It is also interesting to note the
close agreement, in this example, between D_H and MGD_H, and the
subpanels which are picked out as sensitive by these two scores.
It is important to remember the complementary relationship of these
scores. D_H scores subpanel selectivity relating to differences
in response at a fixed dose, while MGD_H scores subpanel selectivity relating to differences in dose required to achieve a fixed
level of response.

REFERENCES

1. National Cancer Institute planning to switch drug development
   emphasis from compound to human cancer-oriented strategy.
   Cancer Lett. 10(41):1-2, 1984.
2. Division of Cancer Treatment Board approves new screening program, natural products concepts. Cancer Lett. 11(9):4-5,
   1985.
3. Division of Cancer Treatment gets okay to proceed with human
   cell line drug screening. Cancer Lett. 13(25):1-2, 1987.
4. Reviewers report progress in new drug prescreen system development. Cancer Lett. 15(48):1-5, 1989.
5. Workshop on "Disease-oriented Antitumor Drug Discovery and
   Development", NIH, Bethesda, MD, January 9-10, 1985.
6. Ad Hoc review committee proceedings for National Cancer Institute _In Vitro_/_In Vivo_ Disease-oriented Screening Project.
   NIH, Bethesda, MD, September 23-24, 1985.
7. Ad Hoc review committee proceedings for National Cancer Institute _In Vitro_/_In Vivo_ Disease-oriented Screening Project.
   NIH, Bethesda, MD, December 8-9, 1986.
8. Ad Hoc review committee proceedings for National Cancer Institute _In Vitro_/_In Vivo_ Disease-oriented Screening Project.
   NIH, Bethesda, MD, May 19-20, 1988.
9. Ad Hoc review committee proceedings for National Cancer Institute _In Vitro_/_In Vivo_ Disease-oriented Screening Project.
   NIH, Bethesda, MD, November 13-15, 1989.
10. Kolberg RJ: Casting a wider net to catch cancer cures. J.
    NIH Research 2(April):82, 1990.

11. Boyd MR: National Cancer Institute drug discovery and development. In: Accomplishments in Oncology, E.J. Frei, E.J. Freireich (eds.), J.B. Lippincott Co., Philadelphia, pp. 68-76, 1986.
12. Jefford CW, Rinehart KL, Shield LS: Pharmaceuticals and the sea. Technomic Publishing AG, Lancaster, 1988.
13. Boyd MR, Shoemaker RH, McLemore TL et al: New drug development. In: Thoracic Oncology, J.A. Roth, J.C. Ruckdeschel, T.H. Weisenburger (eds.), W.B. Saunders Co., Philadelphia, pp. 711-721, 1989.
14. Boyd MR: Status of the NCI preclinical antitumor drug discovery screen. In: Cancer: Principles and Practice of Oncology Update, V.T. DeVita, S. Hellman, S.A. Rosenberg (eds), J.B. Lippincott, Vol. 3(10), Philadelphia, pp. 1-12, 1989.
15. Alley MC, Scudiero DA, Monks A et al: Feasibility of drug screening with panels of human tumor lines using a micro-culture tetrazolium assay. Cancer Res. 48:589-601, 1988.
16. Shoemaker RH, Monks A, Alley MC et al: Development of human tumor cell line panels for use in disease-oriented drug screening. In: Prediction of Response to Cancer Chemotherapy, T. Hall (ed), Alan Liss, New York, pp. 265-286, 1988.
17. Stinson SF, Alley MC, Kenney S et al: Morphologic characterization of human carcinoma cell lines. Proc. AACR 30:613, 1989.
18. Scudiero DA, Shoemaker RH, Paull KD et al: Evaluation of a soluble tetrazolium/formazan assay for growth and drug sensitivity on culture. Cancer Res. 48:4827-4833, 1988.
19. Vistica DT, Skehan P, Scudiero DA et al: Tetrazolium-based assays for cellular viability: A critical examination of parameters which affect formazan production. AACR 30:612, 1989; Cancer Res., in press.
20. Vistica DT, Scudiero DA, Skehan P et al: Development and evaluation of a CO_2-independent culture medium for use in a high-flux _in vitro_ anticancer drug screen employing a broad panel of human tumor cell lines. JNCI in press.
21. Skehan P, Storeng R, Scudiero D et al: Evaluation of colorimetric protein and biomass stains for assaying _in vitro_ drug effects upon human tumor cell lines. JNCI, in press.
22. Monks A, Scudiero D, Skehan P, Boyd M: Implementation of a pilot-scale, high flux anticancer drug screen utilizing disease-oriented panels of human tumor cell lines in culture. Proc. AACR 30:607, 1989; JNCI, in press.
23. Rubinstein LV, Paull KD, Shoemaker RH et al: Correlation of screening data generated with a tetrazolium assay (MIT) versus a protein assay (SRB) against a broad panel of human tumor cell lines. JNCI, in press.
24. Paull KD, Shoemaker RH, Hodes L et al: Display and analysis of patterns of differential activity of drugs against human tumor cell lines: Development mean graph and COMPARE algorithm. JNCI 81:1088-1092, 1989.

25. Paull KD, Hodes L, Plowman J et al: Reproducibility and re-
     sponse patterns of IC_{50} values and relative cell line sen-
     sitivities from the NCI human tumor cell line drug screening
     project. Proc. AACR 29:488, 1988.

3

DISCOVERY OF SOLID TUMOR ACTIVE AGENTS USING A SOFT-AGAR-COLONY-FORMATION DISK-DIFFUSION-ASSAY

Thomas H. Corbett, Frederick A. Valeriote, Lisa Polin, Chiab Panchapor, Susan Pugh, Kathryn White, Nancy Lowichik, Juiwanna Knight, Marie-Christine Bissery, Antoinette Wozniak, Patricia LoRusso, Laura Biernat, Daniel Polin, Lentawn Knight, Sandra Biggar, Darrell Looney, Lisa Demchik, Julie Jones, Lynne Jones, Scott Blair, Kerry Palmer, Sandra Essenmacher, Loretta Lisow, Ken C. Mattes*, Paul F. Cavanaugh*, James B. Rake*, and Laurence Baker

INTRODUCTION

The history of antitumor drug discovery has essentially been the use of two lymphocytic leukemias of mice as selection funnels through which all agents needed to pass in order to advance toward clinical development (L1210 prior to 1975 and P388 after 1975). It is thus not surprising that agents in the clinic are highly active against these tumor systems. However, none of the agents discovered by these leukemias are tumor specific (i.e., active against all tumors), and none of the agents are broadly active against solid tumors of either rodents or humans (1-3). An example contrasting the responsiveness of transplantable solid tumors of mice and the two leukemias is shown in Table-1. The lack of responsiveness of these solid tumors of mice is not unlike those seen in human lung, pancreatic, colon, and prostate tumors. The point to emphasize is that the lack of solid tumor activity of available antitumor agents is not species related. The fault does not lie with the omission of human tumors in the initial selection process, but rather with the omission of solid tumors.

Toward an effort to rectify this omission, we, NCI, Eli Lilly, Eastman Kodak/Sterling, Upjohn, Rhone-Poulenc, and others have moved solid tumors into primary screening for new drug discovery. We begin our search with a tissue culture screen, in which each agent is tested simultaneously against solid tumors (mouse and human), a leukemia (L1210), and normal cells (CFU-GM

* Eastman Kodak Co./Sterling Drug Inc.

36

Table 1

Spectrum of Response of Transplantable Tumors of Mice

	P388	L1210	Panc 02	Colon 51	Mamm 16/Adr	Colon # 38	Panc # 03
Actinomycin D	+++	++	-	-	-	+	NA
Adriamycin	++++	++	-	±	-	++	++
Cytosine Arabinoside	++++	++++	-	-	±	+	-
5-Fluorouracil	+++	+	-	-	++	+++	-
Methotrexate	++	+	-	-	-	-	-
Phenylalanine Mustard	++++	++++	-	-	++	-	NA
Cyclophosphamide	++++	++++	-	+	+++	+	++
BCNU	++++	++++	-	++	-	-	-
Cis-Platinum	+++	+++	-	++	+	±	+
Vincristine	+++	+	-	-	-	-	-

Activity Rating	P388 Leukemia Gross Log Kill	Solid Tumors Gross Log Kill
Inactive -	<1.5	<0.5
+	1.5 -> 2.9	0.5 -> 0.8
++	3.0 -> 4.4	0.9 -> 1.5
+++	4.5 -> 5.9	1.6 -> 2.6
Highly Active ++++	6 -> 7.5	>2.6

Note that less of a $\log_{10}$ cell kill is required to obtain a given +, ++, +++ rating in the solid tumors than for the leukemias. If we used the same scale the solid tumors would appear to be totally unresponsive.

and a fibroblast). We hypothesize that in order to have broad solid tumor activity _in vivo_, it will be necessary to have solid tumor selectivity at the cellular level. Besides testing this hypothesis, there are two additional reasons for beginning a drug discovery search at the cellular level. The first is a humane consideration. Researchers can not justify primary screening in laboratory animals since the identification of active agents through primary _in vivo_ screening has been established to be exceptionally low (based on the many years of screening with leukemias at NCI). In our assay, the agent must have solid tumor selectivity over leukemias or normal cells in order to advance it to animal investigation. This represents less than 2% of the random materials screened. The second reason is cost; primary screening in mice approaches $1,000 per agent and often requires up to 700 mg of the test agent. The tissue culture assay, however, is less than 1/20 this cost and requires a maximum of 10 mg of material.

We have previously published brief descriptions of the disk-diffusion soft-agar colony-formation assay (1,4-11). However, we have not published the detailed laboratory method suitable for the acquisition of needed supplies and appropriate instructions for the research support staff. This is provided in Appendix-1 together with reasons for several design aspects of the assay. This helps the research support staff understand the function of the various components of the assay and thus serves as an incentive not to deviate from the protocol.

We have also provided a brief description of the _in vivo_ evaluation of agents selected by the disk-diffusion assay (Appendix-2). This is a description of _in vivo_ testing methods, and mainly written for a new research assistant with limited experience. The reader should note that this is a highly flexible testing approach, which is intended to obtain an adequate _in vivo_ efficacy trial with a limited supply of drug and limited funding. With the methods of testing described in Appendicies-#1 and #2, and the large numbers of diverse materials examined (over seven thousand per year), we have been successful in discovering limited numbers of solid tumor active agents that will receive clinical evaluations.

We have also investigated certain aspects of the tissue culture assay that allow us to partially evaluate its predictive value in the selection of _in vivo_ active agents. The following are discussions of these investigations and the progress in finding clinical candidates for the treatment of solid tumors.

DRUG DISCOVERY PROTOCOL

The protocol and decision points in our drug discovery program is shown in Figure 1. Test samples are first examined _in vitro_ for cytotoxicity against murine L1210 leukemia, a murine solid tumor (usually Colon 38 or Pancreas 03) and a human solid tumor cell line (usually one of four: CX-1, HCT8, H116 or H125). Based on both absolute and differential cytotoxicity between the solid tumor cells and the L1210 leukemia, the test substance is categorized into one of four groups. If the differential between

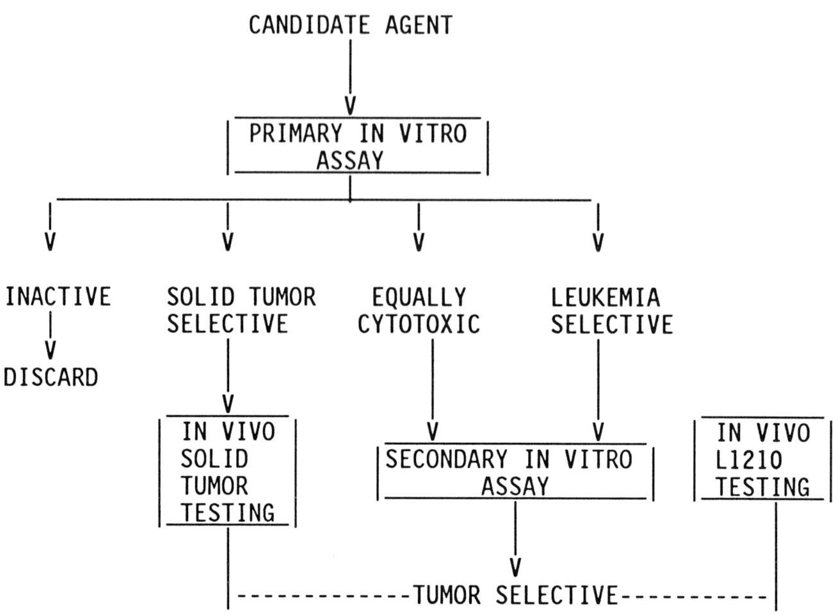

Figure 1: Flow diagram for drug discovery program.

the solid tumors and L1210 is equal to or greater than 250 zone
units, the test agent is classified as either solid tumor- or
leukemia-selective. If the differential is less than 250 zone
units and the absolute cytotoxicity is greater than 200 zone units
for any cell type, the test agent is termed equally active. All
other outcomes, usually zone units of 0 for all cell types, are
relegated to a discard (inactive) status.

Those agents that are solid tumor selective move directly
into _in_ _vivo_ trials against the appropriate solid tumor, either
murine or human xenograft.

Leukemia selective or equally active agents are subsequently
tested in a secondary _in_ _vitro_ assay which compares leukemias
L1210 and AML to a normal cell, CFU-GM (the progenitor of the
granulocyte/macrophage of the hematopoietic tissue). Agents which
yield a zone differential equal to or greater than 250 units in
favor of the leukemias are termed tumor specific: Such agents
which were originally leukemia selective are then tested _in_ _vivo_

against either the L1210 or the C1498 AML leukemia. Tumor selective agents which were initially equally active can be tested _in vivo_ against either a leukemia or the appropriate solid tumor.

For agents which demonstrate _in vivo_ activity, a set of internal criteria exist related to scope of activity, toxicity and other factors which determine whether and at what priority they are moved to clinical trial. This is discussed separately below.

HOW MANY TUMORS ARE NEEDED IN THE PRIMARY DISCOVERY ASSAY? ARE WE MISSING LARGE NUMBERS OF POTENTIALLY USEFUL AGENTS?

In the sequential method of testing, an agent must be active in some first assay (e.g., tissue culture antitumor cytotoxicity) to reach some second assay (e.g., an antitumor efficacy evaluation in mice). It must then be active in the second assay to reach a third assay, and so on. In our tissue culture disk diffusion assay, only one leukemia, one mouse solid tumor and one human solid tumor are evaluated (in comparison with a normal cell). Due to financial limitations, both solid tumors in our assay come from the same tissue type (colon) for most agents evaluated. We have thus been concerned that tumors of some other organ system may be very sensitive to the agents screened, whereas the colon tumors are unresponsive, and we may be missing potentially useful agents. However, at our current level of testing (approximately seven thousand agents per year), the addition of one more plate (e.g., a pancreatic tumor) to answer the question in our general screening operation, would add $60,000 to the cost. As an alternative approach, we selected a few agents that had clear selective cytotoxicity against Colon #38 (compared to L1210 leukemia) in the initial screen and retested them against both Colon-#38 and Panc-#03 in comparison with L1210 (Table-2). As can be seen, only one of eight agents failed to be detected by both solid tumors. We have also used Panc-#03 for a portion of our initial drug screening. Thus, we also selected agents that had clear selective cytotoxicity against Panc-#03 (compared to L1210) in the initial screen and retested them against both Panc-#03 and Colon-#38 (Table-3).

Table 2

**Agents Originally Found to be Selectively Cytotoxic
Against Colon-#38: These Were Retested Against Both
Colon-38 and Panc-03 in the Disk-Diffusion Assay**

Zone Units 200 = 6.5 mm
(The larger the zone, the greater the cytotoxicity)

Agent	ug/Disk	L1210	Colon-38	Panc-03	Selected By	In-Vivo
71316	1000	100-250	580	600	Both	I
175966	500	0	600	700	Both	A
183365	500	0-450	900	780	Both	I
53256	500	30-50	900	830	Both	TNR
183450	62	200-330	850	800	Both	I
72194	250	300-430	>950	>950	Both	TNR
72204	125	80	500	700	Both	NT
150857	500	50-240	430-500	0-200	C38 only	I

I = Inactive, A= Active (T/C < 42%), TNR = Toxicity Not Reached,
NT = Not Tested

Table 3

**Agents Originally Found to be Selectively Cytotoxic
Against Panc-03: These Were Retested Against Both
Colon-38 and Panc-03 in the Disk-Diffusion Assay**

Zone Units 200 = 6.5 mm
(The larger the zone, the greater the cytotoxicity)

Agent	ug/Disk	L1210	Colon-38	Panc-03	Selected By	In-Vivo
118470	160	400-430	860	920	Both	I
131379	500	0	400-700	550	Both	I
21673	500	100-240	920	600-800	Both	TNR
11910	170	0	450	300-400	Both	A
183551	450	150-400	700	750	Both	A
174447	100	400-700	>950	>950	Both	A
119234	41	300-400	330	>950	PO_3 only	A

I = Inactive, A= Active (T/C < 42%), TNR = Toxicity Not Reached

The results were similar; only one of seven agents failed to be detected by both solid tumors. The conclusion of this analysis is obvious: whereas potentially useful solid tumor active agents could be missed, the percent will be relatively low (less than 15% in the studies shown in Tables 2,3).

HOW PREDICTIVE IS THE IN VITRO DISK-DIFFUSION-SOFT-AGAR-COLONY-FORMATION ASSAY IN SELECTING IN VIVO ACTIVE COMPOUNDS?

As we have often emphasized, drug discovery is a "numbers-game"; the more agents tested, the more "actives" will be found; at least, against the primary screening tumor (1). Our data from a single inventory is instructive. In the last thirty-two months, we have tested 16,895 agents from the Kodak/Sterling inventory in the disk-diffusion assay. Initially the inventory was divided into 1,100 chemical categories and we received representatives of each. As active agents were identified, analog searches produced a steady increase in the percentage of submissions. In one case alone, over 1,000 analogs were tested from a single hit. From the 16,895 agents screened, 830 were found to be selective in vitro. These were then tested in mice. One hundred-fifteen of these in vitro selective agents were analogs of some of our previously identified compounds within the Kodak inventory. Sixty-six (of the 830) agents were found to be at least modestly active in the first in vivo test (T/C < 42%). Of these, twenty-nine were analogs of previously identified compounds. Thus, excluding analogs, approximately one agent in twenty that entered mouse testing was found to be at least modestly active (i.e., a 5% in vivo discovery-rate). Obviously, only a small portion of these are found to be of interest in secondary evaluation and will become clinical candidates.

The probability of finding an in vivo active is markedly different for analogs of a solid tumor selective agent for which a "critical active core molecule" has been identified. In this case, the disk-diffusion assay is highly predictive, and 25% to 40% of the analogs that are found selective by the tissue culture assay actually have antitumor activity in mice. The reason for the markedly higher prediction rate for analogs is obvious. One must first consider the limitation of the disk diffusion assay: 1) there is no liver to metabolize the drug and no kidney to eliminate the drug. Approximately 35% of the materials (from random screening) that are tested in mice are non-toxic because they are metabolized and/or excreted before a meaningful concentration x time profile can be obtained. 2) There is no need for an agent to cross multiple physiologic barriers to reach the tumor cell in the tissue culture assay. On the other hand, the ability to cross such barriers is essential for activity in the whole animal. 3) There is no ability to control for all normal cells in a tissue culture assay. Thus, it is common to find some normal tissue (not controlled for in the disk assay) that is as sensitive to the test-drug as the tumor (i.e., the agent is toxic at the dose that is cytotoxic for the tumor).

In the case of analogs of an active agent, the core molecule can usually overcome the three problems; that is, 1) it will not be destroyed by the liver and/or excreted before a meaningful concentration x time is obtained; 2) it can cross multiple physiologic barriers; and 3) normal cells in the body are less sensitive to the agent than the tumor cell population.

One would obviously wish to improve the predictive nature of the assay for random materials, and efforts in this regard are ongoing. Our current approach is to add other normal and "normal-like" cell types to the assay. At the present time we have obtained some success in the use of an "immortal" fibroblast that will not grow in the host of origin with 2×10^7 cell implants. However, a normal cell of ectodermal or entodermal origin would be more desirable considering the origin of the solid tumors that we are using (i.e., colon, pancreas, lung, mammary).

THE SEARCH FOR AGENTS ACTIVE AGAINST A TRUE CANCER TARGET: IS THERE SUCH A TARGET OR TARGETS AND HOW WOULD ONE APPROACH THE SEARCH?

We, like others, have long dreamed of the possibility of discovering an agent that is truly cancer specific (i.e., having

43

some degree of activity against all malignant tumors) and have
both discussed how past screening practices could have overlooked
such an agent and suggested strategies for a more reasonable
search (1). There are several parts to our overall strategy:

1) We begin with the premise that a true cancer target (or
targets) exists and that it (they) is not present in any adult
normal mammalian cell. Thus, destroying the target should have
insignificant toxicity to any normal cell population.

2) The tissue culture prescreen must then contain a normal
cell population for reference. Thus, the agent would be cytotoxic
for the various tumor cell populations, and would have no toxicity
for the normal cells. In our case, we use the CFU-GM from the
bone marrow as the normal population.

3) The solid tumors used have as few vulnerabilities as
possible to the currently available agents. Thus, the tumors will
not signal a response to the currently available antiproliferative
agents and we would not be plagued with the rediscovery of agents
with the mechanisms of actions that are already available. For
example, some agents (such as cytosine arabinoside) are markedly
more cytotoxic for the leukemia models than for the CFU-GM
population.

4) We have constructed the _in_ _vivo_ testing protocol to avoid
the discovery of agents with delayed toxicity, and also agents
that lack the ability to cross physiologic barriers. These types
of agents were routinely discovered as "actives" (actually false
positives) by the IP-IP leukemia screens used between 1955 and
1984 (1). These previously used screening methods unnecessarily
diverted attention, effort, and resources to materials that were
not worth following.

We have incorporated these "cancer-target" strategies into
our search for solid tumor active agents (under the premise that
if you do not specifically search for a desired activity you are
not likely to find it). Up to the present time, we can make no
claim that we have identified any agent with the desired set of
properties. None-the-less, as an example, in Table 4 is shown an
agent that has activity for both drug insensitive solid tumors as

well as L1210; it is significantly more active against the solid
tumors. Further, it is without meaningful cytotoxicity against
the CFU-GM population in the disk-diffusion soft-agar assay. The
agent has modest _in vivo_ activity (Table-4) but is without any
toxicity to the host. To date, analog searching of the parent has
failed to detect any other lead. This may be due to the limited
number of analogs.

AGENTS FOUND TO HAVE SOLID TUMOR SELECTIVITY IN THE DISK-DIFFUSION
ASSAY

Although our drug discovery effort is still in its infancy, a
few agents have been identified that have solid tumor selectivity
in the assay and also have meaningful solid tumor activity in
mice.

Table 4

CANCER TARGET ACTIVITY

Primary Assay Zone Units		Secondary Assay Zone Units	
L1210	0	L1210	800
Panc 03	800	CFU-GM	50
HCT 8	200-300		

In Vivo Pancreatic Ductal Adenocarcinoma 03

OD3-9 SC 1350 mg/kg Total   15% T/C
                   Not Toxic

As might be expected, most are still discrete. We have, however,
published on several that are not discrete (7,9-11). Very few
blanket statements can be made concerning the mechanisms of action
or structural features of agents with solid tumor selectivity.
All of these active agents have been within a molecular weight
range of 120 to 500. Most have belonged to schedule category #3
(7,12-14) (also see Appendix-#2 for definitions of schedule cate-

gories). Cummulative dose limiting toxicities have varied, with liver toxicity, GI toxicity and leukopenia being the most common.

CRITERIA USED FOR ADVANCING AN AGENT TOWARD CLINICAL DEVELOPMENT

Over the last 40 years a large number of "antitumor agents" have been advanced to clinical trials and have failed to be useful. Indeed, we ourselves have advocated an agent that has failed to have a meaningful therapeutic index in humans (i.e., flavone acetic acid) (7). Learning from both the clinical successes as well as the failures, we have drafted a set of preclinical criteria that we hope will improve the chances for clinical success. We wish to emphasize that these criteria are only guidelines, and we would clearly forgo the need for criteria #6 in selected circumstances, while remaining relatively inflexible with the first five.

1. Selective cytotoxicity for solid tumors over leukemia L1210 or normal cells at the cellular level. A zone differential of >250 units is required for meaningful selectivity (see Appendix-#1). This requirement is consistent with our hypothesis that broad solid tumor activity _in vivo_ will be attended by solid tumor selectivity at the cellular level.

2. Activity (<42% T/C) against one or more human tumors in nude mice is desired. The human tumor trials are conducted in the same fashion as the mouse tumor trials: bilateral SC tumor implant of 30 to 60 mg fragments, with the agent injected IV (see Appendix-2). We use the following: Lung H125; Colon CX-1, H116, H8; Mammary MX-1, and Lung LX-1; certainly a large number of other drug insensitive human tumors could be used. The first four were chosen because they are routinely used in the _in vitro_ disk diffusion assay. We especially favor the use of H125 since it is extremely drug insensitive.

3. At a non-toxic dosage level (LD_{10} or less and body weight loss less than 20%), the agent should produce greater than a $2\text{-}log_{10}$ tumor cell kill in two tumor systems from a single course of treatment (10 days or less) with the drug and the tumor administered by a different route, thus requiring the

46

drug to cross multiple physiologic barriers. It must be verified that the responses were obtained in a non-immunogenic
tumor model system (e.g, cured mice reimplanted with 60 mg
tumor fragments will regrow with no substantial alteration in
the Td value). The following tumors are considered acceptable: Pancreatic Ductal Adenocarcinoma #02 or #03; Colon
Adenocarcinoma #38, #51, #07; Undifferentiated Colon Tumor
#26; Mammary Adenocarcinoma #16/C, #16/C/Adr, #17/C/Adr, #13,
#25, #44. The methods for _in_ _vivo_ evaluation and quantifica-
tion of tumor cell kill have been previously published (2,
7-19).

4. In the evaluation of seven tumor systems (from the list given
   in Criteria #3), we require _in_ _vivo_ activity _at two non-toxic_
   dosage levels (0.62 decrements) _in three tumor models_, with
   the drug administered by a route different than the tumor.
   Activity defined as T/C values of <42% (see Appendix #2). It
   should be noted that two tumors are already highly responsive
   in Criteria #3, and it is usually expected that they will
   have responded at two dose levels. This however, is not
   always the case; e.g., Flavone Acetic Acid which is often
   active at only one dose level. The "two-dose-level" requirement is included to exclude agents with exceptionally steep
   dose response cures (where only the maximum tolerated dose
   (MTD) is active). In clinical trials, an agent is rarely
   escalated to a dose that is similar to an MTD in a healthy
   young mouse.

5. In normal, non-tumor mice treated with maximum tolerated dosages of the agent (i.e., no lethality within fifteen days of
   last treatment), there should be no long delayed lethality
   (e.g., twenty to one hundred eighty days post last treatment)
   and a reasonable host recovery time (M/S >2) (14). If the
   agent has an adequate host recovery time, animals treated
   with a MTD should regain their pretreatment weights within
   fourteen days post treatment and continue to gain both weight
   and skeletal size thereafter.

6. Activity against one or more tumors with the multidrug resistant phenotype; e.g., P388/Adr, Mammary Adenocarcinoma 16/C/Adr or Mammary Adenocarcinoma 17/A/Adr is also desired.

In addition to the criteria discussed above, there are several other properties that we consider to be important in the development of a new agent:

1. IV formulation possible. If an agent is water insoluble, it
   is usually possible for the chemists to design water soluble
analogs. An example of some commonly used groups are: $-NH-CH_2-CH2-N(CH3)_2$ or $-CH2-CH2-CH2-N(CH3)_2$ or $-CH2-CH2-N(CH2CH3)_2$.

It would be possible to develop a water insoluble agent for clinical trials if it had oral activity and dependable and consistant absorption. However, if at all possible, it is better to wait for a water soluble analog because IV delivery reduces the number of physiologic barriers the agent must cross, and usually produces a better therapeutic index as a result.

2. Good stability in solution. A half life of at least thirty
   minutes in solution at room temperature is considered necessary for ease of handling and consistent dose delivery. Obviously, the greater the stability, the better.

3. Dosage levels within the limits of the 1100 mg/kg rule.

Over the last forty years, a large number of potentially useful cytotoxic antitumor agents have received clinical trials. In that time, it has been noted that agents with a very large dosage requirement have almost universally failed to be of value (with the exception of hydroxyurea). An analysis of the clinically useful agents has revealed that all (except hydroxyurea) were effective in tumor bearing mouse trials with a total dose of <1,100 mg/kg on an optimum schedule for one course of treatment (i.e., less than twelve days of treatment). This has become known as the 1,100 mg/kg rule. One suspects that agents with a very high dosage requirement simply lack sufficient specificity for whatever target is being hit, and thus have a poor therapeutic index. Whereas it is obvious that one should not be totally bound by the 1,100 mg/kg rule, it is difficult to ignore the failures of nearly all agents that have violated the rule.

4. The agent can be made available in necessary amounts for a reasonable cost.

In drug development, these problems have delayed development of some agents for many years, (e.g., taxol), but have rarely terminated development for highly active agents.

5. Patent protection possible.

Companies are usually unwilling to put up developmental costs unless they can obtain patent protection. Several potentially promising agents in the public domain will probably never be developed.

ACKNOWLEDGEMENTS

Supported by: Natural Products NCDDG CA-53001, Program
Project Project CA-46560
Colon NCDDG 45962
Eastman Kodak Co./Sterling Drug Inc.
Wayne State University Ben Kasle Trust for Cancer
Research
CA-12623
CA-43886

REFERENCES

1. Corbett TH, Valeriote FA and Baker LH: Is the P388 murine tumor no longer adequate as a drug discovery model? Invest. New Drugs 5:3-20, 1987.
2. Corbett TH, Roberts BJ, Leopold WR et al: Induction and chemotherapeutic response of two transplantable ductal adenocarcinomas of the pancreas in C57BL/6 mice. Cancer Res. 44:717-726, 1984.
3. Skipper H: Drug evaluation in experimental tumor systems: Potential and limitations in 1961. Cancer Chemother Rep. 16:11-19,1962.
4. Corbett TH: A selective soft agar assay for drug discovery. Proc. Am. Assoc. for Cancer Res. 25:325, 1984.
5. Corbett TH: A selective soft agar assay for drug discovery. Proc. Am. Assoc. for Cancer Res. 26:332, 1985.

6. Corbett TH, Wozniak A, Gerpheide S and Hanka L: A selective two-tumor soft agar assay for drug discovery. In: In Vitro and In Vivo Models for Detection of New Antitumor Drugs: Proceedings 14th International Congress of Chemotherapy. LJ Hanka, T Kondo, and RJ White (eds) Univ. of Tokyo Press. pp. 5-14, 1986.

7. Corbett TH, Bissery M, Wozniak A et al: Activity of flavone acetic acid (NSC-347512) against solid tumors of mice. Invest. New Drugs 4:207-220, 1986.

8. Corbett TH and Valeriote F: Rodent models in experimental chemotherapy. In: The Use of Rodent Tumors in Experimental Cancer Therapy. RF Kallman (ed), Pergamon Press, pp. 233-247, 1987.

9. LoRusso PM, Polin L, Bissery MC et al: Activity of batra-cylin (NSC-320846) against solid tumors of mice. Invest. New Drugs 6:295-306,1989.

10. LoRusso PM, Polin L, Biernat LA et al: Activity of detallip-tinium (NSC 311152) against solid tumors of mice. Invest. New Drugs 8:253-261, 1990.

11. LoRusso PM, Wozniak AJ, Polin L et al: Antitumor efficacy of PD115934 (NSC 366140) against solid tumors of mice. Cancer Res. 50:4900-4905, 1990.

12. Corbett TH, Leopold WR, Dykes DJ et al: Toxicity and anti-cancer activity of a new triazine antifolate (NSC-127755). Cancer Res. 42:1707-1715, 1982.

13. Pazdur R, Redman BG, Corbett T et al: Phase I trial of spirohydantoin mustard (spiromustine/NSC 172112) and eval-uation of toxicity and schedule in a murine model. Cancer Res. 47:4213-4217, 1987.

14. Corbett TH, Bissery MC, LoRusso PM, Polin L: 5-Fluorouracil containing combinations in murine tumor systems. Invest. New Drugs 7:37-49, 1989.

15. Corbett TH, Griswold DP Jr, Roberts BJ et al: Evaluation of single agents and combinations of chemotherapeutic agents in mouse colon carcinomas. Cancer 40(5):2660-2680, 1977.

16. Corbett TH, Roberts BJ, Trader MW et al: Response of trans-plantable tumors of mice of anthracenedione derivatives alone and in combination with clincally useful agents. Cancer Treat. Rep. 6:1187-1200, 1982.

17. LoRusso PM, Polin L, Aukerman SL et al: Antitumor efficacy of interleukin-2 alone and in combination with adriamycin and dacarbazine in murine solid tumor systems. Cancer Res. 50:5876-5882, 1990.

18. Corbett TH, Griswold DP, Roberts BJ et al: Biology and thera-peutic response of a mouse mammary adenocarcinoma (16/C) and its potential as a model for surgical adjuvant chemotherapy. Cancer Treat. Rep. 62(10):1471-1488, 1978.

19. Griswold DP Jr, Corbett TH, Schabel FM Jr: Clonogenicity and growth of experimental tumors in relation to developing resistance and therapeutic failure. Cancer Treat. Rep. 65(2):51-54, 1981.

APPENDIX 1

GENERAL STRATEGY FOR DISCOVERY OF NEW ANTITUMOR AGENTS

Historically, the primary screening models (_in vitro_ and _in vivo_) are always the most critical in any drug discovery effort. Secondary evaluation is of reduced value since these assays can rarely detect new mechanisms of action. In our strategy, we begin with drug insensitive solid tumors in the primary _in vitro_ screen and in the primary _in vivo_ screen. We believe that it is critical to start a drug discovery effort _in vitro_ (at the cellular level): Solid tumor selectivity over leukemia cytotoxicity; malignant cell toxicity over normal cell toxicity. We believe that cellular selectivity will be the key first step to discovery of broadly active antitumor agents. Based on our own experience (and others), it is clear that cell culture assays will generate a percentage of false positives but very few false negatives if designed correctly. The false positives occur because the same tumor cell exposure conditions can not be achieved in the whole animal or because some normal tissue (that is not monitored in the _in vitro_ assay) has a vulnerability to the agent similar to the target tumor.

The _in vitro_ soft agar, disk-diffusion assay is cell-proliferation dependent. We wish to emphasize that multiple cell divisions are necessary to see the colonies. Furthermore, the essence of the assay; i.e., comparison of the cytotoxic activity of drugs against a leukemia, drug insensitive solid tumors, and normal cells (at the same time) presupposes that cellular selectivity exists. The validation studies have been done and are available.

Operational Characteristics of the Disk-Diffusion-Assay Growth Conditions for Assay

It is well known from bacterial zone of inhibition sensitivity assays (e.g., Kirby-Bauer Disk Diffusion) that a number of factors (e.g., content and % of agar; type of media; inoculum size; replication rate of bacteria; diffusion behavior of the antibiotic; etc.) can influence results. Many of these same types of factors clearly influence the results of the multiple tumor zone of inhibition assay. Standardization of agar, media, gas phase and supplements have eliminated much of the experimental variability. The assay is designed to determine qualitatively <u>large differences</u> in the relative sensitivity of a leukemia, two solid tumors and a normal cell with the same drug. Preferably, one wishes to see either a very large zone or total elimination of the solid tumor colonies from the plate and only minor toxicity for the leukemia (or normal cells).

Disks

6.5 mm disk (standard hole punch of Whatman #1 filter paper). Wash the filter paper disks in water (three times) and then etha-nol. Autoclave. Allow to stand in ethanol.

Compounds

Compounds are initially evaluated at 250 μg/disk. The drug is placed on the disk in solution (ethanol, dH_2O, DMF depending on solubility; 5mg/ml). The soluble agent is delivered onto the disks and allowed to dry. The disks are then placed on the plates that have been prepared within the previous 24 hours.

Cell Preparation and Treatment Conditions

Most mouse tumors give a reasonable cell suspension yield with mechanical disruption. A perfect single cell suspension is not only impossible but unnecessary in the disk-diffusion assay. Colonies arise from varying numbers of cells (1 to 20 cell clumps are common). Tumors which fail to disrupt with mechanical proce-dures are digested with type II collagenase (1%) and DNAase (0.005%). The quality of the cell suspension is followed micro-scopically to judge the degree of disruption. The following is a general procedure for the mechanical disruption.

Mechanical Disruption Technique for Easy to Disrupt Mouse Tumors (e.g., Colon-#38, #9, #7, Panc-03, B-16 melanoma, L1210)

The tumor (1000-1500 mg) is cut up into 200-300 mg fragments in 10-15 ml of saline on ice. Smaller tumors give a poor cell yield and a decreased plating efficiency. This material is poured through a 100 mesh sieve; residual material is forced through (by finger with two sterile gloves), and the sieve is rinsed twice with cold HBSS. It is centrifuged at 150G for 5 min, and resuspended in 15 ml HBSS and again centrifuged. Finally it is resuspended in 10 ml of cold CMRL/Fishers (50:50 proportions).

The leukemia (a culture adapted line of L1210) is also maintained in SC passage in mice and is prepared as for the solid tumor.

Mechanical Disruption Technique for Difficult to Disrupt Mouse Tumors (e.g., Colon-#26, Panc-02)

The tumor (800-1400 mg cut up into 200-300 mg fragments in 10-15 ml of saline on ice) is disrupted using a Stomacher-80 for 20 sec. Smaller tumors give a poor cell yield and a decreased plating efficiency. This material is poured through a 45 mesh sieve; residual material is forced through (by finger with two sterile gloves), and the sieve is rinsed twice with HBSS. The material poured through and forced through the sieve is repeatedly (10 times) drawn up (rapidly) and pushed down (slowly) in a 5 cc glass syringe (without a needle), and again poured through a sieve (100 mesh, without forcing material through) with two HBSS rinses, centrifuged at 150G for 5 min, resuspended in 15 ml HBSS and again centrifuged. Finally it is resuspended in 10 ml of cold, 1:1 CMRL/Fishers.

CFU-GM from Bone Marrow as the Normal Cell Control

The femurs are removed from 3-5 mice, and cleaned with sterile gauze. The joints are clipped from both ends. The marrow is flushed with 1 ml of 1:1 CMRL/Fisher's media, using a 3 ml syringe with a 23 gauge needle. Remove the needle and draw the marrow up (rapidly) in the syringe and push down (slowly) three times to disperse the cells. The cells are counted and volume adjusted with either CMRL/Fisher's supplemented with 15% Dunn Osteogenic Sarcoma conditioned media or a-MEM media supplemented with 10% L-cell conditioned media to give 3×10^6 cells per dish.

Cell Counting (Hemocytometer)

Add 0.1 ml cell suspension to 0.9 ml HBSS + 1 drop of 0.4% Trypan Blue (Gibco #630-5250). Further dilution may be necessary for counting (dye excluding cells only). The volume of the preparation is adjusted appropriately with HBSS. 1 ml of packed cells (solid tumor) will make approximately 30 plates (volume adjusted with 50/50 CMRL/ Fishers so that one tube contains enough media and cells for 3 plates; 2.7 ml/plate, 8 ml/tube). 0.1 ml of leukemic cell stock will make 10 plates (volume adjusted as for the solid tumors).

Bottom Layers

a.   Put a bottle of 3.6% Noble-agar (Difco D-0142-01) in a beaker with water and heat to boiling until melted. <u>Do not microwave heat the</u> <u>agar</u>.

b.   Bring a bottle of media to 37°C in a warm bath. One bottle contains 160 ml of a 1:1 mixture of Fishers - CMRL 1066 (each of these already contain the required serum and antibiotics).

c.   Add 40 ml of 5% TSB (Tryptic Soy Broth Sigma T-8261) which has been autoclaved.

d.   Add a sterile stirring-bar and start mixing in a beaker containing hot water.

e.   Add 55 ml of the hot Noble-agar and pipet the mixture up and down a few times to make sure it is mixed.

f.   Keep the mixture at approximately 50°C.

g.   Add 3ml to each 60 mm dish, in stacks of 3 dishes (per 10 ml pipet); then swirl each stack to distribute the agar over the entire plate surface. Use a 10 ml plastic pipet attached to the automatic pipetter; a glass pipet will not stay warm and will plug up. Avoid bubbles (suck any big bubbles off the agar plate with the pipet). One or two pipets can be used to make the entire batch. One bottle will make approximately 80 plates.

h. Usually, 160 plates (two bottles) or 240 plates (three bottles) are made at one time.

i. Allow the bottom layers to harden before placement in a 5% CO_2 incubator. Use the bottom layers between 2 and 9 days after preparation. Do not use before day 2.

Calculations for the Number of Tumor Cells to be Used and Preparation of the Top Layer

The plating efficiency of the tumors being used is determined (in soft agar), and the titers adjusted to produce approximately 400 colonies of the leukemia and 400 colonies or greater (up to 800) for the solid tumor (per 60 mm dish). Other cell types (e.g., CFU-GM, human tumors) can be prepared in separate dishes and run in parallel.

Top Layer

The top layer is made by adding 1.2 ml of 3.6% Noble-agar (maintained at 46 to 48°) to a tube containing 8 ml of the cells plus media; pipetting this up and down once; and then pipetting 3 ml onto the top of the already prepared bottom layers. A new pipet is used for the preparation of each 3 plates. Special note: _Do not add more than 1.2 ml or less than 1.0 ml of Noble agar. If too much is added the leukemias will not grow well, if too little is added, the plates will be excessively soft. Keep the temperature of the agar below 50°C._

Human Cell Lines-Cell Preparation

Human tumors (e.g., H-125 lung, Colon #116, #8, CX-1, Panc-#1) are maintained in tissue culture. Both mechanical and enzymatic methods have been used for the dispersal of cells for the disk diffusion assay. We favor the mechanical method since this may impose less selective pressure on the cells.

For trypsinization, the cells are removed from the surface of the flasks prior to reaching saturation density. The following method is used: Remove the media. Add 37^{0}C trypsin (0.25%) prepared in 0.02% EDTA in Phosphate Buffered Saline. Allow to stand for 1 min. Remove the trypsin solution and allow the flask to stand for an additional 5 to 10 min. until the cells detach (they can be observed to round-up under microscopic examination). Add fresh media and pipet to suspend the cells. Plate the cells 2 x 10^5 or fewer/60 mm plate to obtain 300 to 1000 colonies per plate.

For the mechanical method, media is removed from the T-75 flask. 10 ml of fresh media is added and the cells scraped from the surface. The cells and media are placed in a 100 mm petri dish and repeatedly (10 times) drawn up (rapidly) and pushed down (slowly) in a 5 cc syringe (without a needle).

Media:
Fishers's
400 ml deionized water (d-H_2O) Sterile (Autoclaved)
 50 ml Fishers's 10X Concentrate (Gibco 330-1735 AJ)
  7.5 ml of 7.5% $NaHCO_3$ Sterilize by filtration
      Adjust pH to 7.1 to 7.2
      Bring Volume up to 500 ml with d-H_2O
  0.05 ml Garamycin (80 mg/2ml Schering)
 55 ml Horse Serum (Fetal Bovine Serum for some tumors)

CMRL-1066 - Enriched
400 ml d-H_2O Sterile (Autoclaved)
 50 ml CMRL-1066 10X Concentrate (Gibco 330-1540 AJ)
 15 ml of 7.5% $NaHCO_3$ Sterile - Add slowly
      Adjust pH to 7.2 to 7.3
      Bring volume up to 500 ml with d-H_2O
 20 ml $CaCl_2$ (100 mM) 1.47 g/100 ml Gibco #895-1110
  0.25 ml Pen-Strep (10,000 units PNC/ml/10,000 ug strep) Gibco
      #600-5140
 10 ml L-Glutamine 100X (200 mM) Gibco #320-5030 Store frozen
  0.05 ml Garamycin (80 mg/2ml Schering)
 75 ml Horse Serum (Fetal Bovine Serum for some tumors)

<u>HBSS</u> (Modified Hank's Balanced Salt Solution
Media for Cell Preparation
 50 ml (10x) Hanks (Gibco #310-4180)
400 ml sterile dH_2O
 50 ml Horse serum
  0.5ml Pen-Strep (10,000 units PCN/ml, 10,000 ug strep)
  4 ml $NaHCO_3$ (7.5% solution)

The assay can also be used to detect antifungals and antibacterials. After the plates are examined for the zones of inhibition of the tumors and normal cells, two plates are set aside from each drug tested. We use one set to evaluate Candida and the other to evaluate Pseudomonas. One drop of media containing Candida (approximately 5×10^8 cells/ ml) or Pseudomonas (approximately 2×10^8 cells/ml) is placed close to the disk. The Pseudomonas plates are stored at room temperature for two days before they are examined for zones. The Candida plates are incubated at $37^\circ C$ for one day before they are examined for zones. Data is recorded only for those producing a zone (which are few). Materials producing a differential zone for Candida compared to the mammalian cells are reevaluated for activity against Aspergillus molds.

Zone Assay Methodology

A volume of 0.05 ml of each drug dilution is dropped onto a 6.5 mm disk (standard hole punch of Whatman #1 filter paper). The disks are allowed to dry and then placed midway between the center and the edge of the dishes containing various tumors. The plates are incubated for 6-10 days and examined on an inverted microscope (10x eyepiece with micrometer scale, 4x objective) for measurement of the zone of inhibition of both tumors. A zone of inhibition (measured from the edge of the disk to the first colony) of less than 75 units (1 unit = 25 micron) of the solid tumor with a concentration of 5 mg/ml (0.05 ml on disk) for the synthetic agent or 0.05 ml for the fermentation is considered to indicate an agent of insufficient cytotoxic activity to be of interest. A difference of 250 or more units between the zone for any solid tumor and the leukemia indicates a significant differential effect (2). This defines the solid tumor selective category of agents. Agents with >250-zone-unit differential represent < 2% of the random samples tested. Agents with greater than a 500 zone differential represent less than 0.1% of the materials evaluated.

Drug Solubility

We have found that the candidate agents do not need to be totally soluble for assessment of activity. Because we prepare a high concentration of the compound (in Ethanol, dH_2O, or Dimethylformamide), we occasionally end up with a fine suspension which is placed on the filter disk. Even for very water insoluble compounds, we often obtain large zones and even significant differences between the tumor types. Our experience to date is that over 90% of the random synthetic compounds provided are fully soluble at the starting concentration in either ETOH, dH_2O or DMF.

Initial Drug Concentration Evaluated

The weakness of a single tumor _in_ _vitro_ assay system is the lack of selectivity: elevate the dose high enough and all the cells die. With our multiple tumor-disk-diffusion-assay, we are seeking a _differential_ _cytotoxicity_. The absolute degree of toxicity at any particular µg/ml concentration is not important. The sensitivity or insensitivity of the solid tumor is automatically evident in its relationship to the material's activity against the leukemia and normal cells. However, one does not wish to set the dosage used for the first trial too low. If an agent with the desired solid-tumor activity (but with very little cytotoxicity) was tested at a low dosage level, it would be missed (clearly undesirable since the desired activity is likely to come along only rarely). One can always go back and retest any agent that was excessively toxic against both tumors in the first trial (at a series of lower dosages), however, an agent that produces no toxicity against the solid tumor at the initial test level would never be tested again.

We have chosen a dose level for an initial trial of 250 µg for the synthetic on the disk. This level was selected because all clinically available cytotoxic antitumor agents were found to be cytotoxic at 1/5 or less of this concentration (except PALA; NSC-224131, which required the full 250 µg/disk level to produce cytotoxicity). For this, synthetics are prepared at a concentration of 5 mg/ml. A volume of 0.05 ml is placed on the 6.5 mm filter paper disk and allowed to dry. In the case of fermentation materials, 0.05 ml of the undiluted material is used for the initial test (50 ug).

Control disks, damp or wet with the various solvents used were found to produce zones of inhibition of less that 50 units (One unit = 25 microns); dry disks alone produced no zones.

If the material is not toxic for either the solid tumors or the leukemia at the starting dose, it is considered to be of no interest. If the test material is excessively toxic at the first dosage, it destroys the colony formation for both tumors and one then retests a range of dilutions of the agents (often at 1/2 $\log_{10}$ decrements) against the same tumors. At one of the dilutions, appropriate toxicity is invariably obtained.

APPENDIX 2

<u>IN VIVO EVALUATION OF PREVIOUSLY UNTESTED CYTOTOXIC AGENTS FOR
ANTITUMOR ACTIVITY AGAINST TRANSPLANTABLE TUMORS OF MICE</u>:
STANDARD EFFICACY TRIAL

Experiments are given in the following format:

Group	# of BDF_1 Mice/group	Bilateral Trocar Colon #38 on day 0	Agent	mg/kg/inj	Schedule	Drug Route
1	5	Yes	No Treatment Control			
2	5	Yes	K207324	160	QD*3-14	IV or SC
3	5	Yes		80		
4	5	Yes		40		

*QD means one injection per day (in this case every day from day
three through day fourteen).

Normally, about five different agents are tested in a single
trial. In the example shown above, we will provide several possible scenarios for this one compound. As various conditions are
encountered, the treatment conditions are altered appropriately.
The reason a fixed protocol is not given is simple: It is impossible to design a single protocol that will give every drug a meaningful evaluation because of widely differing physical properties
and widely differing biologic effects. Furthermore, most of the
drugs being tested are in limited supply. Often, only enough drug
is available to carry out one test. If not given an adequate
test, it is unlikely that the agent will ever get another chance
since it is usually too expensive to resynthesize more compound.
Thus, only agents that have meaningful activity in a first test
will be resynthesized for additional trials in other tumors (and
to reconfirm the activity against the first tumor).

The goal is to inject as much drug (total) as possible, without killing the mice. This may take anywhere from five to thirty
injections. Antitumor activity for cytotoxic agents is related to

the total dosage that can be administered (with only a couple of exceptions that we will explain later). Thus, the more drug injected into the mouse, the more antitumor activity should be seen (if the agent is active). Dose/response curves are very steep. Doubling the dose does not simply double the tumor cell kill. It will often increase the kill by 10- to 1000-fold. This being the case, even 15% to 20% more drug will often mean the difference between detecting activity and failing. In order to assure that the maximum amount of drug is being given, one is attempting to see some evidence of toxicity at the top dose level (e.g., weight loss of greater than 2.5 g/mouse). An excessively toxic dose is considered to be one that causes $\geq$ 20% body weight loss or $\geq$ 20% drug induced deaths from cumulative toxicity. There are three dose levels to work with. Thus, if toxic limits are exceeded in the top dose (or even the top two doses), there is still the dose below to evaluate for efficacy. Deaths within a few minutes or hours of injection do not count in evaluating the toxic limit of the drug. This will be discussed later. It simply means that the dose injected was too high. Frequently, splitting the dose and giving it multiple times per day for many days in a row, will allow deliverance of 10- to 20-fold more drug than a poorly chosen schedule. Compounds with immediate toxicity (called schedule category three, and discussed later) are the most likely compounds to be missed in any antitumor drug discovery program and require extra care in their study design.

<u>STABILITY</u>

Unless it is specifically noted, assume that the agent is stable for less than seven hours. Prepare the drugs for the experiment and inject them immediately (i.e., within 90 minutes of preparation). If the protocol is altered (or designed) for two injections per day, prepare the drug for both injections. Store the drug at room temperature between injections. If the drug is frozen or stored in the refrigerator, the agent is often difficult to resuspend, requiring warming and regrinding in a homogenizer. Incidentally, warming of any agent, if needed, should not exceed

45°C and should be for no longer than two minutes at this temperature. Each drug is prepared fresh daily. If very small dosages are being injected, for which it is difficult to weigh out the very small quantities, a stock may be prepared in ethanol or other suitable solvent and stored in the freezer. If a compound has been found to be active in a first test, it will be evaluated in several more trials; and thus it is useful to obtain a stability estimation. This can be done using the disk diffusion assay. Since the agent produces a characteristic toxicity profile (with selectivity) against a set of tumors and normal cells, it is easy to see if the degree of cytotoxicity and selectivity is maintained over time. Prepare the drug as for a mouse injection (aqueous). Store the sample in a 37°C incubator. At some time interval (e.g., four days) prepare another aqueous sample and store it in the incubator. The next day prepare the last sample and test all three in the disk diffusion soft agar colony formation assay. The one day and five day stability is then known. Drugs are rarely prepared for more than five days of injection even if they are stable.

INJECTION ROUTES

Compounds are usually injected by one of four routes. The volumes delivered and the size of the needles are as follows: Intravenous (IV): 0.2 ml volume, 0.5 inch needle, 27 g 1 ml syringe (BD9623 preferred). In some cases, volumes up to 0.4 ml can be injected, and other needle sizes are satisfactory, e.g., 26 gauge. The mice are warmed under infrared lamps before they are injected IV in either tail vein. The heat expands the veins and makes them easier to see. Since the mice are usually injected multiple times, it is better to begin toward the tip of the tail and work up on successive days. Bruising from repeated injections, or tail vein damage from drug-induced-necrosis will eventually cause the route to be changed (to SC). If the drug induces tail vein damage (necrosis), the alternate route should never be IP because it will often cause sterile peritonitis, pain and death at subtherapeutic dose levels.

<u>Subcutaneous</u> (SC): 0.2 ml volume, 1 inch needle 23 g. In some
cases in which the suspension is poor a 21 g needle can be used,
and a larger volume will usually improve the ability to deliver
the drug (e.g., 0.3 ml). However, the bigger the needle, the more
leakage will occur. In some cases, drugs cannot be prepared in an
aqueous media because they produce "gums" or "glues". These can
usually be prepared in sesame or peanut oil. The plunger on a
plastic syringe will not work with oil. Thus, a glass syringe with
a LeurLok needs to be used.   The site of SC injection is behind
the neck. The mouse is held down on the counter (or screen) with
the nape of the neck pinched between the thumb and the forefinger.
The needle is then slipped between the thumb and the finger so
that the needle and the material being injected can be felt going
in. Pinch the site after removal of the needle to reduce leakage.
SC injections can also be made along the side, low near the inguinal region. The mouse is held as for an IP injection. This
site (the side of the mouse) is usually not an option in our
trials because the solid tumors are transplanted bilaterally in
these regions.

<u>Intraperitoneal (IP)</u>: 0.5 ml volume, 0.25 inch 23 g needle
(Monoject Catalog #8881-250271). A 3, 5 or 6 ml plastic syringe
is used (depending on the number of mice to be injected). Use
only these needles. Smaller gauges or longer needles will express
the fluid too rapidly in a hydraulic action, causing bowel perfora-
tions. A longer needle is also likely to cause damage to vital organs and perforate the bowel. We never inject new, previously untested materials by this route. The reason is simple; some of the
agents will be necrotizing or produce pain. These are best injected IV. There are no intravenous pain receptors, and the rapid
dilution of the agent by the blood will render necrotizing agents
harmless. Many agents of this nature would cause sterile peritonitis if injected intraperitoneal, with deaths at subtherapeutic
dose levels. Several highly useful antitumor agents cause sterile
peritonitis with IP injections (e.g., Adriamycin, VP-16, mitoxantrone). If the agents are not water soluble they are given SC.
Necrotizing agents are usually evident after a few days. In many

cases it is possible to give the drug an adequate trial if the tissue damage is not severe. However, if the agent is very damaging, one will need to discontinue injections SC. <u>Oral</u> (PO): 0.1 ml with a special 1.0 inch 18 g blunt needle with a silver solder ball at the end is used. We custom make these needles as we have not found a satisfactory commercial needle for this purpose. PO injections are required in the secondary evaluation of water insoluble active agents (route studies). Previously untested agents are not evaluated by this route, although it would seem reasonable to do so for water insoluble agents. The reason is due to the fact that the digestive enzymes, or pH conditions rapidly degrade many chemical classes. In primary drug discovery, we are interested in seeing if an agent is active (without creating unnecessary barriers). It is a relatively easy job for a chemist to make an agent water soluble (by adding certain functional groups).

RANDOMIZATION, MOUSE SELECTION AND CONTROLS

Randomization is a critical step in assuring that all the groups are as uniform as possible. The mice should be a single sex, from a single-source, and close to the same size (within 5 g). The mice should be a minimum of 19 g. This assures that the mice are healthy at the start of the experiment. Smaller mice can often have intercurrent infections or be too young to withstand the stress of treatment. After the mice are trocared with the tumor they are put in a single tub and mixed. Mice are then removed <u>unselectively</u> and placed in the various treatment and control groups. This technique is known among statisticians as "casual randomization" and is the method specified in NCI protocols.

Note that there is only a single control in the testing of new agents (and this receives no treatment). This is because several drugs are tested in the same experiment, and we have never seen a case in which they are all active. Thus, the low dosage groups of the inactive agents can serve as a "diluent treated control" to verify that the untreated control is valid in its tumor growth behavior.

SOLUBILITY

Note that the trial initially shown is designed for either IV (intravenous) or SC (subcutaneous) injection. Thus, the solubility of the agent is unknown. Although more time consuming and requiring greater technical skill, we would prefer that an agent be tested IV if at all possible. There are two reasons for preferring the IV route. The first reason for an IV injection is the obvious fact that one has reduced the number of physiologic barriers the agent must cross to reach the tumor cell. Thus, the drug has been given a better chance to be active and the process has simulated the clinical situation (where most antitumor agents are given IV). If the agent is given SC, it will need to be absorbed into the circulation before it can be distributed to the tumor (one extra barrier compared to IV). The second reason the IV route is favored is because some of the drugs will cause tissue damage or pain. This is minimized if they can be injected IV.

However, many agents are not water soluble and must be injected by some other route; in our trials SC.

To determine the solubility, place a few small crystals on a microscope slide, add a drop of water and mix with a spatula. If insoluble, try a few more crystals with 0.001 N HCl and 0.001 N NaOH. Unless the crystals go into solution within a few seconds, assume the agent is water insoluble and proceed as follows.

Place a few crystals at various locations on a microscope slide and check the solubility in various organic solvents (e.g. ethanol, DMSO, and propylene glycol). Repeat the process with various carriers (e.g., Tween 40, carboxymethyl cellulose, and polyethyleneglycol). As an example, we will assume that the agent was soluble in ethanol and Tween-40. The following toxicity test can then be carried out.

TOXICITY TEST

Weigh out approximately 30 mg of compound and put it into a small (2 ml) test tube. Add four drops of ethanol, one drop of POE40 (Tween-40) and mix with a spatula (mash crystals). Add 0.3 ml of H_2O and mix with a spatula. Attach a 1 inch needle 23 g and draw up as much as possible into the syringe (some will be wasted). Inject approximately 0.05 ml of the suspension SC into one mouse (approximately 20 g size, earpunch #1, approximate dose = 200 mg/kg) and the rest of the material (approximately 0.2 ml, earpunch #2, approximate dose = 800 mg/kg) into another mouse. If the material is water soluble, inject it IV. Weigh the two mice (separately) the day of injection and every other day until it is clear that they are gaining weight. This simple toxicity test with only two mice (carried out about four or five days prior to injecting the efficacy trial), provides a wealth of information, for example:

a) If the agent is water soluble, or can not be prepared in an aqueous media.

b) If the agent will cause immediate toxicity (seconds to hours post injection).

c) If the agent is not toxic at high dosages, or if toxicity is somewhat delayed.

d) If the agent is tissue damaging.

Thus, depending on the results of the toxicity trial there may be a desire to adjust the written protocol. Several examples are as follows:

1) If the agent was not toxic and the mice gained weight, elimi-nate the bottom dose (third dose level). It may be desirable to reduce the number of mice to four in each of the remaining groups if the amount of drug is limited (e.g., less than 400 mg). Escalate these remaining dosages more aggressively than usual (e.g., 50% per day instead of 20% to 30%). Eventually, the second dose may be eliminated (e.g., after five or six days of injection) and continue only with the top dose. This allows maximization of the total dose that can be delivered with a limited drug supply.

2) If the agent causes immediate deaths in the toxicity trial carry out a second toxicity test to better locate the level at which the immediate toxicity occurs. The immediate deaths are usually caused by the peak plasma level of the drug, and are most often due to neurologic, respiratory or cardiac

toxicity. Anything that will reduce the peak level of the drug will allow more drug to be administered. Our usual technique is simply to inject the agent multiple times per day (for 7 to 12 days in a row) at levels below those causing the immediate toxicity.

3)   If the agent was water soluble and caused immediate deaths when injected IV, the second toxicity test should include a determination of the lethal level both SC and IV. If the lethal level SC is greater than 4-fold the lethal level of the IV injection, the efficacy protocol should be altered to SC administration of the drug. The SC route simply reduces the peak plasma level of the drug (thus reducing the immediate toxicity and allowing administration of more drug). If the difference in immediate lethality between the SC and IV route is less than or equal to 4-fold, the agent should be given IV twice per day in the efficacy protocol. With this technique, we can usually obtain a true cumulative toxic dose level by the preferred route of administration (i.e., IV). With drugs that cause immediate lethality, dosages are escalated only very slowly (if at all). The way to increase the total dose is to increase the number of injections per day and to increase the number of days of injection.

4)   If weight loss or deaths were delayed in the toxicity test (three or more days post injection), lower the starting dosages and escalate slowly on successive injection days in the efficacy trial.

<u>PREPARATION OF THE DRUG FOR THE EFFICACY TRIAL</u>
<u>Scenario #1</u>

The toxicity test was performed and the agent was found to be water insoluble. The route is now defined as SC. The data from the two toxicity mice are as follows: The mouse given the 800 mg/kg dose died two days post treatment. The mouse given the 200 mg/kg dose lived with no weight loss. Thus, the doses in the protocol above are satisfactory and the experiment can be carried out as written.

67

Batch weigh the mice in each cage and record. Calculate the
mean (average) weight of the mice in each cage. On the computer,
Type <u>basica</u> then load (push <u>F3</u> and enter). Type <u>Drug2</u> and enter.
Next push F2 and enter. Follow the instructions on the screen.
This is the program to calculate the amount of drug to be weighed
out and the dilutions required (a copy of the program is at the
end of this appendix). The print-out for the trial shown as
follows:

Groups	Dosage mg/kg per dose	Number in Injec.	# of Mice/Inj.	Total # of mice	Av. Wt. of mice (gm)
1	160.00	1.00	8.00	8.00	22.00
2	80.00	1.00	8.00	8.00	22.00
3	40.00	1.00	8.00	8.00	22.00

Tot. Wt. of All Mice In Groups	Vol. (ml) Per Mouse	Tot. Vol. Needed	mg of Drug Needed	Vol. (ml) of Stock Solution	Vol. (ml) of Diluent to add
176.00	0.20	1.60	28.16		
176.00	0.20	1.60	14.08	0.80	0.80
176.00	0.20	1.60	7.04	0.40	1.20

Amount of drug to be weighed out - 49.28 mg (one will weigh 49 mg,
the extent of accuracy of the balance)
Amount of stock solution to mix up = 2.80 ml

Note that we have entered the drug for only one injection,
since it will be prepared fresh daily. In order to factor in possible wastage of drug during preparation and transfer, we have
entered the drug for eight mice per injection instead of five. If
the drug is in short supply, enter only for seven mice, and take
additional care in the transfer.

Place the drug in a 15 ml homogenizer. Add 100% ethanol (the
organic solvent) in a volume equal to 3% of the final volume (in
this case 0.03 x 2.8 = 0.09 ml). Then add POE40 (the carrier) in
a volume equal to 1% of the final volume (in this case 0.01 x 2.8
= 0.03 ml, one drop). The POE40 can be purchased from: Sigma

Chemical Co. Catalog #P-1504 = Polyoxyethylenesorbitan Monopal-
mitate.

Put in the teflon plunger attached to a steel rod and mash the
crystals by rotating the plunger by hand. Do not hurry, spend a
couple of minutes trying to get the material into solution. A couple of more drops of ethanol may be added to compensate for evap-
oration. It is possible (although usually not necessary) to increase the concentration of ethanol to 8% and the POE40 to 3%
without causing toxicity to the mouse at the volumes used. Getting the drug into solution in the organic solvent/carrier mixture
is the critical step in obtaining the best possible suspension.
The carrier (POE40) is an organic molecule that has a hydrophobic
region (where the drug will attach) and a hydrophilic region
(which will attach to the water when added to it). Thus, the
carrier helps to hold drug to the water molecules, creating a
suspension of very small crystal size. The smaller the crystal
size the larger the surface area of the total drug suspended and
the more rapidly it will be absorbed from the tissues. Note: Do
not add the ethanol, POE40 and water in any other order or a very
poor suspension will be the result. Other carriers can be substituted for POE40: carboxymethylcellulose (1%), Tween-80 (0.5%).
Other solvents can be substituted for ethanol: propylene glycol
(2%), DMSO (2%).

Next, place the plunger rod in the drill-press and start it
rotating very slowly (adjust the transformer to 30 RPM). Add the
needed amount of dH_2O to the homogenizer as the plunger is rotating. Move the plunger up and down and increase the speed of rota-
tion (by increasing the setting on the transformer to 50 to 70
RPM).

Check the pH (with pH paper) and adjust to 6.5 to 7.5 with
0.1 N HCl or 0.1 N NaOH (one drop at a time with swirling). After
the pH is adjusted, pour the stock suspension into a prelabelled
glass bottle. Remove the proper amount of stock and add this to
two more prelabelled glass vials (0.8 ml and 0.4 ml for this experiment). Now add dH_2O in the proper amount to get the dilutions
(0.8 ml and 1.2 ml in this example). Put rubber stoppers and alu-

minum caps on the bottles and crimp with a crimper. The drug at three different dosages is now ready for injection.

From the three dosages that you will be injecting, set the two top dosages aside. Remove only one cage at a time for injection (first, which will be the low dosage). Match the label on the bottle to the label on the cage (exp #, cage #, dose, drug, volume). Attach a 1.5 inch 18 g needle to the 1 cc syringe. Fill the syringe about 2/3 full with air. Invert the bottle. Push the needle through the rubber stopper. Push the air into the vial. Remove the desired amount of drug (1.1 ml if injecting five mice). Change needle to a 1 inch 23 g. Express a small amount of drug from the needle and begin injections. On the first day of drug administration, inject the low dose cage and wait a full ten minutes for any signs of immediate toxicity. If there is any toxicity or no toxicity, note this on the experiment charts. If there are immediate deaths, adjust the dosages on the two remaining cages (to 1/4 and 1/8 of the toxic dose). However, toxicity should not occur based on the toxicity trial that had previously been run. Put this cage back on the rack and remove the cage to receive the middle dose. Again, match the label on the bottle to the label on the cage. Inject this cage and again wait ten minutes before proceeding to the top dose. Check the mice two to four hours post injection for any untoward side effects. Note in the experiment charts if one sees anything unusual. Typical descriptions may be as follows: anesthesia, ataxia, lethargy, seizures, coma, agitation, tremors, shallow respiration, scruffy appearance. Use adjectives (severe, mild) and duration of events (ten minutes, two hours, etc.). A typical notation may be: "Mild lethargy lasting twenty minutes, no other symptoms". Sometimes lethargy and a scruffy appearance are the only clues that the mouse is not feeling well. Normally, he will be constantly grooming (licking) himself which keeps his fur sleek looking (and presumably free of mites). Failure to groom is the main cause of the scruffy appearance, and is a sure sign he is feeling poorly.

The next day batch weigh all the cages. Dosages are escalated 20% on this day if there is no weight loss in the top dose group and the mice look in good condition. On subsequent days the doses may be escalated 25% to 33% daily if there is no weight loss. Based on weight loss and other symptoms, a dosage may be de-escalated (reduced), omitted, kept the same, or escalated. If immediate toxicities are encountered, dosages may be reduced and the drug should be injected twice daily if recovery is rapid and weight loss is minimal. Note any relevant information about the drug, preparation quirks, toxicity behaviors, etc. It will help refine the next experiment in the event the drug turns out to be active. In some cases, unusual or selective toxicities can lead to other uses for the drug.

Overall, keep in mind that the aim is to maximize the total dose delivered without causing death or undue suffering.

Eventually it becomes desirable to stop drug injection. The following reasons are usually the reasons one should note as a justification:

a) The entire drug supply is exhausted.

b) Clear antitumor activity is evident (control tumors measure 10 mm x 10 mm or more and there is no tumor growth in the top dose group). Stop even though frank toxicity (which one is usually aiming at in the top dose) was not reached.

c) Frank toxicity at the top dose (greater than 20% body weight loss, or more than 20% of the mice dead from cumulative toxicity). Remember, immediate deaths do not count in assessing frank toxicity.

d) Adequate toxicity is judged by weight loss (11% to 19%) with no deaths. In some cases it is evident that the mouse will not be able to tolerate any more treatment from his general condition, although his weight loss is minimal. In these cases treatment can be discontinued and restarted if his general condition and weight recovers.

e) An excessively large total dose has been administered (e.g., >2000 mg/kg and there is no toxicity and no efficacy).

<u>Scenario #2</u>: The agent was water soluble but it caused the first mouse to die two minutes after IV injection of the 200 mg/kg dose.

Instead of injecting the 1000 mg/kg dose (which would obviously have killed the next mouse), dilute it to produce a dosage of 200 mg/kg (enough for three mice), 100 mg/kg (enough for three mice), 50 mg/kg (enough for two mice).

Eventually, find the lethal level (immediate deaths) for the IV and SC routes (e.g., 33 mg/kg IV and 100 mg/kg SC). Since the ratio is less than four, make the route IV for the efficacy trial. Now the protocol can be rewritten.

<u>IN VIVO EVALUATION OF PREVIOUSLY UNTESTED CYTOTOXIC AGENTS FOR</u>
<u>ANTITUMOR ACTIVITY AGAINST TRANSPLANTABLE TUMORS OF MICE</u>
Standard Efficacy Trial

Group	# of BDF_1 Mice/group	Bilateral Trocar Colon #38 on day 0	Agent	mg/kg/inj	Sche-dule	Drug Route
1	5	Yes	No Treatment Control			
2	5	Yes	K207324	20	BID*3-14	IV
3	5	Yes		10		
4	5	Yes		5		

*BID means twice a day.

Try to split these injections four to six hours apart. Do not escalate this trial. The only way to increase the total dose is by increasing the number of injections per day (e.g., three), or by increasing the duration of treatment (e.g., injecting through day twenty-two). In rare cases the mice will adapt to the toxicity. If the mice continue to gain weight after five days of injection, take the bottom dose (Cage-4) and inject it with 30 mg/kg BID. If these die, one can not escalate Cage-2. If they live, slowly escalate it (20% per day) and gradually move the dose up for Cage-2 and Cage-3 (by less than or equal to 20%). A great

deal of caution must be used in trials of this nature. This type
of drug is most often missed in drug discovery programs.

If an immediate-toxicity-drug is water soluble and toxic at a
very low dose, an infusion with a Harvard pump or Alzet pump may
be appropriate.

Scenario #3

The agent was water insoluble and did not cause any deaths or
weight loss in the toxicity mice.

Do not lose faith in drugs of this nature. Remember a drug
active against a true cancer-target would be non-toxic for the
host, and selectively toxic for all tumors.

Start the beginning dosages somewhat higher than written, for
example, adjust the protocol as follows:

IN-VIVO EVALUATION OF PREVIOUSLY UNTESTED CYTOTOXIC AGENTS FOR ANTITUMOR ACTIVITY AGAINST TRANSPLANTABLE TUMORS OF MICE
Standard Efficacy Trial

Group	# of BDF$_1$ Mice/group	Bilateral Trocar Colon #38 on day 0	Agent	mg/kg/inj	Sche-dule	Drug Route
1	5	Yes	No Treatment Control			
2	5	Yes	K207324	300	QD*3-14	SC
3	5	Yes		150		SC
4	5	Yes		75		SC

*QD means one injection per day (in this case every day from day
three through day fourteen).

Dosages can be escalated 30 to 50% per day rather than the
usual 20% to 30%. There is however a practical limit of approximately 500 mg/kg/injection that can be administered SC. If there
is a limited drug supply, stop the bottom dose after four or five
days of injection. The number of mice per group can be reduced if
the supply is limited (e.g., < 400 mg). This type of drug is

usually injected until the drug supply is exhausted (or one has exceeded 2000 mg/kg total).

Other Scenarios

A large number of other scenarios could be developed. In each case it is necessary to adjust the protocol with the changing conditions of host toxicity, efficacy, and physical properties of the drug. Weight changes determined daily, as well as general appearance, are the best guide to toxicity. Sometimes it is useful to assess performance status (e.g., prod the mouse with a finger to see how he moves and check his temperament). If his movements seem uncoordinated (e.g., duck walk), he may have peripheral neuropathy. Also, place him on a pencil to see if he can walk on it or at least hold on without falling off. Other toxicities need to be specifically looked for [e.g., diarrhea, stomatitis (for stomatitis examine the gums for ulcers)]. If either diarrhea or stomatitis is noted, treatment should be stopped. If the toxicities resolve, treatment can be reinitiated.

NECROPSIES

If death occurs during the first three days of injections, virtually nothing is seen on necropsy (unless there was some pathology prior to treatment). Thereafter, necropsy findings are highly useful in determining dose limiting toxicities. Look for deposits of the drug (if any) at the SC injection site, and tissue damage or edema at the site. Open the mouse midline and pin the skin flaps to the board. First examine the size of the spleen. A small spleen is an indication that the mouse died from leucopenia. Next look at the liver for reduced size and rounded lobes, indicating liver damage. Also note the color of the liver (if unusual). Next look for diarrhea and stomatitis. Next, examine the other organ systems, (e.g., kidneys, lungs) and note anything unusual. Fix anything that is very unusual in 10% formaldehyde.

EVALUATION OF AGENTS FOR ACTIVITY AGAINST TRANSPLANTABLE SOLID TUMORS IN MICE
[DEFINITIONS, AND IN VIVO CHEMOTHERAPY PROTOCOL DESIGN, DATA ANALYSIS]

I. Solid Mouse Tumors

The initial trial with a new drug will be done in the tumor in which selective cytotoxicity was seen in the disk diffusion assay (usually Colon-38, Panc-03). A large number of other tumors in secondary evaluation studies will be encountered. These include: Colon Adenocarcinomas 51, 09; Colon Carcinoma 26 (un-differentiated); Pancreatic Ductal Adenocarcinoma 02; Mammary Adenocarcinoma 16/C, 16/C/Adr (to determine the activity of each agent against the multi-drug-resistant phenotype), Hormone Dependent Mammary Ductal Carcinoma, MXT; Mammary Adenocarcinomas 44, 13, 17, and 25; Squamous Cell Lung tumors LC12, and ASB, Lewis Lung carcinoma (Wilkoff subline); B16 melanoma; and M5076 ovarian tumor (actually of RES origin). These tumors are used because they represent a broad spectrum of biological and drug response characteristics.

II. Leukemias

L1210 (a number of different induced resistant sublines are also available for cross-resistance studies). P388/0 and P388/Adr are evaluated to determine the activity of each agent against the multi-drug resistant phenotype (if the agent is active against P388).

III. Human Tumors

Human Colon CX-1, H116, H8; Human Pancreatic P-1, P-2; Mammary MX-1; and Human Lung H125.

IV. Tumor and Animal Maintenance

Mouse tumors are maintained in the mouse strain of origin and are transplanted into the appropriate F_1 hybrid (or the mouse of origin) for therapy trials. _Never_ use the F1 hybrid mice for passaging the tumors; such practice will alter the biologic behavior

of the tumor. Individual mouse body weights for each experiment
are within five grams and all mice are over nineteen grams at
the start of therapy. The mice are supplied food and water <u>ad
libitum</u>. In addition, place some food in the bottom of the cages
of the mice being treated with chemotherapy. The food is "breeder
chow" that is soft and easy to eat (higher in fat).

V. <u>Chemotherapy of Solid Tumors</u>
   The animals are pooled, implanted subcutaneously bilaterally
with 30 to 60 mg tumor fragments by 12 gauge trocar, and again
pooled before unselective distribution to the various treatment
and control groups. For early stage treatment, chemotherapy is
started within one to three days after tumor implantation while
the number of cells is relatively small (10^7 to 10^8 cells).
If the tumor is rapidly growing (e.g., Lewis Lung, Colon 26, Panc
02, Mamm 16/C, Mamm-44) begin treatment the day after implant (day
0 is the day of implant). For slower tumors (Colon 38, Panc 03,
Colon 7), begin treatment three days after implant. Tumors are
measured weekly (or twice weekly for the more rapidly growing
tumors) with a caliper . Mice are sacrificed when their tumors
reach 1500 mg (i.e., before they can cause the animal discomfort).
Tumor weights are estimated from two-dimensional measurements:
   <u>Tumor Weight (in mg)</u> = $(a \times b^2)/2$, where a and b are the
tumor length and width (mm), respectively.

VI. <u>End Points for Assessing Antitumor Activity</u>
   The following quantitative end-points are used to assess
antitumor activity:
A.   <u>Percent Increase in Host Life Span</u> (%ILS) = 100 x MDD (median
     day of death of the treated tumor-bearing mice) - (MDD of the
     tumor-bearing control mice)/MDD of the tumor bearing control
     mice. %ILS is only used for leukemia trials.

B.   <u>Tumor Growth Delay</u> (T-C value), where T is the median time
     (in days) required for the treatment group tumors to reach
     750 mg. C is the median time (in days) for the control group

tumors to reach 750 mg. Time to 1000 or 1250 could be appropriate tumor sizes in selected cases. Cures are excluded in the determination of T and C values.

C. <u>Calculation of Tumor Cell Kill</u>

For subcutaneously (SC) growing tumors, the $\log_{10}$ cell kill/dose is calculated from the following formula:

$$\text{Log}_{10} \text{ kill/dose} = \frac{T-C}{(3.32)\ (Td)\ (\text{Number of Doses})}$$

Td is the tumor volume doubling time (in days), estimated from the best fit straight line from a log-linear growth plot of the control-group tumors in exponential growth (100 to 800 mg range). The conversion of the T - C values to $\log_{10}$ cell kill is possible because the Td of tumors regrowing post treatment (Rx) approximates the Td values of the tumors in untreated control mice.

$$\text{The Log}_{10} \text{ Cell Kill Total (gross)} = \frac{T - C}{(3.32)\ (Td)}$$

$$\text{The Log}_{10} \text{ Cell Kill Net} = \frac{(T - C)-(\text{Duration of Rx in days})}{(3.32)\ (Td)}$$

If the $\log_{10}$ cell kill (net) value is positive, there are fewer cells present at the end of therapy than at the start. If, on the other hand, the value is negative, the tumor grew under treatment. A positive gross value with a negative net value indicates inhibition of growth of the tumor cell population during drug treatment.

The $\log_{10}$ kill value is converted to an arbitrary activity rating. It has been our experience that if this conversion is not used, a single injection will invariably appear superior to longer treatment regimens when net cell kills are compared. Likewise, therapies of greater than twenty days will appear superior to

single injection schedules if gross tumor cell kills are evaluated
and compared.

<u>CONVERSION OF LOG_{10} TUMOR CELL KILL TO AN ACTIVITY RATING</u>

Antitumor Activity	Duration of Rx <5 days Log_{10} Kill (Net)	Duration of Rx 5 to 20 days Log_{10} Kill (Net) (Gross)		Duration of Rx >20 days Log_{10} Kill (Net) (Gross)	
Highly Active ++++	>2.6	>2.0	>2.8	>0.8	>3.4
+++	1.6 - 2.6	0.8 - 2.0	2.0 - 2.8		2.5 - 3.4
++	0.9 - 1.5		1.3 - 1.9		1.7 - 2.4
+	0.5 - 0.8		0.7 - 1.2		1.0 - 1.6
Inactive -	<0.5		<0.7		<1.0

An activity rating of +++ to ++++ is needed to effect partial
(PR'S) or complete regressions (CR'S) of 100 to 300 mg size masses
of most transplanted solid tumors of mice. Thus, an activity rating of + or ++ would not be scored as active by usual clinical criteria.

D.   <u>Non-Quantitative Determination of Antitumor Activity by Tumor</u>
     <u>Growth Inhibition (T/C VALUE)</u>

The treatment and control groups are measured when the control group tumors reach approximately 800 to 1100 mg in size (Median of Group). The median tumor weight of each group is determined (including zeros). The T/C value in percent is an indication of antitumor effectiveness: A T/C equal to or less than 42%
is considered significant antitumor activity by the Drug Evaluation Branch of the Division of Cancer Treatment (NCI). A T/C
value of less than 10% is considered to indicate highly significant antitumor activity (and is the level used by NCI to justify a
clinical trial if toxicity, formulation, and certain other requirements are met: termed DN-2 level activity). A body weight loss

nadir (mean of group) of exceeding 20%, or greater than 20% drug deaths is considered to indicate an excessively toxic dosage in most single course trials.

Laboratory researchers should be familiar with the methods used and the more important aspects of data collection so that evaluations of efficacy and toxicity can be carried out with fidelity. The following considerations should be kept in mind:

1) For T/C calculations the aim is to measure all the tumors in all cages when the control group tumors are in the 800 to 1200 mg size (median of the group). This size range is selected because the tumors are still in exponential growth (the only time at which the T/C calculation method is valid). It is very important that the evaluation not be carried out at a size larger than this because the tumors will begin to have a progressively longer tumor-volume-doubling-time due to the fact that the tumor will be invading and destroying its own blood supply, thus limiting the food and oxygen supply to the tumor cells. Measurements at these larger sizes will make a moderately active drug appear to be inactive.

2) For tumor growth delay calculations (T-C values), the tumors will need to be measured multiple times. If the tumor is rapidly growing (e.g., Mammary Adenocarcinoma 16/C, which has a Td of one day) all the tumors will need to be measured three times per week starting as soon as the control tumors can be detected as approaching 400 to 500 mg (usually about day seven). In addition, two measurements of the control group need to be obtained as soon as the tumors (60 mg to 150 mg) can be felt. These very early measurements of the control group are needed to obtain an accurate exponential doubling time of the tumor. This is necessary for the Log Kill calculation. For slow growing tumors (Td values of 2.5 to 3.5 days), measurements twice a week are sufficient.

3) It is important to carry out all measurements by one person on a given experiment if at all possible.

VII. <u>Leukemias</u>

An LD_{10} value is determined in other testing or in non-tumor normal mice before leukemia testing is undertaken. Dosages used are 1.6 x LD_{10}, the LD_{10} and 0.62 x LD_{10}.

Tumor Implantation: Hemocytometer counted L1210 cells (10^5/mouse) are implanted IV on day zero. A 10^3 and a 10^1 titer is implanted into 5 mice each to verify take-rate and cell doubling time. Cell doubling time, take rate and cell kill are well known and very reproducible for this tumor. The test agents are injected IP, IV, SC or PO (depending on the experimental design, usually IV for new materials if solubility permits) starting day one for early stage disease or day three or day four for more advanced stage disease.

Cause of death is determined by examination of spleen size and the appearance of the liver (large and mottled in the event of a leukemic death). This simple necropsy procedure overcomes one of the classical defects of leukemia screening; i.e., being unable to separate delayed drug deaths from tumor deaths. Antitumor activity is determined by %ILS. Quantification of tumor cell kill is similar to that outlined for solid tumor testing. The T-C value is the survival time in days (tumor free survivors excluded) for the treatment group (T) minus the survival time for the control group (C). The Td value is obtained from a plot of the median day of death (tumor-free survivors excluded) against the $\log_{10}$ dilutions of the tumor cells in untreated mice. With these values, the $\log_{10}$ cell kills (per dose, gross, and net) are calculated as for solid tumors.

VIII. <u>Schedule Trials</u>

The determination of the optimum schedule depends on the toxicity behavior of the agent under evaluation.

We have invariably found that cytotoxic agents fall into one of four different categories. It should be emphasized that the distinction in the first two categories is <u>not</u> made on comparisons of antitumor efficacy for various schedules but rather on toxicity only (although we and others carry out the schedule trials in tumor bearing animals for efficacy evaluation). Efficacy evaluation has recently become important in schedule trials because of the discovery of Flavone-Acetic-Acid (FAA), which does not fall into the historic categories. Efficacy is the best endpoint to separate category 3 from category 4 (see below).

In <u>Category 1, (schedule dependent for lethal toxicity),</u> the schedule markedly influences the total dosage that can be administered. This occurs for most antimetabolites (S-phase specific; e.g., 6-thioguanine, cytosine arabinoside, methotrexate). The total dosage (at the maximum tolerated level) markedly decreases (usually by a factor of 3 to 30, depending on the half-life of the agent) as the number of injections increase within a ten day treatment period. The reason for the marked change is well understood. Cytotoxicity (for normal and tumor cells) from these drugs occurs because of inhibition of critical enzymes necessary for DNA synthesis during S-phase (or because of DNA synthesis itself if the agent is incorporated into the DNA, which obviously occurs only during S-Phase). In the case of enzyme inhibition, the first dosage of the drug binds all of the enzyme that is already present in the cell (and the cell will die if it enters S-phase at this time). However, new enzyme is constantly being synthesized and the drugs usually have short half-lives (five to twenty minutes). If the cell is not in S-phase, and the intracellular concentration of the drug falls to a negligible level, the enzyme newly synthesized prior to S-phase can rescue the cell from death. Cell killing is thus a function of time (T) above a minimum cytotoxic concentration (i.e., that concentration necessary to bind all the existing enzyme and any new enzyme being synthesized). This can be accomplished by extended infusions (at a low level, but above the minimum cytotoxic concentration) or by high intermittent bolus injections (which will take many half-lives of the drug to drop below the minimum cytotoxic concentration after each injection). The use of high intermittent bolus injections is, however, ill advised for human therapy, since the half-life of the drug will often vary markedly from patient to patient. Thus, a given dose will become life-threatening in some patients (in which metabolism and elimination is slow), and markedly suboptimal treatment in other patients in which metabolism and elimination is rapid. In Category 1, efficacy (for a sensitive tumor) correlates predominantly with <u>Time</u> above a minimum cytotoxic concentration of the drug. Interestingly, if an agent has a very long half-life (e.g., palmo-Ara-C, a depot form of Ara-C that has a twenty-seven hour half-life), the behavior in schedule trials is very similar to a Schedule-Category-2 agent (see below).

In <u>Category 2, (schedule independent for lethal toxicity)</u>, the schedule does not appreciably influence the total dosage that can be administered. Examples include: mitotic inhibitors, DNA-binders, alkylating agents, DNA-scission agents that produce repairable lesions (VP-16), and some antimetabolites (FUra). The maximum tolerated total dosage (MTTD) does not change significantly as the number of injections increase in a ten day time period. In Category 2, the antitumor activity (for a sensitive tumor) correlates with the total dosage (actually the area under the concentration x time curve) that can be administered and dose-splitting does not appreciably change efficacy.

In <u>Category 3, (schedule independent with a peak plasma problem)</u>, the total dosage at the apparent maximum tolerated level appears to increase as the number of injections increase within the ten day period. This phenomenon is usually caused by an intolerance to a high plasma level of the drug and results in immediate post-injection deaths and an erroneous assignment of the maximum tolerated total dose. The schedule producing the immediate deaths is not satisfactory for the evaluation of antitumor activity. In these cases, efficacy and the MTTD can only be determined with a schedule utilizing more frequent injections of lower dosage levels (i.e., individual dosages just below those causing immediate toxicity problems, or a prolonged low dose infusion schedule) as shown below where the total dose at the "apparent" HNTD appears to increase as the number of injections increase with a ten day period.

Schedule Category #1: Schedule-dependent. Infulence of schedule on toxicity: LD_{100} total dosage in mg/kg in BDF_1 mice (IP injections)

| | MAXIMUM TOLERATED TOTAL DOSAGE FOR THE THREE SCHEDULES | | | | | Ratio of LD_{10} values: |
Agent	Single injection mg/kg	Q4days X 3 inj. mg/kg total dosage	Daily X 9 mg/kg total dosage	3hr X 8 days 1,5,9,13 mg/kg total dosage	Q3hr X 16 mg/kg total dosage	<u>Single injection LD_{10}</u> Multiple Injection $\overline{LD}_{10}$
Cytosine Arabinoside (NSC63876)	2049 (116)*	5751 (4)*	414 (16)*	416 (253)*	94.4 (50)*	22
Methotrexate (NSC740) (Amethopterin)	178 (18)*	54 (56)*	15.3 (59)*	5.7 (26)*	NA	31
6-Thioguanine (NSC752)	52 (80)*	23.7 (15)*	15 (28)*	12.8 (100)*	NA	4.1

* Data of NCI; Numbers in parenthesis are the number of separate trials used to obtain median LD_{10} values in BDF_1 mice.

Schedule Category #2: Schedule independent. Lack of influence of schedule on toxicity LD_{10} total dosage in mg/kg in BDF_1 mice (IP-injections).

	Single injection mg/kg	Q4day X 3 mg/kg total dosage	Daily X 9 mg/kg total dosage	Q3hr X 8 days 1,5,9,13,mg/kg total dosage
Cytoxan (NSC26271)	253 (1535)[a]	329 (4)[a]	315 (4)[a]	320 (29)[a]
Adriamycin (NSC123127)[b]SC	12 (65)[a]	18.9 (8)[a]	19.8 (25)[a]	11.2 (5)[a] (Q3hrX8, day 1 only)
Vincristine (NSC67574)	3.1 (214)[a]	3.3 (105)[a]	2.8 (35)[a]	3.1 (9)[a] (Q3hrX8, days 1,5,9)
5-FUra (NSC19893)	193 (276)[a]	231 (49)[a]	243 (67)[a]	288 (5)[a] (Q3hrX8, days 1,5,9)

[a]Data of NCI; Numbers in parenthesis are the number of separate trials used to obtain LD_{10} values in BDF_1 mice
[b]Subcutaneous administration

Schedule Category #3:

Total Dose in mg/kg at HNTD

Agent	Single Injection	Multiple (# of injections)
Spiromustine	12	33 (4-same day)
NSC-127755	3.7	243 (27)
S-183577	40	480 (3 hr infusion)

Frequently, it is necessary to extend the treatment duration (e.g., three times per day for twelve to fifteen days in a row) in order to obtain meaningful toxicity. Category 3 agents are often encountered in new-drug-discovery programs.

We find that many solid tumor selective materials are in this category. Historically, agents in Category 3 are rarely evaluated adequately. Very few have reached clinical trials. The problem is mainly a mouse problem. In the human, the drug will produce a much lower peak plasma level at an equivalent area under-the-plasma-curve. The difference is the 10-fold slower transit time through the liver and kidneys of the human, and the resulting longer half-life. In Category 3, the antitumor activity (for a sensitive tumor) correlates with the total dosage (area under the concentration x time curve) that can be administered. Dose splitting allows higher total dosages to be tolerated, and thus an improvement in efficacy in a responsive tumor. There is a sub-category of agents that cause toxicities to which that the mouse adapts (e.g., glaucarubinone). In these cases the mice adapt to the dose limiting toxicity over a period of several days, and levels can be markedly increased (often > 6-fold above a dosage that is lethal in unadapted mice). Increased metabolism is a common suspected mechanism, although others are possible (e.g., the target for the cytotoxic antitumor activity is an inducible enzyme).

FAA is in a category by itself (Category 4). For <u>Category 4</u>, the total dose (at the apparent MTTD levels) increases with the dose-splitting (opposite Category-1), whereas efficacy decreases

with dose-splitting (unlike Categories 2 and 3). As we now understand, this is due to non-linear pharmacokinetics and the fact
that the agent has peak-plasma-problems similar to the standard
Category 3 drug.

Once the various categories are understood, and the fact that
schedules producing immediate injection deaths can <u>not</u> be used to
assign the MTD value, schedule trials are rather easy to design
and interpret. The first step is to determine if the agent produces immediate post injection deaths. If it does not, a split
dose schedule (e.g., twice per day for seven days) versus an intermittent schedule (e.g., Q7dx2) will allow placement of the agent
into Categories 1 or 2. If done in tumor bearing mice, this same
protocol will separate Category 3 from 4 since the BID schedule
will have more antitumor activity than the Q7d x 2 schedule in
Schedule Category 3 but less activity in Schedule Category 4. In
many cases, it is necessary to include an infusion schedule to define the severity of the immediate toxicity problem for both Category 3 and Category 4. We usually carry out infusions with either
a modified Harvard pump or implantable Alzet pumps.

IX. <u>Host Recovery Time</u>

Once an optimum schedule and route are determined, it is
often useful to determine the host recovery time and the long term
cumulative toxicity (14). Assistance can be provided in an estimation of the host recovery time of a drug by simply continuing to
weigh the mice frequently (e.g., twice per week after treatment
has been stopped; continuing to weigh the mice until the pretreatment weight is reached). This will give a very good idea of the
degree of irreversible damage to the host. Recovery of weight
within five or six days of the weight loss nadir is a good indication of rapid host recovery. Recovery of longer than fourteen
days is an indication of slow host recovery and probably some organ damage of an irreversible nature. Agents with slow host recovery will have more cumulative toxicity with repeated courses of
treatment.

85

The following is the program used to calculate drug dilutions and the amount drug that one will need to weigh out.

```
LIST :drug2
10 CLS : KEY OFF : PRINT "Drug Program " : PRINT
20 PRINT "If more than 1 group at each dose, separate by '/',
e.g.,"
30 PRINT "2/4/7."
40 PRINT "In order to stop, hit <return> when the computer asks
for"
50 PRINT "the group number." : PRINT
60 OPTION BASE 1
70 DIM TABLE(100,11),G$(100)
80 MAXD = 0 : ND = 1 : ID=1
90 OPEN "LPT1:" FOR OUTPUT AS #1 : OPEN "SCRN:" FOR OUTPUT AS #2
100 INPUT "Do you want the output to go to the Screen or Printer
(S/P) ",ID$
110 IF ID$="S" OR ID$="s" THEN ID=2
120 LINE INPUT "Group number(s) ",G$(ND)
130 IF G$(ND) = "" THEN 280
140 FOR J=1 TO 7
150 ON J GOTO 160,180,200,250,220,250,240
160 INPUT "Dosage(mg/kg/dose) = ",TABLE(ND,1)          'A
170 GOTO 250
180 INPUT "Number of injections = ",TABLE(ND,2)        'B
190 GOTO 250
200 INPUT "Number of mice/injection = ",TABLE(ND,3)    'C
210 GOTO 250
220 INPUT "Avg. Wt(gm) of mice in group = ",TABLE(ND,5) 'E
230 GOTO 250
240 INPUT "Volume(ml)/mouse = ",TABLE(ND,7)            'G
250 NEXT J
260 PRINT
270 ND = ND + 1 : GOTO 120
280 ND = ND - 1
290 IF ND<1 THEN 730
```

```
300 '
310 ' Calculation of results
320 '
330 SUMI = 0
340 FOR I=1 TO ND
345 IF TABLE(I,1)>=MAXD THEN MAXD=TABLE(I,1)
350 TABLE(I,4) = TABLE(I,2) * TABLE(I,3)                'D
360 TABLE(I,6) = TABLE(I,4) * TABLE(I,5)                'F
370 TABLE(I,8) = TABLE(I,4) * TABLE(I,7)                'H
380 TABLE(I,9) = TABLE(I,1) * TABLE(I,6) / 1000         'I
390 SUMI = SUMI + TABLE(I,9)
400 NEXT
410 L = SUMI
420 FOR I=1 TO ND : IF TABLE(I,1)=MAXD THEN M = L * TABLE(I,8) /
    TABLE (I,9) : GO TO 440
430 NEXT
440 FOR I=2 TO ND
450 TABLE(I,10) = M * TABLE(I,9) / L                    'J
460 TABLE(I,11) = TABLE(I,8) - TABLE(I,10)              'K
470 NEXT
480 '
490 'Print out results
500 '
505 IF ID=2 THEN CLS
510 PRINT#ID, TAB(12);"Dosage"
520 PRINT#ID, TAB(12);"mg/kg ";TAB(22);"Number";TAB(32);"# of
    ";TAB(42);"Total #
    ";TAB(52);"Avg.Wt of"
530 PRINT#ID, "  Groups";TAB(12);"per dose";TAB(22);"of
    injec.";TAB(32);"mice/in
    j";TAB(42);"of mice";TAB(52);"mice(gm)"
540 FOR I=1 TO ND
550 PRINT#ID, USING "  \        \"; G$(I);
560 FOR J=1 TO 5 : PRINT#ID, USING "#####.##  ";TABLE(I,J); : NEXT
    J
570 PRINT#ID,
```

```
580 NEXT I
590 PRINT#ID, : PRINT#ID,
600 PRINT#ID, "Tot.Wt.of";TAB(32);"mg of";TAB(42);"Vol
    (ml)";TAB(52);"Vol (ml)"
610 PRINT#ID, "all mice";TAB(12);"Vol.(ml)";TAB(22);"Tot.Vol";
   TAB(32);"Drug";TAB(42);"of Stock";TAB(52);"of Diluent"
620 PRINT#ID, "in grps.";TAB(12);"per mouse";TAB(22);"needed";
    TAB(32);"needed";TAB(42);"solution";TAB(52);"to add"
630 FOR I=1 TO ND
640 FOR J=6 TO 11
650 IF (I=1) AND (J>9) THEN 680
660 PRINT#ID, USING "#####.##   ";TABLE(I,J);
670 NEXT J
680 PRINT#ID,
690 NEXT I
700 PRINT#ID, : PRINT#ID,
710 PRINT#ID, USING "Amount of drug to be weighed out   =#####.##
    mg";L
720 PRINT#ID, USING "Amount of stock solution to mix up =#####.##
    ml";M
730 END
Ok
*
```

4

THYMIDYLATE SYNTHASE INHIBITION OF MODIFIED QUINAZOLINE
ANTIFOLATES

A.J. Barker, L.R. Hughes, P. Warner, K. Burrows and A.L. Jackman

Thymidylate synthase (T.S.) is a pivotal enzyme in pyrimidine
biosynthesis. The enzyme catalyses the conversion of deoxyuridine
monophosphate (dUMP) to deoxythymidine monophosphate (dTMP) and represents the only _de novo_ source of this nucleotide required for
DNA synthesis. The co-factor 5,10-methylenetetrahydrofolate (<u>1</u>)
supplies the one-carbon fragment required for the reaction and
also acts as a reducing agent. Regeneration of the co-factor is
achieved in a cycle of reactions catalysed by the enzymes dihydrofolate reductase (DHFR) and serine hydroxymethyl transferase
(SHMT) (Figure 1). Whilst SHMT has received little attention,
many antifolate approaches to cancer chemotherapy have been based

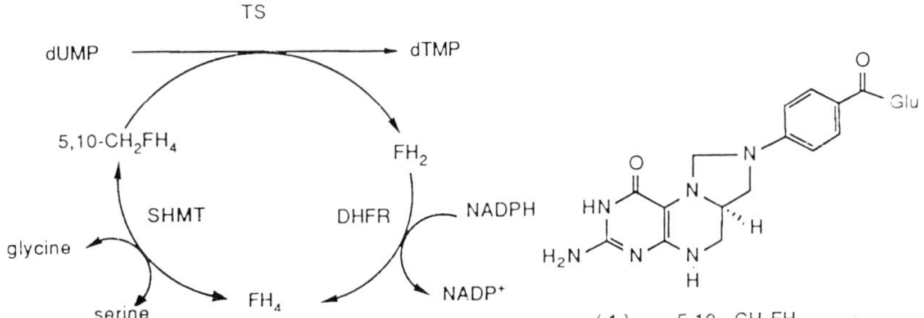

Figure 1.

upon the inhibition of DHFR (1). In turning our attention to T.S.
as a target for antifolate chemotherapy we anticipated several potential advantages over inhibition of DHFR. Principal among these
was that inhibition of T.S. should not affect purine biosynthesis,
protein synthesis or RNA synthesis and in this respect may avoid
some of the side effects associated with DHFR inhibitors such as
methotrexate (2,3).

The discovery of the quinazoline antifolate N^{10}-propargyl-
5,8-dideazafolate (2, Table 1) at the Institute of Cancer Research

Table 1

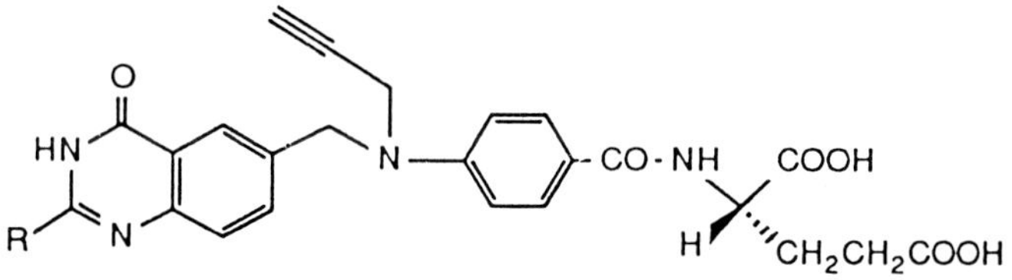

(2) R = NH_2

(3) R = H

(4) R = CH_3

Compound	T.S. (L1210) K_i, nM(30)	DHFR (rat liver) K_i, nM(30)	Solubility (mg/ml) pH 5	pH 7.4
(2)	3	75	0.0086	0.312
(3)	27	2250	0.043	>107
(4)	10		0.15	a

a: solubility at pH 6 _ca_ 50 mg/ml

(4) resulted from a search for an inhibitor of T.S. based upon the
structure of co-factor (1). Compound (2) is an excellent inhibitor of T.S. isolated from both murine and human sources with reported K_i values in the 1-20 nM range (5-9) (Table 1). Although
(2) has activity against isolated DHFR (K_i 14-250 nM) (Table 1)
(4,6,8,10) inhibition of T.S. is the intracellular locus of action

of (2) both *in vitro* (4,6,11,12) and *in vivo* (11-13). The compound is a substrate for folylpolyglutamate synthase (FPGS) (14) and the resultant polyglutamate forms of (2) are retained within cells and show greatly enhanced potency against T.S. (Table 2)

Table 2

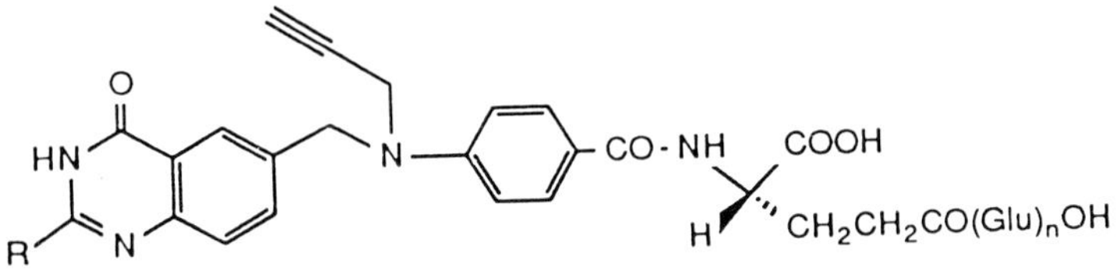

R	n	Fold increase in T.S. inhibition	Fold increase in DHFR inhibition
NH$_2$ (2)	0	-	-
	1	26	3.5
	2	87	2.8
	3	119	5.1
	4	114	3.5
CH$_3$ (4)	0	-	
	1	28	
	2	78	
	3	115	
	4	78	

(6,8,15-17). This feature of compound (2) undoubtedly contributes to its cytotoxicity. The compound exhibits *in vitro* cytotoxic activity against the murine leukemia cell line L1210 (Table 3) and this cytotoxicity is totally prevented by the co-administration of exogenous thymidine indicating that T.S. is the sole locus of action (12). *In vivo* activity in mice was observed with the L1210:CBR1 tumour and against a human hepatoma xenograft (4,12, 18).

Table 3

Compound	L1210, IC_{50}, $\mu M(31)$	L1210:1565, IC_{50},μM	FPGS,KM,μM
(2)	3.4	3.6	40
(3)	0.36	4.1	56
(4)	0.09	8.2	40

In collaboration with ICI Pharmaceuticals N^{10}-propargyl-5, 8-dideazafolate (2) progressed to the clinic and in trials exhibited activity against a variety of breast, liver and ovarian tumours (19-22). Further clinical progress of (2) was prevented by unpredictable liver and dose limiting kidney toxicity. The kidney toxicity was believed to be associated with the low solubility of (2) at acidic and neutral pH (Table 1). The observation of crystalline deposits of (2) in the kidneys of mice dosed with the compound (13) reinforced this assumption.

The low solubility of (2) was believed to be the result of the concentration of hydrogen bond donors and acceptors present in the 2-aminoquinazolin-4(3H)-one portion of the molecule (23) and in an attempt to improve solubility a programme to modify this portion of the structure was initiated.

Replacement of the 2-amino group of (2) with either hydrogen, to give (3) (23), or a methyl group, to give (4), significantly improved solubility at acidic and neutral pH (Table 1). Biologically these changes resulted in compounds which were slightly poorer as inhibitors of T.S. but more selective for T.S. over DHFR (Table 1). Surprisingly the _in vitro_ cytotoxicity of these two compounds was superior to (2) with the 2-hydrogen substituted compound (3) being 10-fold and the 2-methyl substituted compound (4) being about 40-fold more potent against the L1210 cell line (Table 3) (23-26). This difference in cytotoxic potency could not be explained by differences in the affinity of the compounds for folylpolyglutamate synthase (FPGS) since all three compounds exhibited similar substrate specificity for this enzyme (Table 3) (24), whilst the synthetic polyglutamates of (4) showed similar increases in activity against T.S. as those observed for (2) (Table 2) (24,25). Differences in transport into the cells of the compounds appear to account for the increased cytotoxic potency of (3) and (4). This can be illustrated by the mutant L1210:1565 cell line which has a reduced ability to actively transport reduced folates (27). This cell line is 10-fold resistant to (3) and 100-fold resistant to (4). There is no cross-resistance to (2) suggesting the former two compounds are actively transported into cells _via_ the reduced folate carrier in contrast to (2) (Table 3). The higher levels of compounds (3) and (4) entering the cells may lead to higher levels of polyglutamates and improved cytotoxic activity. More importantly when the three compounds were administered to mice in doses which resulted in broadly comparable AUC no liver or kidney toxicity was observed for the more soluble compounds (3) and (4) as evidenced by measuring rises in the levels of plasma alanine transaminase and urea, respectively (Table 4); this was in contrast to the observations made with compound (2) (24). Both (3) and (4) have significant antitumour activity against the L1210:ICR tumour in mice (24,25).

Table 4

Compound	Dose (mg/kg)	Plasma AUC (μM.hr)	Plasma urea increase (%)	ALT increase (%)
(2)	100	680	100	4000
(3)	500	208	0	0
(4)	500	390	0	0

These results encouraged us to make further investigations into the structure-activity relationships of modified quinazoline antifolates. Some of this work has already been published (28) and we wish now to report more of our recent results. Our general strategy involved sequential investigation of structural features of molecule (2) important for activity. In this paper we wish to report the results of modification of the quinazoline bicycle and the effects of replacing the glutamic acid moiety with other amino acids.

The absence of renal and hepatic toxicity and encouraging cytotoxicity observed with compounds (3) and (4) led us to consider further modifications of the quinazoline C-2 substituent (26,29). Increases in size of the alkyl group at C-2 from methyl (4) through to phenyl (7) (Table 5) generally resulted in poorer T.S. inhibition presumably reflecting a size restriction on the groups acceptable to the enzyme at this position. The reduced activity of these compounds for the enzyme is reflected in their activity against the L1210 cell line (Table 5). Variation in af

Table 5

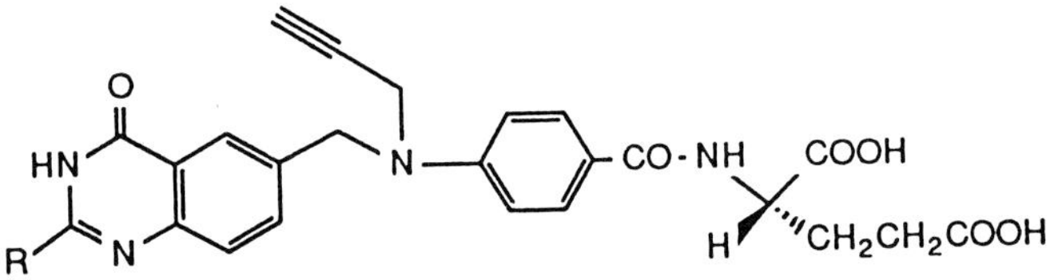

Compound	R	TS, IC_{50}, μM (30)	L1210, IC_{50}, μM (31)
(2)	NH_2	0.02	3.4
(3)	H	0.17	0.36
(4)	CH_3	0.05	0.09
(5)	CH_2CH_3	0.14	2.5
(6)	$CHMe_2$	0.62	48
(7)	Ph	0.22	100
(8)	CH_2OH	0.10	5
(9)	CH_2F	0.10	0.4
(10)	CHF_2	0.58	24
(11)	CF_3	5.70	>100
(12)	$NHCH_3$	0.18	24
(13)	$NHCH_2CH_3$	0.30	>100
(14)	$NHCOCH_3$	0.29	50
(15)	OCH_3	0.02	2
(16)	SCH_3	0.12	13
(17)	Cl	0.20	67

finity for the reduced folate carrier and hence transport into
cells and changes in FPGS substrate specificity may also contribute to this reduced activity.

Introduction of polar substituents onto the C-2 methyl group
of compound (4) results in compounds of similar T.S. activity (compounds (8), (9), Table 5). However, further substitution with
electron withdrawing groups leads to a rapid fall-off in activity
against both the enzyme and the L1210 cell line. This trend might
appear surprising but the electronic nature of the C-2 substituent
also affects the N^3-H bond, an increase in the electron withdrawing power of the C-2 substituent on going from (9) to (11) results in the increased acidity of the N^3-H bond to the extent
that the trifluoromethyl compound (11) is ionised at physiological
pH. The result obtained with (11) indicates that the enzyme will
not readily tolerate such a build up of charge in this region.

Modification of the amino group present in (2) via alkylation
(12,13) or acylation (14) afforded compounds which were up to 15-
fold poorer against the enzyme and exhibited little activity in
the L1210 cell assay (Table 5).

However, exchanging the heteroatom at the C-2 position from
nitrogen to oxygen giving (15) led to equivalent T.S. inhibitory
potency. Interestingly, although being a poorer substrate for
FPGS (24), the methoxy derivative (15) also showed enhanced cytotoxicity in the L1210 assay (Table 5). If in the enzyme the amino
group of (2) is hydrogen bonded to a carboxylate or amide oxygen
atom then the possibility exists in the case of (15) that a similar interaction may be mediated by a water molecule resulting in a
similar strong interaction with T.S. Exchanging the oxygen atom
of (15) for sulphur to give (16) results in a poorer inhibitor of
T.S. presumably due to the inability of sulphur to enter into a
similar type of hydrogen bonding process.

Similar arguments could explain the lower enzyme activity of
chloro-compound (17) (Table 5) although the chlorine substituent
also affects the N^3-H bond strength and may have similar side
effects to those described for compound (11).

96

The wide range of C-2 substituents accepted by the enzyme and
resulting in good T.S. inhibitory activity and cytotoxicity encouraged us to investigate the quinazoline nucleus in more detail. In
an attempt to quantify the relative importance of the N-1 and N-3
centres of the quinazoline in enzyme binding we modified the heter-
ocycle by removing both nitrogen atoms sequentially.

Removal of N-1 gave the series of isoquinolones the results
of which are summarized in Table 6. All were significantly (up to
250-fold) worse as inhibitors of T.S than the corresponding quin-
azolines and possessed minimal cytotoxicity against the L1210 cell
line. These results clearly emphasise the importance of the N-1
centre of the quinazoline in enzyme binding.

Table 6

Compound	R	TS, IC_{50}, μM	L1210, IC_{50}, μM
(18)	Cl	1.5	ca 54
(19)	H	4.1	ca 200
(20)	Ph	4.6	ca 80
(21)	CH_3	12	>100
(22)	CF_3	19	>100

Removal of N-3 from the quinazoline nucleus results in 4-qui-
nolone (23) which again showed modest enzyme inhibitory properties
and resulted in no cytotoxic activity against L1210. However, in
removing N-3 we have radically changed the nature of the N-1 centre converting it from an H-bond acceptor into an H-bond donor.

In returning to an aromatic basic nitrogen at N-1 we removed the carbonyl oxygen at C-4. We initially investigated the effect of different C-4 substituents in a series of 2-methylquinolines (Table 7). The hydrogen (<u>24</u>) and methoxy-substituted compounds (<u>25</u>) were similar in activity to (<u>23</u>). Better activity against the enzyme was observed with the methyl (<u>26</u>) and cyano-substituted (<u>27</u>) quinolines whilst the halogen substituted compounds (<u>28</u>) and

Table 7

X, CH$_3$, N, N, CO NH, COOH, H, CH$_2$CH$_2$COOH

Compound	X	TS, IC$_{50}$, μM	L1210, IC$_{50}$, μM
(<u>23</u>)	OH	6.3	>100
(<u>24</u>)	H	7.9	>100
(<u>25</u>)	OCH$_3$	6.0	>100
(<u>26</u>)	CH$_3$	0.8	>100
(<u>27</u>)	CN	1.5	75
(<u>28</u>)	Br	0.54	23
(<u>29</u>)	Cl	0.25	8

(<u>29</u>) were only some 5-10 fold poorer as inhibitors of T.S. than the 2-methylquinazoline (<u>4</u>). 4-Chloroquinoline (<u>29</u>) also exhibited interesting cytotoxicity and confirmation that T.S. remained the sole locus of action was obtained when this cytotoxicity was prevented by co-administration of thymidine in the cell assay.

Modification of the methyl group of (<u>29</u>) resulted in two excellent enzyme inhibitors (Table 8). The 2,4-dichloro (<u>30</u>) and 2-amino-4-chloroquinoline (<u>31</u>) exhibit similar T.S. inhibition to that shown by 2-methylquinazoline (<u>4</u>). The cytotoxicity exhibited by these compounds though good is somewhat disappointing. We are unable to rationalize this result since the evidence we have suggests that the compounds are substrates for the FPGS enzyme.

In contrast to these two compounds the introduction of an acid group at the C-2 positon of the quinoline to give (<u>32</u>) results in a large loss of activity against the enzyme. We speculate that this is the result of the ionised carboxylate group of (<u>32</u>) entering into an unfavorable interaction with the T.S. enzyme complex.

Table 8

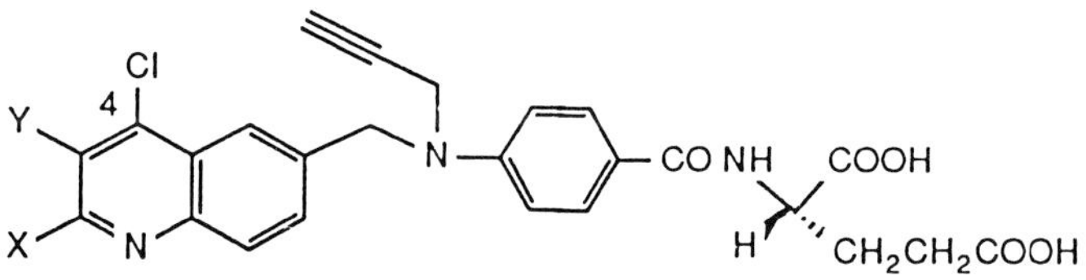

Compound	X	Y	TS, IC_{50},μM	L1210, IC_{50},μM
(<u>30</u>)	Cl	H	0.064	8.6
(<u>31</u>)	NH_2	H	0.096	11
(<u>32</u>)	COOH	H	31	>100
(<u>33</u>)	H	Cl	0.50	>100
(<u>34</u>)	H	NH_2	0.04	1.6
(<u>35</u>)	H	COOH	21	>100
(<u>36</u>)	Cl	Cl (4-H)	6.6	>100

Repositioning of these three substituents into the 3-position of a 4-chloroquinoline leads to broadly similar results (Table 8). However, whilst the 3-amino compound (34) still gives good T.S. inhibition and <u>in vitro</u> cytotoxicity against the L1210 cell line superior to (<u>2</u>), the 3,4-dichloroquinoline (<u>33</u>) is 8-fold worse against T.S. than the 2,4-dichloroquinoline isomer (<u>30</u>) and is devoid of <u>in vitro</u> cytotoxic activity. A further 13-fold loss of enzyme activity is seen with the 2,3-dichloroquinoline (<u>36</u>) (Table 8). We are forced to conclude that the presence of a chlorine substituent in the 3-position of the quinoline nucleus is detrimental to enzyme binding and this may be because the chlorine atom is occupying the position normally occupied by the N^3-H group, a hydrogen bond donor, and consequently enters into an energetically unfavorable interaction with the enzyme.

The quinoline SAR emphasise the importance of the N-1 centre in enzyme binding whilst suggesting that the N-3 centre is not so crucial.

In turning our attention away from the heterocyclic portion of the molecule we next focussed on the glutamic acid moiety. Replacement of glutamic acid in compound (4) with a series of α - amino acids bearing different length alkyl chains resulted in optimal enzyme activity when an n-propyl (40) or n-butyl (41) side chain replaced the carboxyethyl portion of glutamic acid. _In vitro_ cytotoxicity against L1210 was significantly diminished compared to (4) (Table 9) presumably because the former compounds are incapable of polyglutamation. Branching of the alkyl chain as in compounds (43) and (44) (Table 9) also gave excellent T.S. inhibi

Table 9

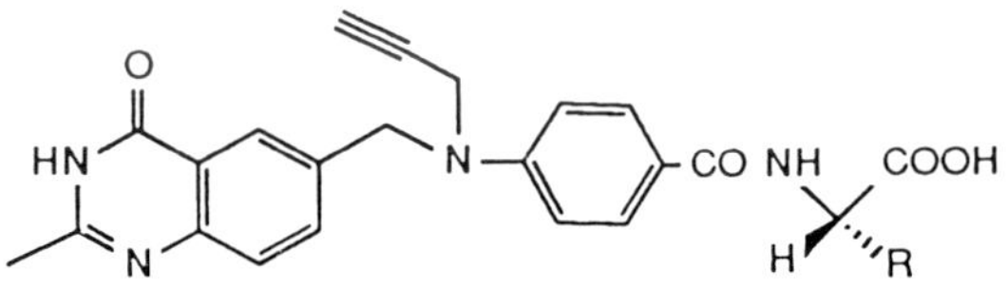

Compound	R	TS, IC_{50}, μM	L1210, IC_{50}, μM
(37)	H	0.52	>100
(38)	CH_3	0.15	25
(39)	CH_2CH_3	0.09	4.3
(40)	n-Pr	0.04	2.5
(41)	n-Bu	0.05	6.6
(42)	n-C_5H_{11}	0.35	
(43)	$CHMe_2$	0.06	0.96
(44)	CMe_3	0.06	0.45
(45)	Ph	0.03	15
(46)	CH_2Ph	0.17	41
(47)	CH_2CH_2Ph	0.08	ca 20

tors which also possessed good _in vitro_ cytotoxic activity. These results suggest that whilst the enzyme undoubtedly possesses a site capable of strong interaction with the α-carboxyl group of the amino acid there also appears to be a size-limited lipophilic pocket in the same region capable of significant interaction with a suitable side-chain. This conclusion is further supported by the phenylglycine derivative (45) which is also an excellent enzyme inhibitor. However, making this group larger as in derivatives (46) and (47) results in some loss of activity against the enzyme. Nevertheless these amino acid derivatives form an interesting class of compounds which cannot be substrates for FPGS. The cytotoxicity exhibited by compounds such as (43) and (44) suggests that they are substrates for the reduced folate carrier transport system.

In making the modifications to our basic quinazoline antifolate (2) we have been able to draw several conclusions. The N-1 centre of the quinazoline appears more important than N-3 for interaction with the enzyme. The enzyme is relatively tolerant of substituents at the C-2 position of the quinazoline but small and/or polar groups are preferred. Suitably substituted quinolines provide a good replacement for the quinazoline nucleus in designing T.S. enzyme inhibitors. In the glutamate portion of the molecule, additional enzyme-inhibitor binding is available by interacting with an apparent lipophilic pocket also present in this region. This information will no doubt allow us to design better inhibitors of the T.S. enzyme.

REFERENCES

1. Hitchings GH: Selective inhibitors of dihydrofolate reductase. Angew. Chem. Int. Ed. Eng. 28:879, 1989.
2. Martin DS: Enhancement of 5-fluorouracil chemotherapy with emphasis on the use of excess thymidine. Cancer Bull (Texas) 30:219, 1978.
3. Harrap KR, Taylor GA, Browman GP: Enhancement of the therapeutic effectiveness of methotrexate and protection of normal proliferating tissues with purines and pyrimidines. Chem. Biol Interac. 18:119, 1977.

4. Jones TR, Calvert AH, Jackman AL et al: A potent antitumour
    quinazoline inhibitor of thymidylate synthetase: Synthesis,
    biological properties and therapeutic results in mice. Eur.
    J. Cancer 17:11, 1981.
5. Jackman AL, Calvert AH, Hart LI, Harrap KR: In: Purine
    Metabolism in Man - IV, 165B: C.H.M.M. DeBruyn. HA Simmonds,
    M Muller (eds), New York and London, Plenum Publishing Corp,
    pp. 375-378, 1984.
6. Jackson RC, Jackman AL, Calvert AH: Biochemical effects of a
    quinazoline inhibitor of thymidylate synthetase, N-(4-(-((2-
    anino-4-hydroxy-6-quinazolinyl)methyl)prop-2-ynylamino)ben-
    zoyl)-L-glutamic acid (CB3717), on human lymphoblastoid
    cells. Biochem. Pharmacol, 32:3783, 1983.
7. Pogolotti AL, Danenberg PV, Santi DV: Kinetics and mechanism
    of interaction of 10-propargyl-5,8-dideazafolate with thymidy-
    late synthase. J. Med. Chem. 29:478, 1986.
8. Cheng Y-C, Dutschman GE, Starnes MC et al: Activity of the
    new antifolate N10-propargyl-5,8-dideazafolate and its poly-
    glutamates against human dihydrofolate reductase, human thy-
    midylate synthetase, and KB cells containing different levels
    of dihydrofolate reductase. Cancer Res. 45:598, 1985.
9. Cheng Y-C, Ueda T, Dutschman GE et al: In: Proceedings of
    the Second Workshop on Folyl and Antifolyl-polyglutamates.
    ID Goldman (ed), Praeger Scientific, NY, 1985.
10. Jones TR, Calvert AH, Jackman, AL et al: Quinazoline anti-
     folates inhibiting thymidylate synthase; variation of the N10
     substituent. J. Med. Chem. 28:1468, 1985.
11. Jackman AL, Jones TR, Calvert AH: In: Experimental and
     Clinical Progress in Cancer Chemotherapy. FM Muggia (ed),
     Martinus Nijhoff, Boston, pp. 155-210, 1985.
12. Jackman AL, Taylor GA, Calvert AH, Harrap KR: Modulation of
     anti-metabolite effects: Effects of thymidine on the
     efficacy of the quinazoline based thymidylate synthetase
     inhibitor CB3717. Biochem. Pharmacol. 33:3269, 1984.
13. Jackman AL, Calvert AH, Taylor GA, Harrap KR: In: The
     Control of Tumour Growth and its Biological Basis. W Davis,
     C Maltoni, S Tanneberger (eds), Berlin, Akademie-Verlag, pp.
     404-410, 1983.
14. Moran RG, Colman PD, Rosowsky A et al: Structural features
     of 4-amino antifolates required for substrate activity with
     mammalian folylpolyglutamate synthetase. Mol. Pharmacol.
     27:156, 1985.
15. Sikora E, Jackman AL, Newell DR, Calvert AH: Formation and
     retention and biological activity of N10-propargyl-5,8-
     dideazafolic acid (CB3717) polyglutamates in L1210 cells in
     vitro. Biochem. Pharmacol. 37:4047, 1988.
16. Sikora E, Jackman AL, Newell DR et al: In: Chemistry and
     Biology of Pteridines. BA Cooper, VM Whitehead (eds), de
     Gruyter, Berlin, pp. 675-679, 1986.
17. Pawelczak R, Jones TR, Kempny M et al: Quinazoline anti-
     folates inhibiting thymidylate synthase: Synthesis of four
     oligo(L-γ-glutamyl) conjugates of N10-propargyl-5,8-dideaza-
     folic acid and their enzyme inhibition. J. Med. Chem.
     32:160, 1988.

18. Curtin NJ, Harris AL, James OFW, Bassendine MF: Inhibition of the growth of human hepatocellular carcinoma _in vitro_ and in athymic mice by a quinazoline inhibitor of thymidylate synthase, CB3717. Br. J. Cancer 53:361, 1986.
19. Calvert AH, Alison DL, Harland SJ et al: A Phase I evaluation of the quinazoline antifolate thymidylate synthase inhibitor, N10-propargyl-5,8-dideazafolic acid, CB3717. J. Clin. Oncol. 4:1245, 1986.
20. Bassendine MF, Curtin NJ, Loose H, Harris AL: Induction of remission in hepatocellular carcinoma with a new thymidylate synthase inhibitor, CB3717; a Phase II study. J. Hepatol. 4:349, 1987.
21. Vest S, Bork E, Hansen HH: A Phase I evaluation of N10-propargyl-5,8-dideazafolic acid. Eur. J. Cancer Clin. Oncol. 24:201, 1988.
22. Cantwell BMJ, Macaulay V, Harris AL et al: Phase II study of the antifolate N10-propargyl-5,8-dideazafolic acid (CB3717) in advanced breast cancer. Eur. J. Can. Clin. Oncol. 24:733, 1988.
23. Jones TR, Thornton TJ, Flinn A et al: Quinazoline antifolates inhibiting thymidylate synthase: 2-desamino derivatives with enhanced solubility and potency. J. Med. Chem. 32:847, 1989.
24. Harrap KR, Jackman AL, Newell DR et al: Thymidylate synthase: A target for anticancer drug design. Adv. Enz. Regulation 29:161, 1989.
25. Jackman AL, Newell DR, Jodrell DI et al: In: Chemistry and Biology of Pteridines. H Curtius, S Ghisla, N Blau (eds), de Gruyter, Berlin (in press).
26. Jackman AL, Marsham P, Hughes LR et al: Analogues of 2-desamino-2-CH3-dideazafolates as inhibitors of thymidylate synthase; substitution on the benzene ring. Proc. Am. Assoc. Cancer Res. 30:1892, 1989.
27. Fry DW, Besserer JA, Boritzki TJ: Transport of the antitumour antibiotic CI-920 into L1210 leukemia cells by the reduced folate carrier system. Cancer Res. 44:3366, 1984.
28. Marsham PR, Chambers P, Hayter AJ et al: Qunazoline antifolate thymidylate synthase inhibitors: Nitrogen, oxygen, sulfur and chlorine substituents in the C2 position. J. Med. Chem. 32:569, 1989 (and references cited therein).
29. Jackman AL, Taylor GA, O'Connor BM et al: Activity of the thymidylate synthase inhibitor 2-desamino-N10-propargyl-5, 8-dideazafolic acid and related compounds in murine (L1210) and human (W1L2) systems _in vitro_ and in L1210 _in vivo_. Cancer Res. 50:5212, 1990.
30. Enzyme assays were performed as described in ref. (4).
31. Cell growth inhibition assays were performed as described in: Chemistry and Biology of Pteridines. BA Cooper, VM Whitehead (eds), Walter de Gruyter, Berlin, pp. 645, 1986.

31. Cell growth inhibition assays were performed as described in
"Chemistry and Biology of Pteridines". BA Cooper, VM Whitehead (eds), Walter de Gruyter, Berlin, pp. 645, 1986.

5

DNA-MINOR GROOVE BINDING ANTICANCER AGENTS

Wendell Wierenga, Ph.D.

INTRODUCTION

The B form of DNA is distinguished by two grooves called the major and the minor groove. These grooves represent the key loci for information transfer between DNA and molecules that interact with it. A simplified diagram of the key contact atoms for hydrogen bonding or pole/dipole interactions is shown below for both the GC and AT pairs.

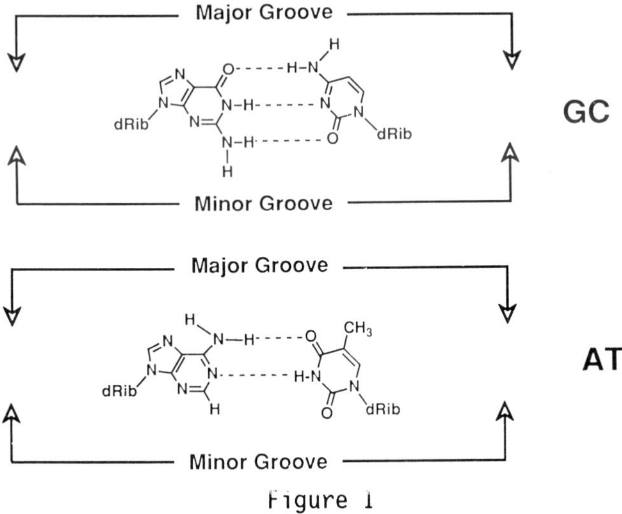

Figure 1

Important positions in the minor groove of GC pairs include the 2-amino group of guanine and the 3-oxygen of cytosine which is contrasted with the minor groove of AT pairs where there is only the 2-oxygen of thymine directed into the minor groove.

Most protein interactions with DNA involve the major groove
by virtue of its width, depth and the complementary size of the
binding region of the proteins. DNA binding proteins are both
regulatory in nature as well as operational. Operationally, they
play key roles in DNA replication, recombination, strand scission
and transcription. In the regulatory sense, they control the expression of key genes. Various structural motifs have been uncovered for protein DNA interactions, including zinc finger, leu-
cine zipper, EF domains and an alpha helix, usually exemplified in
a helix turn helix motif (1,2).

Agents that interact in the minor groove of DNA include low
molecular weight agents that are either natural products or synthetic in origin. They were usually uncovered due to certain
biological activity manifested through their relatively unique
interactions with DNA. These agents include the netropsin/dista-
mycin-like compounds, the CPI compounds (based on the structure of
the novel antibiotic CC-1065), anthramycins, bleomycins, bis-qua-
ternary ammonium heterocycles, phthalanilides, bis-guanylhydra-
zones, diarylamidines, mithromycin, chromomycin, and olivomycin
(Figure 2) (3,4). The compounds that have received the most extensive structural studies involving complexation with DNA include
netropsin/distamycin, CC-1065, and the fluorescent dye Hoechst
22258. Hoechst 33258 binds very tightly to DNA and is a potent
carcinogen. DNA footprinting studies as well as analysis of the
crystal structure of its DNA complex show it prefers AT-base pairs
in its binding site (5,6).

Similarly, footprinting and x-ray crystallographic analysis
of the structures of netropsin and distamycin binding to DNA have
revealed a high specificity for AT-base pairs (7,8). This binding
to minor groove, B-form DNA is distinguished by bifurcated hydrogen bonds of netropsin involving the amide hydrogens with opposite
strand pairs such as the O2 of thymine and the N3 of adenine. The
binding is high affinity (K=10^9 at 25°C) and is enthalpy
driven (9).

Various structural modifications of the netropsin/distamycin
molecule have been made to both improve its biological activity

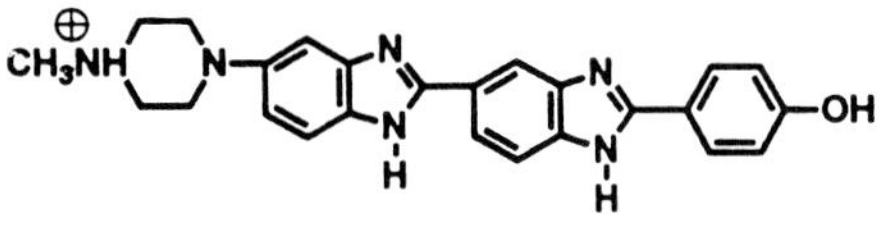

Hoechst 33258

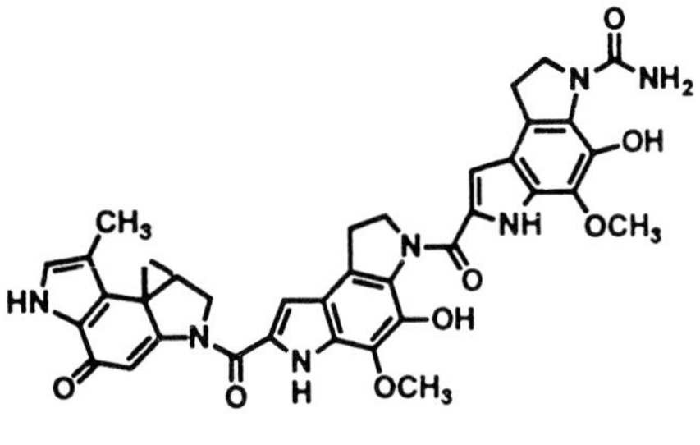

CC-1065 (U-56,314)

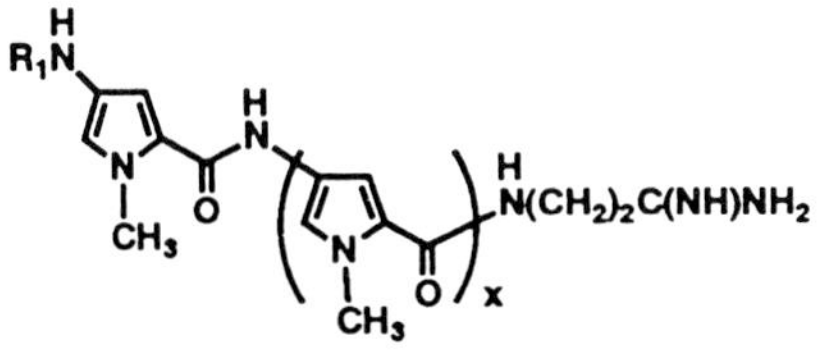

Distamycin/Netropsin Family

Figure 2

(principally antitumor) as well as modify its sequence selectivity. For example, the N-methyl pyrrole was replaced by an
N-methyl imidazole to accommodate hydrogen binding to the 2-amino
group of guanine and thus provide for some GC selectivity. This
novel class of molecules was concomitantly conceived by J.W. Lown
and R.E. Dickerson and termed "lexitropsins" (Figure 3) (10,11).

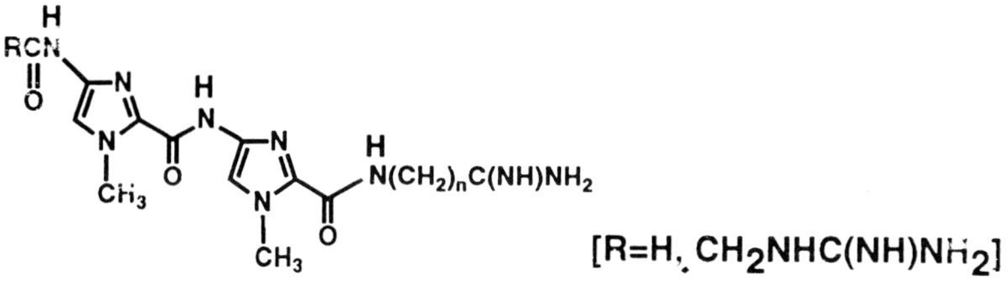

$[R=H, CH_2NHC(NH)NH_2]$

Figure 3

In addition, various alkylating moieties have been appended to
this structural class to enhance antitumor activity (12,13,14).
The two most interesting compounds appear to be the distamycin
analogs (structure shown below, Figure 4) to which have been appended either the 2-dichloroethyl amino group or the 2-chloro-
ethylaminobenzoyl group.

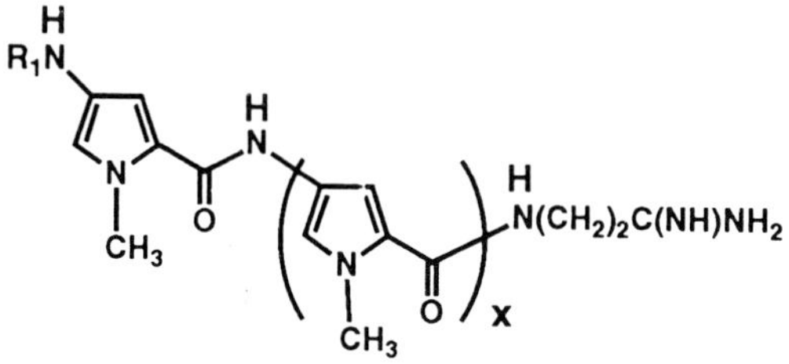

$$R_1 = CO\text{-aryl-}N(CH_2CH_2Cl)_2$$
$$N(CH_2HC_2Cl)_2$$

Figure 4

These compounds exhibit _in vivo_ antitumor activity against
the murine leukemia L1210 with increase in life spans of about 80%
at optimum doses of 0.4 and 0.3 mg/kg and also exhibit activity in
the melphalan resistant L1210 line. Researchers at Farmitalia
have further characterized these distamycin analogs in terms of
their DNA binding effect on key regulatory proteins such as OTF-1,
the transcriptional activator for histone H2B and found that FCE
24517 inhibits the binding of OTF-1 to DNA as well as reduces
message RNA of histone H2B in L1210 leukemia cells by 90% (no
effect on histone H4 or actin mRNAs) (15).

<u>CPI Analogs</u>

CC-1065 (structure shown below) is a fermentation product of
Streptomyces zelensis (16). It was discovered at the Upjohn laboratories in the late 1970's under a contract with the NCI involving screening of soil microorganisms for antitumor antibiotics
(17). It exhibited modest antitumor activity (DN2 level versus
B16). Initially a decision was made at the NCI to develop CC-1065

as an anticancer agent, but this was reversed when Upjohn scientists determined that CC-1065 exhibited delayed and irreversible toxicity in mice at therapeutic doses (18,19). There were however several unique features of CC-1065 that prompted an effort to invest further research in this molecule. One unique feature, of course, is its unusual structure incorporating a trimeric pyrolloindole distinguished by the cyclopropylpyrrolindole (CPI) on the left hand side of the molecule (20). In addition, it exhibited unusual potency. For example CC-1065 shows 1-2 nM level inhibition of B16 melanoma cell growth and DNA synthesis as well as 10-50 µg/kg/day optimum doses for _in vivo_ antitumor activity (21,22). Lastly, and probably most interestingly, was its putative, unusual mechanism of action involving binding in the minor groove of DNA in an irreversible, sequence selective fashion. In collaboration with the Hurley group at the University of Texas, the Upjohn group determined that CC-1065 selectively alkylated the N-3 of adenine in the minor groove of DNA within two 5-base pair consensus sequences, a polyA sequence and a PuNTTA sequence (23). Furthermore, this alkylation was unique, involving site specificity on the cyclopropyl ring at the methylene group. The mechanism most probably involves a push-pull mechanism of AR-1,5 alkylation, presumably utilizing a phosphate protonation of the quinone carbonyl followed by SN2' attack on the methylene group of the cyclopropane ring by the unpaired electrons of the N3 nitrogen of adenine (24,25). Molecular modeling shows that CC-1065, whose x-ray crystallographic structure has been determined (26), exhibits a natural ellipticity which fits very nicely into the DNA minor groove helix. Unfortunately, attempts to co-crystallize DNA CC-1065 have been without success to date.

Molecular modification using synthetic chemistry began with the left-hand segment or CPI part of the molecule (U-62736) (27). It was intriguing to us that the CPI molecule itself exhibited antitumor activity although the potency was several orders of magnitude different from the natural product. However, we quickly ascertained that further elaboration of the CPI template with groups mimicking the pyrroloindole structures afforded a dramatic

P388
(ip/ip)

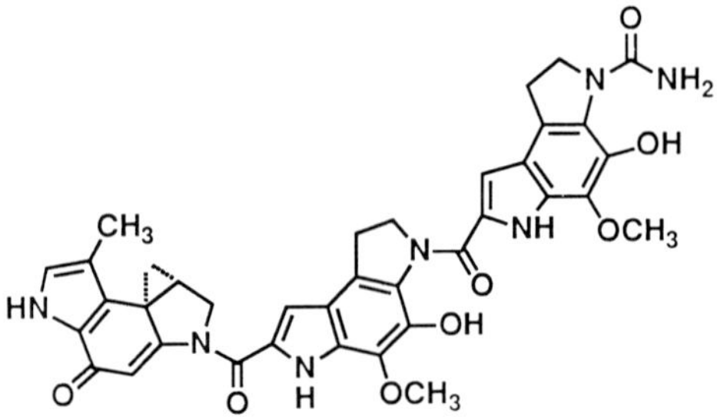

T/C =164
at 0.012 mg/kg

CC-1065 (U-56,314)

(L.J. Hanka, D.G. Martin, et al, J. Antibiot. 31:124, 1978)

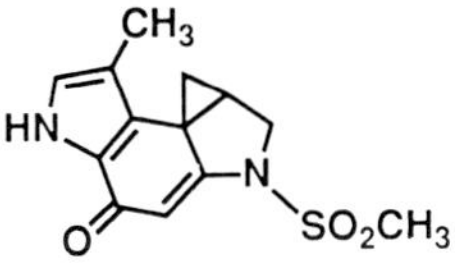

T/C = 164
at 25 mg/kg

U-62,736
(W.   Wierenga, JACS 103:5621, 1981)

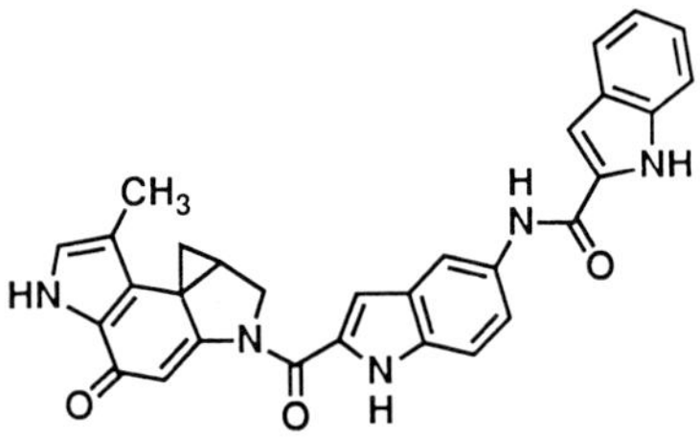

4/6 cures
at 0.050 mg/kg

U-68,415
(M.A. Warpehoski, et al, Proc. AACR 26:870, 1985)

Figure 5

increase in potency rivaling the natural product.   In addition
there was a parallel improvement in antitumor activity (28).

A synopsis of the molecular modification, engineered through
total syntheses, is graphically depicted in the Figure 6.   We were
able to determine which portions of the molecule were critical for
biological activity, for DNA interaction, and ultimately, differen-
tiate delayed toxicity from therapeutic activity (29,30,31).

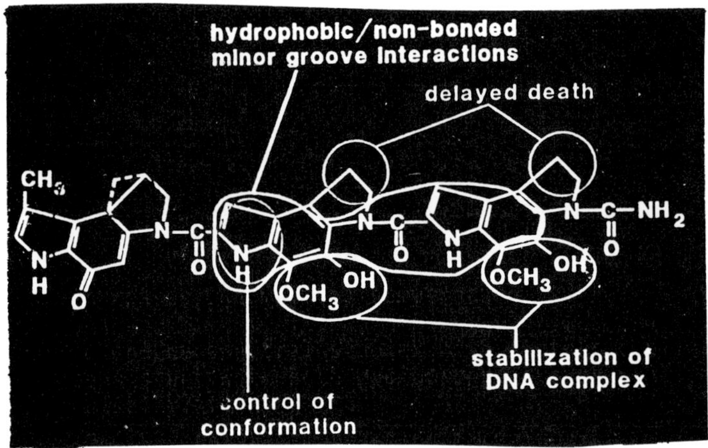

Figure 6

The first generation clinical candidate generated from this exciting work was U-73975. This optically active molecule is prepared by total synthesis (18 steps) and exhibits comparable potency to CC-1065, albeit with much more effective antitumor activity as is evident in Figure 7.

Site	Tumor	Response	Route
ip	P388 leukemia	curative	ip
ip	L1210 leukemia	curative	ip
ip	L1210 leukemia	100% increased lifespan	iv
ip	B16 melanoma	190% increased lifespan	ip
iv	Lewis lung	74% increased lifespan	ip
iv	Lewis lung	curative	iv
sc	Colon 38	91% tumor growth inhibition	iv
sc	LX-1 (human xenograft)	90% tumor growth inhibition	iv

Figure 7. U-73975 (Optimum dose 75-100 μg/kg)

It exhibited no delayed or irreversible toxicity in preclinical toxicology and is currently in early clinical studies in cancer patients. It binds in the minor groove of DNA, alkylating on the N-3 of adenine, exhibiting some sequence selective interaction overlapping with CC-1065 but not identical.

U-73975 is a monoalkylating CPI analog. We reasoned that since many clinically useful alkylating agents such as cisplatin, mitomycin, melphalan, and cyclophosphamide cross-link DNA, and it is generally accepted that cross-linked DNA is more difficult to repair in cells, that the sequence selectivity of a CPI dimer, by requiring the correct juxtaposition of two reactive adenine containing sequences on opposite strands, would further enhance the specificity of the "DNA-reading" of these molecules and would be more difficult to repair. This is shown schematically below, wherein two CPI molecules with appropriate stereochemistry are tethered together by group X.

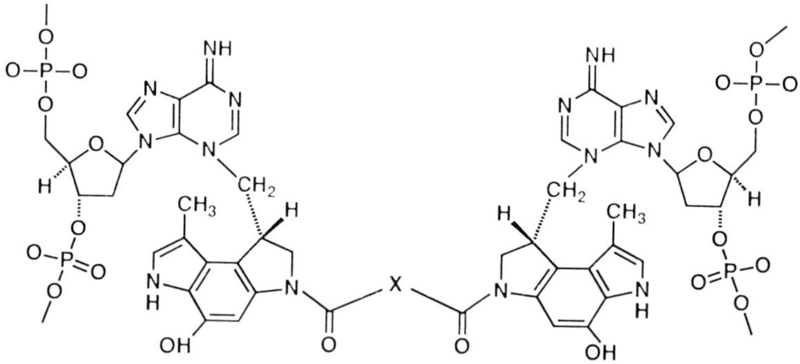

Figure 8.   Interstrand Crosslinking of DNA by U-73975.

As is shown in Table 1, several conclusions are evident. Tethering two CPI molecules with a methylene chain (U-75559) increases the potency by four orders of magnitude (compare U-77991). Secondly, the replacement of X as a methylene chain with various heterocycles such as indoles (e.g. U-77779) affords an even more potent molecule. And thirdly, the stereochemistry of the reactive alkylating group, whether it is the activated cyclopropane or the precursor chloromethylphenol, is critical to the antitumor activity. The analog of most interest, biologically speaking, was U-77779 which exhibited _in vivo_ potency against murine tumors of about 10-fold over U-73975, the monoalkylator.

The in vivo antitumor efficacy is exemplified by Table 2.

That these CPI dimers did in fact interact with DNA was shown by an increase in DNA melting temperature with these analogs. In addition, based on a library of circular dichroism and UV spectral studies with synthetic oligonucleotides and various monoalkylating

Table 1

In Vitro/In Vivo Cytotoxic Potency

Compound	3-day L1210 leukemia cell growth, ID_{50}, pM
CC-1065	30
U-73975	7
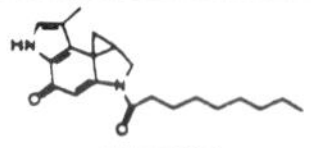 U-77991	60,000
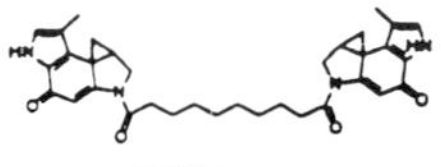 U-75559	5
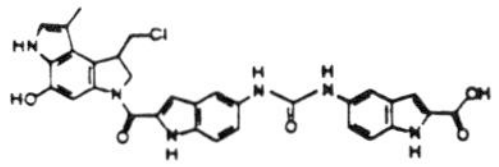 U-85021	10,000
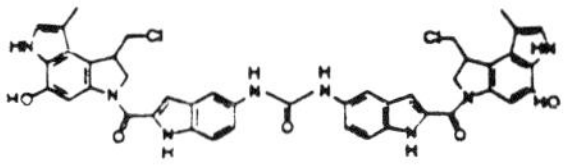 U-77779	1

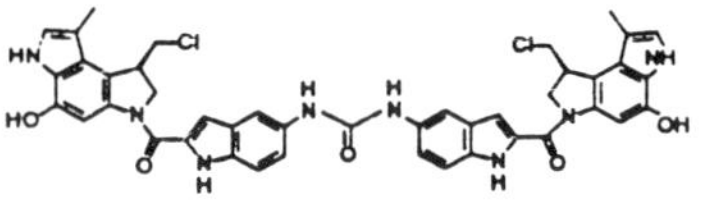

nat U-77779 nat

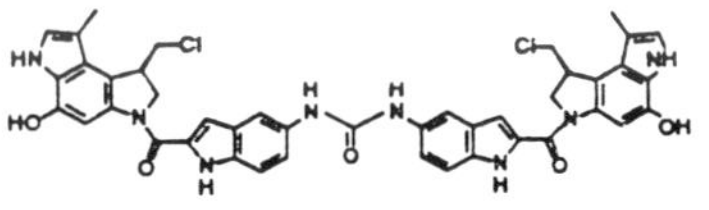

nat U-85054 ent

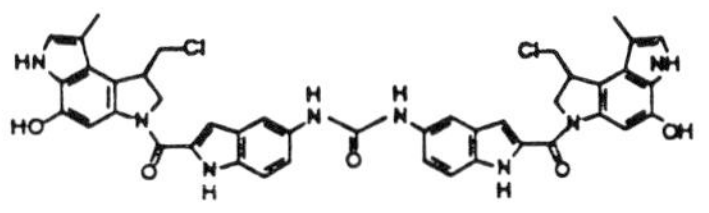

ent U-85605 ent

	ID_{50} 3 day in vitro L1210 10-6 μg/ml	T/C L1210 in vivo ip tumor, iv drug day 1	Dose μg/kg
U-77779	1	3/6	10
U-85054	400	129	160
U-85605	4000	129	800

Table 2

In Vivo Antitumor Efficacy of U-77779, A Rigid CPI Dimer

Tumor		Drug		U-73975		U-77779	
				%ILS[a]	OO[b]	%ILS	OO
Site	System	Route	Schedule	(Cures/total)	mg/kg/day	(survivors/total)	mg/kg/day
ip	L1210 leukemia	iv	day 1	94	0.1	(3/6)	0.01
sc	L1210 leukemia	iv	day 1	(4/6)	0.1	(6/6)	0.01
sc	L1210 leukemia	iv	day 5	70	0.1	90 (1/6)	0.025
ip	B16 melanoma	ip	days 1,5,9	93 (1/8)	0.025	115 (2/8)	0.004
ip	B16 melanoma	iv	day 1	60	0.1	67	0.015
iv	Lewis lung	ip	days 1,5,9	106	0.033	69	0.004

[a]%ILS - percent increase in lifespan of drug-treated virsus control mice (60 day survivors)
[b]OO = optimal dose

Tumor		U-73975			U-7779		
		OO			OO		
Site	System	mg/kg/day[c]	%TGI(day)[d]	%ILS[e]	mg/kg/day	%TGI(day)	%ILS
sc	pancreatic 02	0.05	80 (16)	40	0.01	70 (12)	48
sc	colon 38	0.05	94 (27)	67	0.005	100 (13)	59
sc	colon 38	0.05	99 (13)	36	0.0075	92 (13)	29

[c]Optimal dose; drugs were administered iv on days 2 and 9
[d]Percent tumor growth inhibition relative to control mice (measurement day).
Tumors were measured on days 9,12,14,16 and 18 in the panc 02 experiment and days 13,20,27 and 34 in the colon 38 experiments
[e]Percent increase in life span of drug-tested versus control mice

CPI analogs, the CPI dimers exhibit bisalkylation as exemplified by the scheme below (Figure 9a). In addition, we have analyzed DNA alkylation using the alkaline gel mobility assay. It is evident in Figure 10 that there are slower mobility bands of cross-linked DNA fragments with increasing doses of U-77779 versus the negative controls of solvent and U-73975 (lane 18). The positive control is psoralen followed by a two minute irradiation (U-9721, lane 19). The methylene tethered CPI analog U-75559 shows much less DNA cross-linking at these doses even though it is a potent cytotoxic agent. One can model the CPI dimers on DNA much the same as CC-1065 or the CPI monoalkylating agents such as U-73975, as is shown in Figure 9b where energy minimized structures exhibit a natural ellipticity with crosslinking alkylation of the opposite strand N3's of adenine (Figure 9b).

While U-73975 exhibited excellent broad spectrum _in vivo_ activity and exquisite potency, we noted in pharmacokinetic studies in mice that its elimination phase half-life was relatively short (less than 1 hour by intravenous administration). We therefore

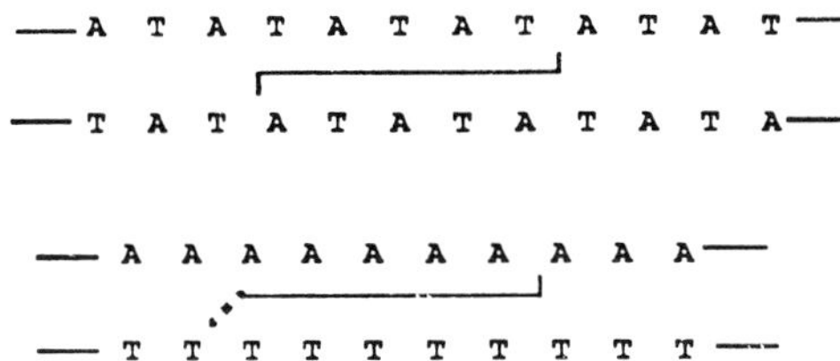

o   increases DNA melting temperature

o   cd and uv spectral studies with synthetic oligos:
    consistent with both cyciopropyl groups reacted
    (bisalkylation)

Figure 9a.   DNA Interaction Studies

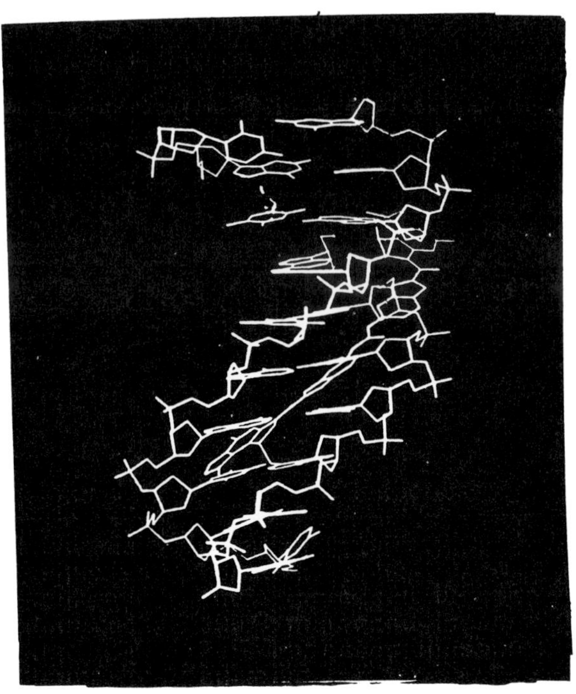

Figure 9b

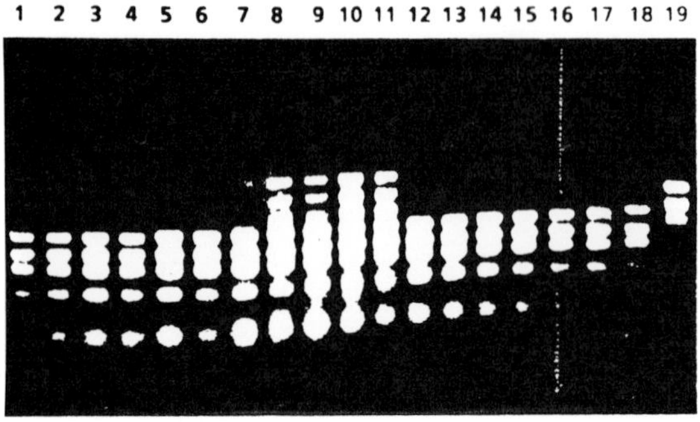

Lane	Agent	Dose*
1	DNA	(untreated)
2	DMA	(solvent control)
3	U-77779	5
4	U-77779	10
5	"	25
6	"	50
7	"	100
8	"	150
9	"	200
10	"	250
11	"	300
12	U-75559	50
13	"	100
14	"	150
15	"	200
16	"	300
17	"	500
18	U-73975	100
19	2 min irradiation with U-9721	

* Drug concentrations are expressed as #Drug/Genome

Figure 10. A Dose Response Comparison of Crosslinking by U-77779 and U-75559.

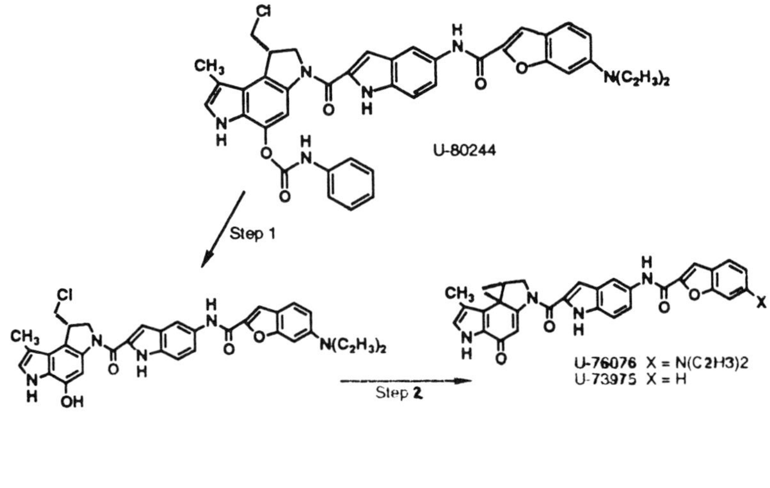

U-80244

Step 1

U-76076 X = N(C2H3)2
U-73975 X = H

Step 2

Hypothesis: U-80244 can act as a slow release form of the biologically active cyclopropyl containing species (U-76074) via the metabolic pathway shown above.

Figure 11. CPI Prodrugs - A New Class of Highly Active Agents explored various molecular modifications to enhance the half-life of the CPI molecule in the form of a prodrug. Various derivatives were made and the agent exhibiting the most interesting efficacy was U-80224 whose structure and putative activation, in a two step sequence, is shown in Figure 11. We anticipate the cleavage of the phenyl urethane to be enzymic either in the liver or in serum and the activation to the cyclopropane to be chemical. It can be seen from Table 3 that U-80244 exhibited excellent _in vivo_

Table 3

Efficacy of U-80244 in Murine Tumor Systems

TUMOR		DRUG		U-80244	
				Optimal Dose	% ILS
Site	System	Route	Schedule	mg/kd/day	(survivors/total)
ip	L1210 leukemia	iv	day 1	0.6	125(2/6)
sc	B16 melanoma	ip	days 1,5,9	0.10	92
ip	B16 melanoma	iv	day 1	0.5	75
iv	Lewis lung	ip	days 1,5,9	0.15	103(2/8)

TUMOR		U-80244 (administered iv on days 2 and 9)		
Site	System	Optimal Dose mg/kg/day	%TGI(day)[a]	%ILS
sc	pancreatic 02	0.4	98(14)	85
sc	colon 38	0.2	90(20)	47
sc	colon 38	0.2	99(27)	38

[a] Percent tumor growth inhibition relative to control mice measurement day. Tumors were measured on days 9, 12,14, 16, and 18 in the Panc 02 experiment and days 13, 20, 27, and 34 in the colon 38 experiments.

118

Table 4

Activity Against a Panel of Tumors in Vivo

| | Tumor Response[a] | | | | | | | |
Agent	L1210 Leukemia (ip)	Lewis Lung (iv)	B16 Melanoma (ip)	B16 Melanoma (sc)	Colon 38 (sc)	Panc 02 (sc)	Human Lung LX-1 (sc)	Human Renal Caki-1 (sc)
Adriamycin[b]	++	++	++	--	+	--	--	
Cisplatin[b]	++	++	++	--	+	--	--	
Cyclophosphamide[b]	++	++	++	+	++	--	+	
U-73975[c]	++	++	++	++	+	+	++	++
U-80244[c]	+++	++	++	++	++	++		+++

[a] - Inactive
+ using NCI DN1 level of activity
++ using NCI DN2
[b] Data generated by NCI testing contractors
[c] Data generated at Upjohn

activity against both the rapidly growing L1210 leukemias as well
as the slower growing subcutaneous solid tumors. As is shown in
Figure 11, it generally exhibits better activity against the colon
38 and Panc 02 carcinomas relative to U-73975. Also, shown for
comparison purposes are the activities of adriamyin, cisplatin and
cyclophosphamide. U-80244 shares with U-73975 essentially a schedule independent antitumor activity with maximum efficacy seen on
single dose administration intravenously, irrespective of the site
and type of tumor inoculation (Table 5). The question remained,
of course, as to whether U-80244 represented a pharmacologically
improved version of the CPI monoalkylator U-73975. As shown in
Table 6, varying the time of administration of U-80244 versus
U-73975, relative to tumor implantation, relative to U-73975, generates a sustained antitumor activity for a longer period of time
for U-80244.

We have continued to evaluate these three classes of molecules against other tumor models including human tumors in culture
and ingrafted into nude mice, and mouse tumors that are at different stages of growth prior to therapy. For example, Tables 7 and
8 show the efficacy of CPI analogs U-73975 and U-80244 versus the

pancreatic O2 carcinoma of Corbett at various time points relative
to chemotherapy. Efficacy of U-73975 falls off with increasing
tumor burden as does U-80244 but at a later time point.

Table 5

Comparison of the Route of Drug Administration
Against Mouse L1210 Leukemia[a]

| | U-73975 | | U-80244 | |
Route	MTD[b] (mg/kg)	ILS (%)	MTD[b] (mg/kg)	ILS (%)
iv	100	75	600	156(2/6)[c]
ip	25	100	600	- (6/6)
sc	250	88	500	82
po	250	31	5000	113

[a] 10^5 cells/mouse, ip
[b] Maximal tolerated or optimal dose was given on Day 1
[c] Number of 30-day survivors/total

Table 6

Effect of Varying the Time of Drug Administration
Relative to Time of Tumor Implantation on Activity
Against L1210 Leukemia

	IV Single Dose, mg/kg	Time of Dosing Relative to Tumor Implant, hr	IV Implant		IP Implant	
			ILS(%)[a]	30 d Survivors	ILS(%)[a]	30 d Survivors
U-73975	100	-24	14		13	
		-6	14		19	
		-4	14		13	
		-2	29		38	
		-1	57		75	
		0	--	5/6	125	2/6
		+24	200	1/6	106	
U-80244	400	-24	14		25	
		-6	79		100	
		-4	100		--	3/6
		-2	--	5/6	--	6/6
		-1	--	6/6	--	5/6
		0	--	6/6	--	4/6
		+24	214	1/6	--	3/6

[a] % ILS = percent increase in lifespan of drug treated over
control mice (7 days for iv tumor, 8 days for ip tumor)

Table 7

Efficacy of CPI Analogs Against Mouse Pancreas 02 Tumor[a]

Agent[b]	Dose (mg/kg/inj)	Schedule	TGI(%)[c]	Score[d]
5-FU	70	Days 2,9	63	+
U-75975	0.03	Days 2,6,10	71	+
	0.03	Days 2,6,10,14	72	+
	0.03	Days 2,9,16	27	
U-80244	0.25	Days 2,6,10	95	++
	0.25	Days 2,9,16	82	+

[a] Inoculated sc (Trocar)
[b] 5-FU (ip), CPI analogs (iv)
[c] Tumor weight of untreated control = 664 mg measured on Day 15
[d] + TGI>58%; ++ >90% (followed the criteria for Colon 38 tumor set by NCI)

Table 8

Comparison of the Efficacy of Delayed Treatment of Mouse Pancreas 02 Tumor[a]

Analog[b]	Schedule	TGI(%)[c]	Scored
U-73975	Days 2,9	48	
(35 μg/kg/inj)	Days 6,15	0	
	Days 10,17	4	
U-80244	Days 2,9	95	++
(400 μg/kg/inj)	Days 6,13	89	+
	Days 10,17	55	

[a] Inoculated sc (Trocar)
[b] Analog injected iv
[c] Tumor weight of untreated control is 847 mg measured on day 19

ACKNOWLEDGEMENTS

This work represents the dedicated effort of many indivi-
duals, including: Paul A. Aristoff, Bijoy K. Bhuyan, Thomas F.
DeKoning, IIse Gebhard, Paul D. Johnson, Robert C. Kelly, Li H.
Li, David G. Martin, J. Patrick McGovren, Mark A. Mitchell, Gary
L. Petzold, David H. Swenson, Martha A. Warpehoski, Nancy
Wicnienski, and Marta G. Williams.

REFERENCES

1. Schlief R: DNA Binding by proteins. Science 241:1182-1187,
    1988.
2. Mitchell PJ, Tjian R: Transcriptional regulation in mam-
    malian cells by sequence-specific DNA binding proteins.
    Science 245:371-378, 1989.
3. Zimmer C, Wahnert U: Nonintercalating DNA-binding ligands:
    specificity of the interaction and their use as tools in bio-
    physical, biochemical and biological investigations of the
    genetic material. In: Progress of Biophysics and Molecular
    Biology, 47:31-112, 1986.
4. Pullman B: Molecular mechanisms of specificity in DNA-
    antitumor drug interactions. In: Advances in Drug Research,
    Vol. 18, B. Testa (ed), Academic Press, London, pp. 2-115,
    1989.
5. Harshman KD, Dervan PB: Molecular recognition of B-DNA by
    Hoechst 33258. Nucleic Acids Research 13:4825, 1985.
6. Dickerson RE, Pjura P, Kopka ML: Rational design of DNA
    minor groove binding antitumor drugs. NATO ASI Ser. Ser. A
    126:209-221, 1987.
7. Kopka ML, Yoon C, Goodsell D et al: The molecular origin of
    DNA-drug specificity in netropsin and distamycin. Proc. Nat.
    Acad. Sci., USA 82:1376, 1985.
8. Portugal J, Waring MJ: Comparison of binding sites in DNA
    for berenil, netropsin and distamycin. A footprinting study.
    Europ. J. Biochemistry 167:282-289, 1989.
9. Marky LA, Breslauer KJ: Origins of netropsin binding
    affinity and specificity: Correlations of thermodynamic and
    structural data. PNAS USA, 84:4359-4363, 1987.
10. Lown JW: Lexitropsins: Rational design of DNA sequence
    reading agents as novel anti-cancer agents and potential
    cellular probes. Anticancer Drug Design 3:25-40, 1988.
11. Krowicki K, Louw JW: Synthesis of novel imidazole-containing
    DNA minor groove binding oligopeptides related to the
    antiviral antibiotic netropsin. J. Org. Chem. 52:3493-3501,
    1987.
12. Krowicki K, Balzarini JL, DeClercq E et al: Novel DNA groove
    binding alkylators: Design, synthesis, and biological
    evaluation. J. Med. Chem. 31:341-345, 1988.

13. Baker BJ, Dervan PB: Sequence-specific cleavage of double-helical DNA, N-Bromoacetyldistamycin. J. Am. Chem Soc. 107:8266-8268, 1985.

14. Arcamone FM, Animati F, Barbieri B et al: Synthesis, DNA-Binding Properties, and Antitumor Activity of Novel Distamycin Derivatives. J. Med. Chem. 32:774-778, 1989.

15. Broggini M, Ponti M, Ottolenghi S et al: Distamycins inhibit the binding of OTF-1 and NFE-1 transfactors to their conserved DNA elements. Nucleic Acids Research, 17(3):1051-1059, 1989.

16. Hanka LJ, Dietz A, Gerpheide SA et al: CC-1065 (NSC-298223), a new antitumor antibiotic. Production in vitro, biological activity, microbiological assays and taxonomy of the producing microorganism. J. Antibiot. 131:1211-1217, 1978.

17. Martin DG, Chidester CG, Duchamp DJ Mizsak SA: Structure of CC-1065 (NSU-298223), a new antitumor antibiotic. J. Antibiot. 33:902-903, 1980.

18. Martin DG, Biles C, Gerpheide SA et al: CC-1065 (NSC-298223), a potent new antitumor agent. Improved production and isolation, characterization and antitumor activity. J. Antibiotic. 34:1119-1125, 1981.

19. McGovren JP, Clarke GL, Pratt EA, DeKoning TF: Preliminary toxicity studies with the DNA-Binding antibiotic, CC-1065. J. Antibiotic. 37:63-70, 1984.

20. Carter P, Fitzjohn S, Magnus P: Studies on the synthesis of the antitumor agent CC-1065. Synthesis of PDE1 and PDE II, inhibitors of cyclic adenosine-3',5'-monophosphate phosphodiesterase. J. Chem. Soc. Chem. Commun. 15:1162-1164, 1986.

21. Li LH, Swenson DH, Schpok SL et al: CC-1065 (NSC 298223), a novel antitumor agent that interacts strongly with double-stranded DNA. Cancer Res. 42:999-1004, 1982.

22. Swenson DH, Li LH, Hurley LH: Mechanism of interaction of CC-1065 (NSC 298223) with DNA. Cancer Res. 42:2821-2828, 1982.

23. Hurley LH, Reynolds VL, Swenson DH et al: Reaction of the antitumor antibiotic CC-1065 with DNA: Structure of 2 DNA adducts with DNA sequence specificity. Science 226:843-844, 1984.

24. Warpehoski MA, Hurley LH: Sequence selectivity of DNA covalent modification. Chem. Res. Toxicol. 1:315-333, 1988.

6

2-((ARYLMETHYL)AMINO)-1,3-PROPANEDIOLS (AMAPS); DISCOVERY,
SELECTION AND DEVELOPMENT OF FOUR CLINICAL CANDIDATES

Kenneth W. Bair

INTRODUCTION

Many compounds that show antitumor activity are known to bind
to DNA (1). In order to rationally design antitumor drugs, we
felt that a greater knowledge of the process was needed. Studies
on a number of natural products with antitumor activity, derivatives of acridine, phenanthridine and other small ring systems had
been conducted over the past three decades, but no definitive overview of this phenomenon existed.

We synthesized a series of simple intercalators to study
their interactions with DNA and to discover structural elements
responsible for antitumor activity about ten years ago. These
studies led to the synthesis of a unique series of molecules collectively denoted 2-((arylmethyl)amino)-1,3-propanediols (AMAPs).
Four of these compounds have been selected for clinical development. In this chapter, I will outline the early work on prototype
derivatives and structure/activity studies on the AMAPs, but spend
most of the time describing some of the preclinical studies on the
four compounds selected for clinical development.

DNA STRUCTURAL CONSIDERATIONS

Before we discuss the prototype derivatives it is important
to first examine the structure and physical properties of the target macromolecule, DNA. These features define the structure of
the molecules that will interact with DNA and hopefully those present in drugs affecting DNA, especially antitumor drugs.

124

DNA, whatever form it is in, can be regarded as a tubular macromolecule with three distinct regions: the base pairs, the edge of the base pairs (the major and minor grooves) and the phosphodiester backbones. These regions differ in relative polarity, but are in close proximity to each other. The relatively planar stacks of hydrogen bonded pairs of purine and pyrimidine bases (adenine-thymine (AT) and guanine-cytosine (GC)) form a relatively hydrophobic region in DNA that is stabilized by van der Waals interactions. The major and minor grooves are higher polarity regions that have structural elements capable of hydrogen bonding with molecules that interact with DNA. The two polyanionic phosphodiester backbones are the most polar regions on DNA. Appropriately, these areas are on the outside perimeter of the macromolecule and as such are most exposed to the polar aqueous environment in which DNA exists.

DRUG/DNA INTERACTIONS

Small molecule/DNA interactions can be divided into two categories: outside (external) or internal (intercalative) binding (Figure 1). The molecules that bind externally to DNA utilize hydrogen and/or electrostatic bonding to form stable drug/DNA complexes. Small molecules that bind DNA externally can mask the more exposed regions of DNA (the major and minor grooves and the

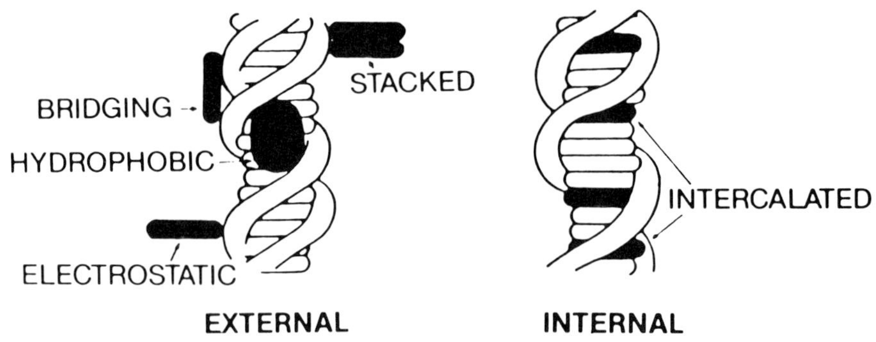

Figure 1. Mechanisms of Small Molecule/DNA Interaction.

phosphodiester backbone) and thus interfere with its normal functioning. Although the externally-bound small molecule/DNA complex is more rigid and stable to thermal denaturation that native DNA, the conformation of DNA is relatively unchanged.

Molecules that bind DNA by intercalation insert relatively planar portions of their structure between the base pairs of DNA, and depending on their structure may also utilize hydrogen and/or electrostatic bonding to enhance the interaction and to create base pair specificity. Intercalation changes the contour length and conformation of DNA. In order to accomodate the additional ring sytem being inserted, DNA must unwind and expand its size. We chose to study molecules of this type.

An examination of clinically active antitumor agents shows that many of these molecules intercalate DNA. All of these molecules share important common structural features. Furthermore, these shared structural elements are complementary to those of DNA. The structures of two such molecules (adriamycin and mitoxantrone) are shown in Figure 2. Each of the molecules has a planar ring system that can be inserted between the base pairs of DNA and a polar side chain that can interact with the elements of both the grooves and phosphodiester backbones.

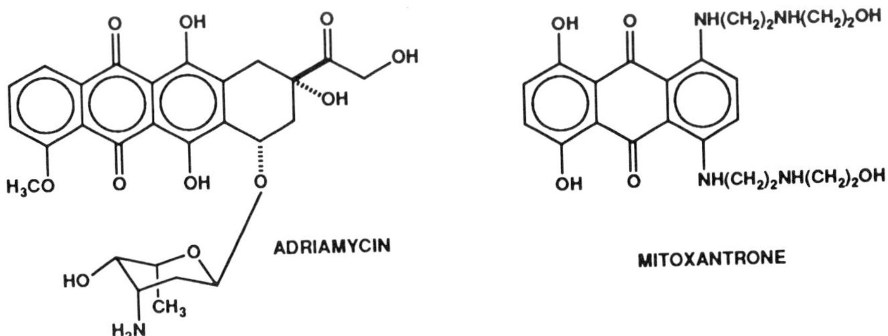

Figure 2. Structures of Adriamycin and Mitoxantrone.

INITIAL STRUCTURAL INVESTIGATIONS

Our first efforts focused on pyrene-containing derivatives with various side chains (Figure 3) (2). A number of compounds

were synthesized from commercially available 1-pyrenecarbaldehyde
and various mono-, di-, tri-, and tetra-amines as exemplified by
the -$CH_2NHCH(CH_3)(CH_2)_3NEt_2$ (the side chain of quinacrine) derivative 911U78. This compound was very H_2O soluble and bound DNA
strongly. Molecules derived from polycyclic systems containing

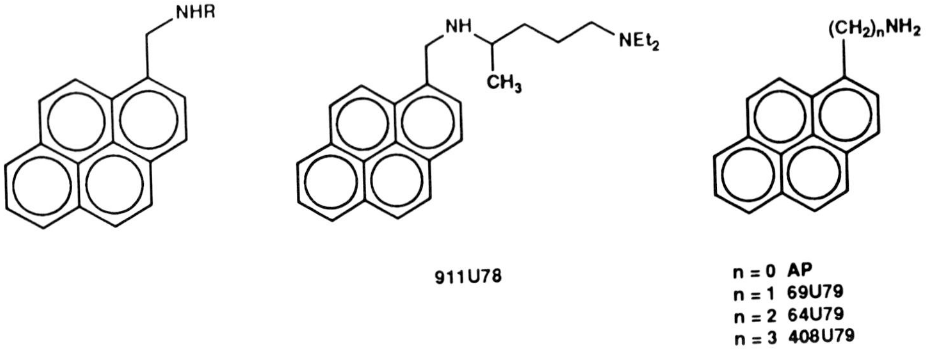

911U78

n = 0 AP
n = 1 69U79
n = 2 64U79
n = 3 408U79

Figure 3.   Early Pyrene Derivatives Examined.

1-5 aromatic rings bearing these amine side chains were studied
extensively. A number of basic rules for DNA binding were determined for these derivatives which are applicable to the AMAP
series and will be discussed later. One important structural
feature that should be mentioned is the separation on the N-atom
directly attached, or 1, 2 or 3 atoms removed from the pyrene ring
system. DNA binding studies (such as the thermal denaturation
($\triangle T_m$) experiments) show that for the polycyclic aromatic ring
systems studied, the optimal separation of the N-atom and the ring
system is one atom (e.g. a benzylic arrangement). As a result, we
have studied mainly $ArCH_2NR_1R_2$ derivatives. Fortuitously, the
chemical synthesis of this type of molecule is easier than other
structural classes. One-carbon functionalization of the numerous
commercially available or easily synthesized polycyclic aromatic
and heteroaromatic ring systems followed by coupling with commercially available amines has provided access to a large variety of
structures for study.

SIDE CHAIN STRUCTURE/ACTIVITY STUDIES

No antitumor activity was seen for these prototype series discussed in the previous Section. Although some antiparasitic activity was seen for some of the congeners with the quinacrine side chain, it was generally observed that these compounds were not bioavailable. We reasoned that the multiply-charged polyamine side chains were responsible for this lack of useful activity. We found that only one basic N-atom is required in the side chain to produce H_2O soluble derivatives with tetracyclic ring systems. As a result, we examined derivatives of 1-(aminomethyl)pyrene (69U79), especially those containing β-OH groups. These side chains (most were commercially available) were expected to enhance the solubility of the resulting compounds as well as potentially increasing DNA binding by hydrogen bonding to structural elements residing in both the grooves and the phosphodiester backbones. These molecules were generally more soluble, but biophysical studies showed that their DNA binding was not increased relative to the parent compound. Most importantly, two of these aminoalcohol-containing derivatives (644U79 and 1139U79) showed the first <u>in vivo</u> antitumor activity in the pyrene series (Figure 4). Space considerations do not permit a full discussion of the structure/

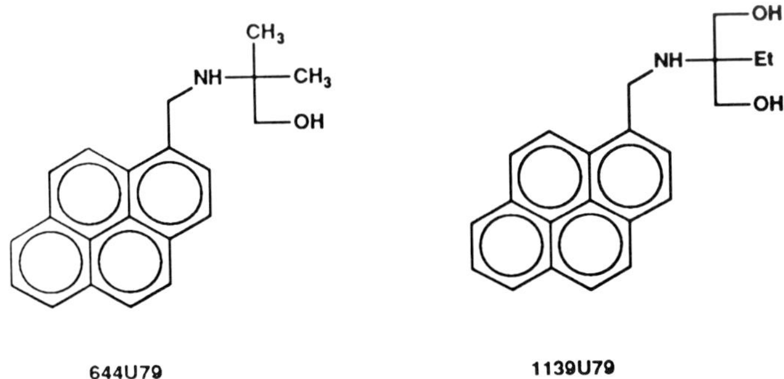

Figure 4. Structures of 644U79 and 1139U79.

activity studies performed on the side chain, but the most important structural features in the side chain that are necessary for, or affect the antitumor activity in the AMAP series are as follows

(Figure 5) (see Reference 2 for more details): 1) The presence of a secondary, benzylic N-atom is absolutely required (i.e. $ArCH_2NHR$).

$$ArCH_2NH-\overset{\displaystyle R_2}{\underset{\displaystyle R_3}{\overset{\displaystyle |}{\underset{\displaystyle |}{C}}}}\begin{matrix} -OH \\ -R_1 \\ -OH \end{matrix}$$

Figure 5. AMAP General Side Chain Structural Features.

2) Two -OH groups in the side chain, each two atoms away from the N-atom are required for optimal antitumor activity. Some anti-tumor activity is seen when only one -OH group is present in the side chain. With three -OH groups in the side chain (i.e. when the amine used is $H_2NC(CH_2OH)_3$) resulting AMAPs have good antitumor activity, though decreased relative to the two-OH-containing side chain congener. 3) Optimal activity is seen when the side chain position substituted by the N-atom (the 2-position) contains a small alkyl group (e.g. R = -H, $-CH_3$, $-CH_2CH_3$, or $-CH_2OH$). 4) The presence of a $-CH_3$ group at the 1- or 3- position (R_2 or R_3) of the 1,3-propanediol group enhances antitumor activity slightly.

AROMATIC RING SYSTEM STRUCTURE/ACTIVITY STUDIES

In addition to the structure/activity studies on the side chain, the effect of variation of the aromatic ring system on anti-tumor activity was studied for compounds of the general structure $ArCH_2NHC(CH_3)(CH_2OH)_2$ (Figure 6) (3). The amine used to synthesize these congeners ($H_2NC(CH_3)(CH_2OH)_2$) is commercially available, not

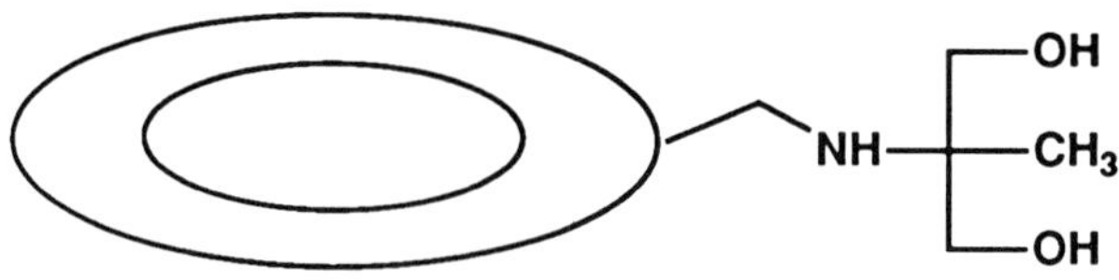

Figure 6. General AMAP Ring Structure.

optically active, and produces compounds with close to the maximum possible antitumor activity in a given ring system. As with the side chain studies, space does not permit full discussion of the work done on the effect of ring system variation on antitumor activity, but the general trends observed are as follows (see Reference 3 for more details): 1) The ring system must be planar or nearly planar. 2) At least three fused aromatic rings are required for antitumor activity. Compounds with smaller-sized ring systems bind poorly to DNA under physiologic conditions. 3) Optimal antitumor activity is seen for compounds containing four fused aromatic rings. 4) Although only a few compounds with five fused aromatic ring systems have been synthesized, they have lower antitumor activity. These congeners, however, bind the strongest to DNA. DNA binding is a necessary, but not sufficient, criterion for antitumor activity in the AMAP series. 5) In the tetracyclic series of AMAPs, the shape of the ring system does not appear to be important, but the position of the side chain affects the antitumor activity tremendously. 6) Carbocyclic and heterocyclic AMAPs appear to have somewhat different profiles of _in vivo_ and _in vitro_ antitumor activity.

AMAP SYNTHESIS OVERVIEW

Over 400 AMAPs have been synthesized in the last ten years, representing 68 different ring systems (21 carbocyclic and 47 heterocyclic ring systems). A total of 114 positional isomers have been made with these ring systems. Eighty five different side chains have been produced. A good number of ring substituents have been examined (31 different groups), mainly in the anthracene ring system. With the exception of the anthracene ring system, the substituted ring derivatives are less active than their parent congeners (Table 1).

SELECTION OF CLINICAL CANDIDATE AMAPs

Four congeners from the AMAP series have been chosen for clinical evaluation thus far (Figure 7). These compounds were selected on the basis of their antitumor spectrum of activity and range

130

Table 1

AMAP Synthesis Overview

Total AMAPs Synthesized	401
Total # of Ring Systems	68
Carbocyclics	21
Heterocyclics	47
Total # of Isomers	114
Total # of Side Chains	84
Total # of Substituents	31

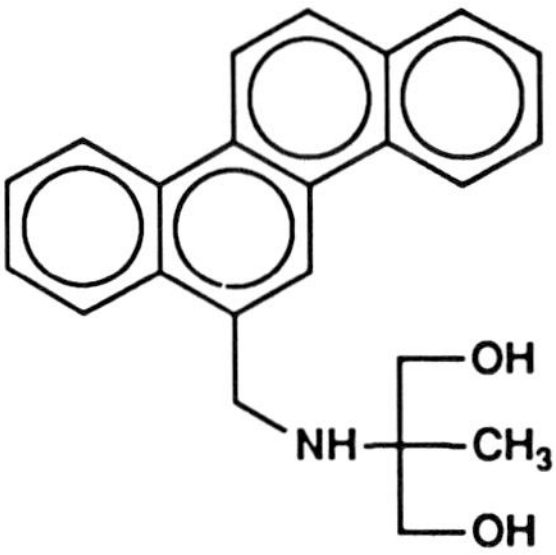

770U82
(CRISNATOL)

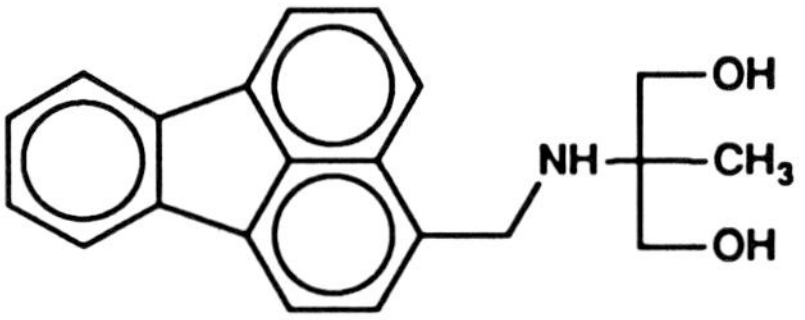

773U82

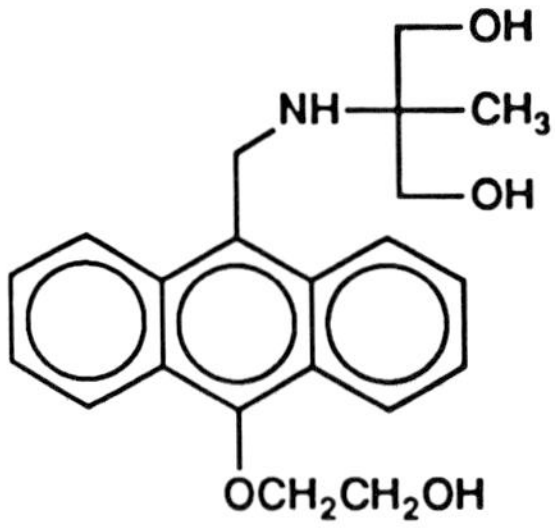

502U83

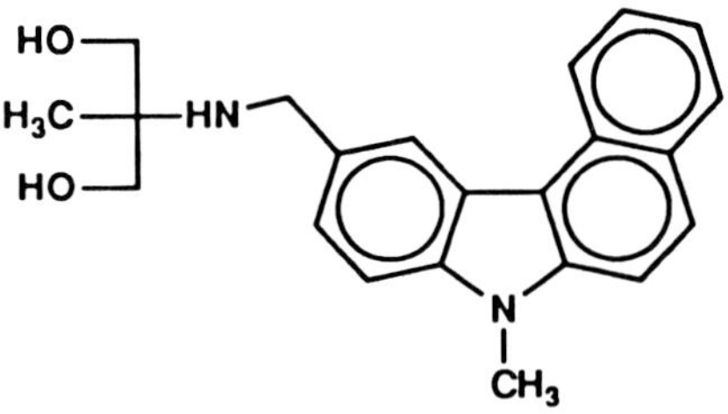

7U85

Figure 7. Clinical Candidate AMAPs.

of physical properties. The compounds selected were the chrysene derivative 770U82 (crisnatol), the fluoranthene derivative 773U82, the anthracene derivative 502U83 and the benzo[c]carbazole derivative 7U85. Selected physical properties of these derivatives are shown in Table 2 (4). The molecular weight of the free bases (FB) of these drugs are similar. The methanesulfonate salts of AMAPs are normally the most soluble and have been used for crisnatol, 773U82 and 7U85. The hydrochloride salt was used for 502U83. The calculated log Ps for the free bases of the four congeners range from 1.90-4.04. The DNA binding parameters also vary considerable for these compounds (5).

Table 2

Physical Properties of Candidate AMAPs.

Cpd. #	MW (FB)	Calc. Log P	HCl Salt H_2O Sol. (mg/mL)	MS Salt H_2O Sol. (mg/mL)	ΔT_m (°C)	Unwinding Angle (°)	Visc. Slope	$k \times 10^3$ (0.15 M NaCl)
770U82	345.446	4.04	2.1	9.8	12.6±0.80	16.9	1.30±0.12	1500±160
773U82	319.407	3.31	4.9	20.9	9.33±0.67	14.2	0.91±0.13	1500±300
502U83	355.438	1.90	125	ND	3.5±0.9	11.5	0.99±0.13	220±50
7U85	348.444	3.49	5.0	27.3	7.4±0.4	20.4	1.45±0.1	900±70

IN VIVO MURINE ANTITUMOR STUDIES

The AMAP series has been extensively evaluated against a wide variety of murine tumors _in vivo_ (6,7). These tumors include the lymphocytic leukemias P388 and L1210, the mastocytoma P815, the melanoma B16, colon 38 adenocarcinoma and the ovarian carcinoma M5076. The antitumor data presented for each of the four compounds shown in Table 3 was obtained in the same experiment for each tumor type using a days 1,5,9 dosing schedule. This schedule was previously shown to be optimal for these compounds against ip P388 with ip drug administration (see the following Section).

Table 3

Response of Several Murine Tumors to AMAPs Administered IP on Days 1,5,9.

AMAP	Tumor	Site	Implant Inoculum	Optimal Dose ($\leq LD_{10}$) (mg/kg/dose)	% ILS ($\pm$ s.e.m.)	60-Day Tumor Free Survivors
Crisnatol MS	P388 leukemia	i p	1×10^6 cells	115	141±7	50/186
773U82 HCl				105	174±9	50/186
502U83 HCl				130	192±24	26/81
7U85 MS				70	170±11	7/132
Crisnatol MS	L1210 leukemia	i p	1×10^5 cells	105	104±12	3/36
773U82 MS				85	155±11	1/36
502U83 HCl				100	250±89	20/24
7U85 HCl				55	190±13	5/30
Crisnatol MS	M5076 sarcoma	i p	1×10^6 cells	90	51±6	1/35
773U82 MS				85	66±6	3/6
502U83 HCl				90	88±10	3/26
7U85 HCl				65	42±6	0/50
Crisnatol MS	B16 melanoma	i p	0.5 mL of 10% brei	105	47±10	3/70
773U82 MS				95	98±5	2/70
502U83 HCl				130	157±19	8/20
7U85 HCl				65	75±7	2/74

AMAP	Tumor	Site	Implant Inoculum	Optimal Dose ($\leq LD_{10}$) (mg/kg/dose)	% T/C	Tumor-Free Survivors on Day of Evaluation
Crisnatol MS	Colon 38	s c	Fragment	105	58±14	0/40
773U82 MS				85	28±6	1/40
502U83 HCl				100	46±14	2/10
7U85 HCl				45	0	58/60

These and other AMAPs of interest showed broad activity against the variety of murine tumor types examined. We have routinely used the number of 60-day tumor-free survivors to aid in evaluating the activity of drugs under investigation, including the AMAPs. For the faster growing murine tumors, %ILS values are sufficient for comparing moderately active compounds where no 30-day survivors are observed. When significant numbers of 30-day survivors are seen in an assay, the %ILS reflects only those animals dying during that period. Extending the evaluation period to 60 days permits those animals surviving more than 30 days, but still bearing tumor (1-100 cells) to die in the second 30-day period. The range of possible %ILS is larger and the number of dying animals that can be evaluated for a given dose in an experiment also increases. Mice surviving 60 days are counted as long term survivors only if dissection shows them to be tumor-free.

The activity of the carbocyclic AMAPs (crisnatol, 773U82 and 502U83) against the tumor types examined was similar. The heterocyclic AMAP (7U85) was somewhat less active than the carbocyclic AMAPs against P388, M5076 and B16 tumors but curative against the solid tumor, colon 38. This high activity against solid tumors appears to be general for heterocyclic AMAPs (Figure 8). P388 activity is further decreased with heterocyclic AMAPs containing two heteroatoms in the aromatic ring. The colon 38 activity of the latter type of AMAP is currently under examination.

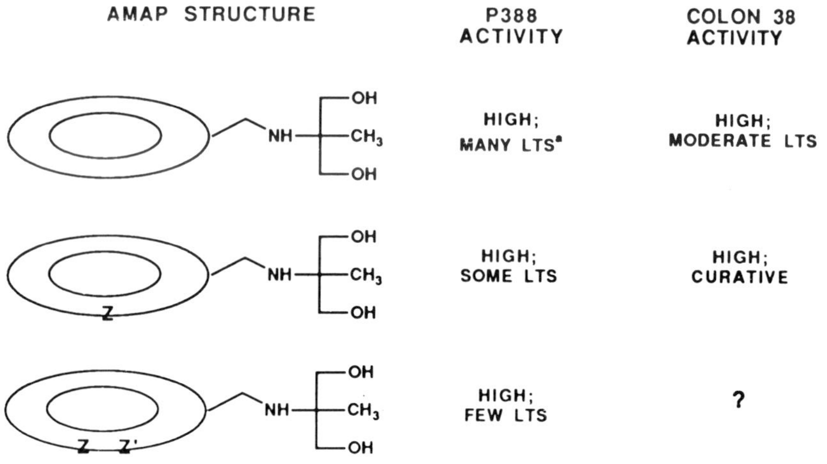

AMAP STRUCTURE	P388 ACTIVITY	COLON 38 ACTIVITY
NH—CH$_3$ (OH, OH)	HIGH; MANY LTS[a]	HIGH; MODERATE LTS
NH—CH$_3$ (OH, OH), Z	HIGH; SOME LTS	HIGH; CURATIVE
NH—CH$_3$ (OH, OH), Z Z'	HIGH; FEW LTS	?

[a]LTS = Long Term Survivors (> 60 Days)

Figure 8. Comparison of Colon 38 and P388 Activities of Three AMAP Ring Structure Types.

DOSING SCHEDULE STUDIES - P388

The effects of dosing schedule and *in vivo* antitumor activity were studied in ip implanted P388 with ip drug administration with each of the four candidate AMAPs (Table 4) (8). Toxicity studies were first conducted on the various schedules for each drug and

Table 4

Effects of Dosing Schedule on the Activity of IP
Administered AMAPs Against IP Implanted P388 Leukemia

Agent	Schedule	Optimal Dosage ($< LD_{10}$) (mg/kg/dose)	Total Dose (mg/kg)	%ILS ($\pm$ s.e.m.)	Total 60 day Survivors
Crisnatol MS	Day 1 only	120	120	59	0/6
	q8h x 2, Day 1 only	110	220	72	0/6
	Days 1-3	80	240	86	0/6
	q8h x 2, Days 1-3	60	360	86	0/6
	Days 1-5	60	300	82	0/6
	Days 1-9	60	540	118	0/6
	Days 1,3,5,7,9	105	525	118	0/6
	Days 1,5,9	110	330	140±4	10/268
	q8h x 2, Days 1,5,9	90	540	160±9	3/72
	q2h x 5, Days 1,5,9	40	600	127	0/6
773U82 HCl	Day 1 only	140	140	44	0/6
	Days 1-5	40	200	71	0/6
	Days 1,5,9	105	315	174±9	50/186
	q8h x 2, Days 1,5,9	60	360	187±12	14/60
	q4h x 3, Days 1,5,9	60	540	208±10	4/12
502U83 HCl	Day 1 only	175	175	63	0/6
	Days 1-3	100	300	91	0/6
	Days 1-5	60	300	109	0/6
	Days 1,3,5,7,9	60	300	86	0/6
	Days 1,4,7,10	100	400	100	0/6
	Days 1,5,9	140	420	247±51	13/28
	q8h x 2, Days 1,5,9	80	480	179±11	82/161
	q4h x 3, Days 1,5,9	70	420	208±3	6/12
7U85 HCl	Day 1 only	105	105	45	0/6
	Days 1-3	35	105	109	0/6
	Days 1-5	20	100	123	0/6
	Days 1-9	15	135	154	0/6
	Days 1,3,5,7	35	140	145	0/6
	Days 1,4,7,10	45	180	145	0/6
	Days 1,5,9	65	195	158±6	5/246
7U85 MS	q8h x 2, Days 1,5,9	40	240[a]	183±14	1/24
7U85 HCl	q4h x 3, Days 1,5,9	10	90	136	0/6
7U85 HCl	q2h x 5, Days 1,5,9	10	150	209	0/6

[a]Equivalent to a total dose of 277 mg/kg of the HCl salt.

the actual assays performed using doses bracketing the LD_{10}. Optimal activity was observed for the AMAPs when dosing was done at 4-day intervals (days 1,5,9). More frequent intervals daily (days 1-3, 1-5 or 1-9), 2-day intervals (days 1,3,5,7) or 3-day intervals (days 1,4,7,10) were less effective for all four compounds although 7U85 activity appeared least affected by schedule variation. Longer dosing intervals and additional doses of AMAP did not increase antitumor activity (data not shown). Additionally, divided dosing (2-5 times daily) of AMAPs on any of the schedules (data not shown) except days 1,5,9 did not enhance antitumor activity. The amount of drug administered in each of the divided doses was less than that given in the single daily dose regimen for all four of the drugs. With crisnatol and 773U82, the total amount of drug that could be administered during the dosing period increased with more frequent administration. Twice daily administration of 502U83 and 7U85 also permitted greater amounts of drug to be given, but greater toxicity was seen with more frequent daily dosing. Unfortunately, multiple daily administration of the four AMAPs on the days 1,5,9 schedule did not appreciably affect the antitumor activity relative to that seen with single daily dosing.

ROUTE OF ADMINISTRATION STUDIES - P388

The bioavailability, distribution and activity of a candidate drug against tumors implanted at various sites is a key consideration of its potential utility. The antitumor activity of the four candidate AMAPs have been examined using P388/BW, a subline that is less responsive to therapy than the one used for screening (Table 5). The four compounds were examined using oral, ip and iv routes of administration against tumors implanted ip, iv, sc, im, id and in the footpad (fp) at doses near the LD_{10}.

Although the AMAPs are active against tumors implanted at the various sites, ip drug administration generally produces the best therapeutic effect. Crisnatol showed no activity via iv administration; CNS-related side effects precluded dosing at higher (presumably more active) levels. Of the four AMAPs, the antitumor act-

Table 5

Effects of Route of Administration on the Activity of AMAPs Against P388/BW Leukemia Implanted at Various Sites

Agent	Optimal Dosage (< LD_{10}) (mg/kg/dose)	Route of Administration	Tumor Implant Site					
			ip %ILS	iv %ILS	sc %ILS	im %ILS	id %ILS	fp %ILS
Crisnatol MS	105	ip	86	122	5	35	29	90
	325 or 400	po	95	71	NT[a]	NT	NT	21
	25	iv	0	0	0	0	0	16
773U82 HCl	85	ip	100	80	41	35	50	95
	250	po	54	40	TOXIC[b]	57	64	76
	75	iv	54	40	38	43	36	76
502U83 HCl	110	ip	78	110	38	73	108	62(1/6)[c]
	350	po	19	110(1/6)	31	53	43	76
	70	iv	33	67	22	50	42	26
7U85 HCl	75	ip	174	107	125	129	100	133(3/6)
	75	po	78	81	106	107	112	157
	55	iv	78	62	69	100	85	79

[a]NT = Not tested.
[b]Toxic at doses tested.
[c]60-Day Survivors.

ivity of 7U85 seemed least affected by route of administration and tumor implant site. Unlike the other candidate AMAPs, the toxicity of 7U85 via ip, po and iv routes of administration was very similar (75, 75 and 55 mg/kg respectively).

CROSS-RESISTANCE PROFILE

The AMAPs have been examined in a series of resistant P388 tumors (Table 6). No cross-resistance has been seen for any AMAPs with P388 strains resistant to alkylating agents [BCNU, cyclophosphamide (CPA), L-PAM, or platinol (cis-DDP)] or antimetabolites [(cytosine arabinoside (ara-C), 5-FUra, methotrexate (MTX)] or to the microtubule inhibitor vincristine (VCR). Mixed AMAP cross-resistance has been seen for drugs that are known to intercalate DNA, although additional mechanisms of action have been demonstrated for a number of these compounds. No cross-resistance was seen with actinomycin D resistant-P388 (a RNA polymerase inhibitor).

Table 6

Cross-Resistance of Drug-Resistant P388 Sublines to AMAPs. Approximate Log_{10} Change in Tumor Burden Following Final Drug Treatment

P388/Resistant Cell Line	Crisnatol MS		773U82 MS		502U83 HCl		7U85 HCl		Parent Drug	
	P388/0	P388/R	P388/0	P388/R	P388/0	P388/R	P388/0	P388/R	P388/0	P388/R
P388/ADR	-4.5	+1.2	ca -6.6	0.0	-6.3	+1.8	-2.3	+2.3	-6.0	-1.0
P388/*m*-AMSA	-5.0	+1.6	ca -6.7	+0.6	ca -6.7	+1.1	-6.7	+1.5	-6.0	
P388/ACT-D	-5.0	-6.8	-6.0	-5.7	ca -6.6	-3.4	-2.3	+2.0	-5.0	-2.0
P388/DIOHA	-3.5	-0.3	-6.4	-4.4	-5.5	-4.4	-5.1	ca -7.2	----	----
P388/*ara*-C	-5.6	-2.4	-6.8	-4.7	-6.8	-6.6	-5.7	ca -6.5	-6.0	-1.0
P388/5-FU	-3.6	-4.0	----	-6.2	----	-4.9	-3.6	ca -6.8	-5.0	+1.0
P388/MTX	-3.6	-1.6	ca -6.7	ca -6.8	ca -6.7	ca -6.8	-2.3	-2.4	-3.0	+3.0
P388/BCNU	-5.0	-5.0	-5.3	-4.2	ca -6.5	-3.6	-2.9	+1.6	-7.0	-1.0
P388/CPA	-5.4	ca -6.6	----	ca -6.6	----	ca -6.6	-3.5	ca +2.3	-7.0	-1.0
P388/L-PAM	-3.6	-2.8	ca -6.6	ca -6.7	ca -6.6	ca -6.7	-2.8	0.0	-7.0	-1.0
P388/VCR	-6.6	-5.7	-5.0	-4.7	-6.6	-5.7	-5.4	ca -6.8	-6.0	+2.0
P388/*cis*-DDPt	-5.0	-3.0	-5.3	-6.7	-3.1	-6.7	-3.1	-4.0	-6.0	+2.0

[a]Log_{10} change = net log_{10} change in tumor stem cell population at the end of treatment as compared to the start of treatment: a -3 log change means that there was a 99.9% reduction and a +3 log change means that there was a 1000-fold increase in tumor burden at the end of R_x.

With P388 strains resistant to intercalators also known to affect topoisomerase II such as adriamycin, m-AMSA and other AMAPs (data not shown) there is generally complete cross-resistance to AMAPs. In addition, complete cross-resistance was seen for AMAPs against an etoposide (also a known topoisomerase II inhibitor that does not intercalate DNA) resistant-P388 strain. With the exception of the lack of AMAP cross-resistance with mitoxantrone (a topoisomerase II inhibitor that also intercalates DNA), the data indicates that AMAPs are not likely to be active against tumors made resistant by exposure to other topoisomerase II inhibitors.

FOOTPAD TUMOR MODELS

Two footpad models (outgrowth and regression) have been used extensively to examine and compare the AMAPs. These models were originally developed to aid in the ranking of the AMAPs during their early development. These models are similar to other typical antitumor screens. A tumor implanted in the footpad is generally more protected from the drug and as a result, the drug must be systemically available to produce an antitumor response. Footpad tumors grow as a solid mass that can be measured with calipers. P388 tumor growth rates in the footpad are slower than those observed with other sites of implantation, but the tumor still metastasizes. As seen in the therapy of tumors implanted at other sites, the parent tumor may disappear from the footpad area after drug treatment, but the mouse may die at some point, presumably due to metastatic tumor. The tumor mass produced in the regression model is qualitatively much closer to that observed in the clinical situation: tumor bulk is significant and metastasis has occured.

Using the normal P388 screen (ip drug administration and ip tumor implantation) over 50% of the 400 AMAPs examined produced significant antitumor effects (>100 %ILS, many with 30-day survivors). The activity of the four clinical candidate AMAPs is basically the same in this assay. Using the outgrowth and regression footpad assays, and employing a number of routes of drug administration, significant differences can be discerned between the more active compounds. In general, 7U85 shows much better activity in these two models than the other three AMAPs. 7U85 produces the lowest percentage of 60-day survivors of the four candidate AMAPs, but the activity of 7U85 against P388 in either of the two models parallels that seen in the standard P388 assay. Typically, in the outgrowth model (using ip drug administration), crisnatol was least active (50 %ILS). 773U82 and 502U83 were moderately active (75-80 %ILS). 7U85 routinely produced 100-150 %ILS with some long term survivors. In the regression model, crisnatol, 773U82 and 502U83 produced significant tumor regression but had little effect on survival. In addition to significant tumor regression, 7U85 also produced 50-100 %ILS but no long term survivors.

The challenge posed by the two assays can also be seen in the responses produced by standard clinical agents. m-AMSA showed minimal activity in the outgrowth model and was not different from control in the regression model. Adriamycin shows good activity in the outgrowth model but little effect in the regression model. The alkylating agent cyclophphosphamide shows excellect activity in both models; this effect may be more related to the extreme general sensitivity of the leukemias P388 and L1210 to this class of compounds.

HUMAN TUMOR XENOGRAFT STUDIES

The four clinical candidate AMAPs have been examined against a variety of human tumors grown as xenografts in nude mice including the small cell lung carcinomas, H-82 and H-69, the lung adenocarcinoma A-549, the lung adenocarcinoma, HT-29 and the mammary carcinoma MX-1. Against the typical 100-200 mg tumors present at the start of treatment in the assays, the four candidate AMAPs showed only transient tumor regressions. The optimal antitumor effect produced by the AMAPs in any of the xenografts was $\approx$ 30 %T/C up to two weeks following the last drug dose. 7U85 showed the best activity of the four candidate AMAPs in four of the five tumors examined in the xenograft studies.

AMAP METABOLISM

Preliminary metabolic studies on crisnatol, 773U82 and 502U83 in animals and man have been performed. Examination of 7U85 is not yet complete in any species. Examination of the general AMAP structure suggests that metabolism could occur via modification of the aromatic ring system or the side chain. Typical oxidation of the ring produces diol- and hydroxylated-derivatives of crisnatol and 773U82 (Figure 9). Although diolepoxides are presumable formed, none of these reactive materials have been isolated from urine or feces for any of the AMAPs. Direct oxidation of the anthracene ring system in 502U83 has not been observed. Although studies on 7U85 are incomplete, it appears that its metabolic profile resembles that of crisnatol and 773U82.

It was originally thought that extensive metabolism of the benzylic -C-N- bond would produce aromatic derivatives at various

140

oxidation states including $ArCH_2OH$ (via hydrolysis) and ArCHO or ArCOOH (via oxidation).

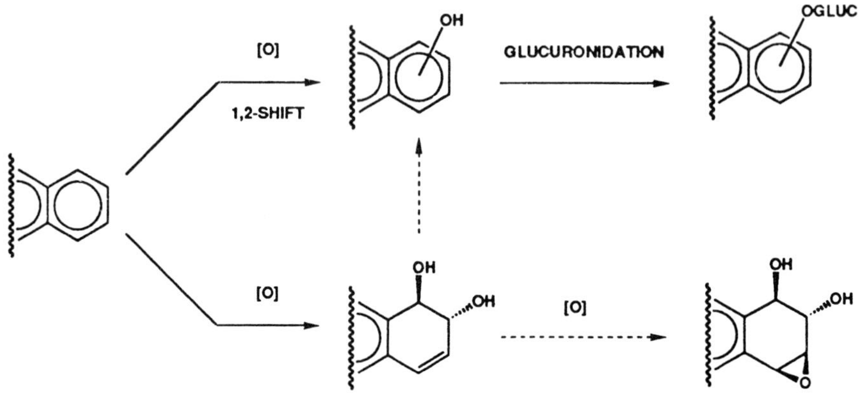

Figure 9.   AMAP Aromatic Ring Metabolism.

These simple materials have not been observed for crisnatol or 773U82. Although sulfation and glucuronidation of the AMAP side chain has been seen, the only side chain modified compound that has been isolated is the amino acid derivative of crisnatol (Figure 10).

502U83 is the only AMAP under clinical development that possesses additional ring functionality. Oxidation of the $-OCH_2CH_2OH$ group to $-OCH_2COOH$ occurs readily, and other than glucuronidation, metabolism of 502U83 in humans occurs mainly via this route.

The levels of glucuronidation that were observed for the candidate AMAPs appears to be related to the relative lipophilicity of the AMAP. The more lipophilic AMAPs, crisnatol and 773U82, are not extensively glucuronidated relative to 502U83. Furthermore, relative amounts of material (parent drug and metabolites) excreted in feces versus urine decreases as the polarity of the AMAP decreases.

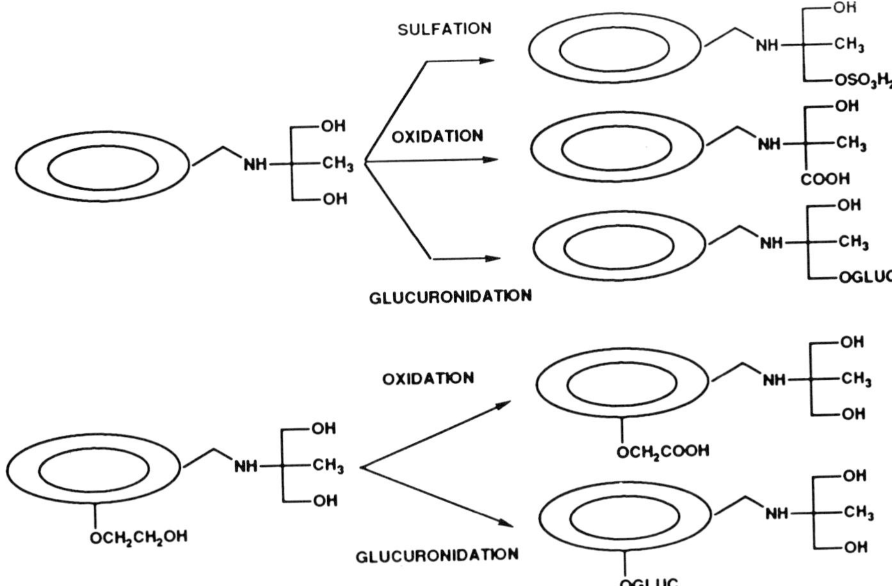

Figure 10.   AMAP Side Chain Metabolism.

HUMAN TUMOR STEM CELL ASSAY (HTSCA)

The four clinical candidate AMAPs have been examined against a variety of tumors in the HTSCA using 1 hour or continuous (7 days) exposures and drug concentrations of 1 and 10 μg/mL (standard screening conditions), by Von Hoff _et al_ (Table 7) (8). Initially, we had hoped that the range of physical properties represented in these compounds might result in distinct profiles of activity in the assay, but this was not observed. All four of the congeners showed significant inhibition of the growth of breast, colon, lung, melanoma, ovarian and kidney tumors at the 10 μg/mL drug concentration and continuous exposure. With a 1 μg/mL drug concentration and continuous exposure conditions, only 7U85 showed good activity. None of the AMAPs showed significant activity when examined using a 1 hour drug exposure at either concentration. Thus, clinical activity of the exposure times and drug plasma concentrations approaching 10 μg/mL. These results are also confirmed by pharmacodynamic studies on the AMAPs. Phase I studies on some of the AMAPs have shown that is is possible to achieve these drug concentrations, but side effects are a problem.

142

Table 7

Human Tumor Stem Cell Assay Data for Candidate AMAPs
Using a Continuous Exposure Screening Mode.[a]

Drug Concentration - 10 μg/mL

Tumor Type	7U85	773U82	502U83	770U82
Breast	14/17	9/13	10/14	3/13
Colon	7/7	7/11	8/13	3/13
Lung (All Types)	14/15	10/13	7/12	8/19
Melanoma	3/3	10/11	7/7	5/7
Ovarian	17/18	12/19	7/21	8/27
Kidney	8/8	8/11	3/7	5/9
Total for Six Tumors	63/68 (93%)	56/78 (72%)	42/74 (57%)	32/88 (36%)
Total for All Tumors	65/70 (93%)	78/121 (65%)	53/152 (35%)	36/109 (33%)

Drug Concentration - 1 μg/mL

Tumor Type	7U85	773U82	502U83	770U82
Breast	8/17	2/7	0/11	1/13
Colon	0/7	1/3	1/11	2/13
Lung (All Types)	6/15	0/3	2/10	5/19
Melanoma	2/3	1/3	0/6	2/4
Ovarian	12/18	5/14	3/12	1/28
Kidney	7/8	0/3	0/5	0/7
Total for Six Tumors	35/68 (51%)	9/33 (27%)	6/55 (11%)	11/84 (13%)
Total for All Tumors	36/70 (51%)	14/44 (32%)	6/64 (10%)	14/103 (14%)

[a]Tumors showing $\geq$50% decrease in colony number.

IN VITRO PHARMACODYNAMIC ASSAY

Adams _et al_. have examined the four clinical candidate AMAPs and a number of their ring positional isomers in an _in vitro_ pharmacodynamic assay using P388 and MCF-7 cell lines (11,12). _In vitro_ activity of the AMAPs examined was found to be a function of both concentration and time (C^nxT) rather than concentration alone. _In vivo_ P388 activity correlated with _in vitro_ P388 activity only at antiproliferative exposures (surviving fraction of tumor >1.0) for each group of isomers. There was no correlation between the two assays when survival fractions in the _in vitro_ assay were in the 0.1-0.001 ranges commonly used as endpoints in cytotoxicity studies. The minimum CxT survival curves for the four clinical candidate AMAPs also confirmed observations from the HTSCA and from Phase I clinical trials of crisnatol, 773U82 and 502U83; the higher exposure levels (CxT) of these AMAPs required to produce meaningful responses will be obtained by longer infusion schedules in order to avoid serious side effects produced by more intensive dosing regimens.

AMAP EFFECTS ON MACROMOLECULAR SYNTHESIS

The _in vitro_ effects of the four candidate AMAPs on macromolecular synthesis have been examined using the murine leukemia P388 and the human mammary adenocarcinoma, MCF-7 under conditions of short-term drug exposure (13). AMAPs that were observed to inhibit macromolecular synthesis produced equipotent inhibition of DNA and RNA synthesis. Equivalent inhibition of protein synthesis generally required significantly greater concentrations of AMAP. A general correlation between inhibition of polynucleotide synthesis and _in vivo_ antitumor activity was observed. The effects of four clinical candidate AMAPs (crisnatol (770U82), 773U82, 502U83, and 7U85) on macromolecular synthesis were further compared with those of actinomycin D, adriamycin, mitoxantrone, etoposide, _m_-AMSA and cisplatin in MCF-7 cells (Table 8). The pattern of AMAP action was the most similar to that observed for adriamycin and mitoxantrone. Finally, the effects of these four AMAPs on the size, specific activity and rate of incorporation of [^{3}H]-dTTP

144

Table 8

IC$_{50}$s (μM) for Candidate AMAPs and Clinically
Established Agents on the Specific Activities
of DNA, RNA and Protein in MCF-7 Cells.[a]

Compound	DNA	RNA	Protein
Crisnatol	5.6 ± 1.1	5.7 ± 1.2	14.9 ± 2.6
773U82	4.4 ± 0.3	7.4 ± 0.5	21.4 ± 3.9
7U85	2.9 ± 0.4	3.9 ± 0.6	13.9 ± 0.9
502U83	30.1 ± 3.2	29.6 ± 3.6	92.9 ± 17.0
Adriamycin	11.4 ± 1.6	11.4 ± 1.9	>40.0
Mitoxantrone	9.2 ± 1.1	10.2 ± 2.1	28.6 ± 5.7
Actinomycin D	>5.0	0.27 ± 0.03	>5.0
Etoposide	47.3 ± 1.4	18.9 ± 0.8	91.5 ± 4.4
m-AMSA	>20.0	13.9 ± 1.5	>20.0
Cisplatin	>200.0	>200.0	>200.00

[a]Agents and radiolabelled precursors added similtaneously to log-
phase MCF-7 cells. Values represent the mean ± standard error for
at least three independent experiments.

into DNA of MCF-7 cells synchronized by pretreatment with hydroxyurea was determined. It was found that DNA synthesis was inhibited by these AMAPs independent of inhibition of the uptake, phos-
phorylation, or retention of the metabolic precursors. These results support the theory that antitumor AMAPs interfere with the
normal functioning of enzymes, such as topoisomerase II or DNA and
RNA polymerases, which interact with DNA.

AMAP EFFECTS ON TOPOISOMERASES

Mechanism of action studies were first concerned with the
interaction of AMAPs with DNA. More recently, efforts have focused on the enzyme topoisomerase II. A large number of AMAPs, including three of the four candidate AMAPs (502U83 is only weakly

active) inhibit the ability of topoisomerase II to unknot DNA and
to inhibit the normal functioning of the enzyme in the cleavable
complex. The cross-resistance studies mentioned previously as
well as the pattern of macromolecular synthesis inhibition both
suggest that the AMAPs are related to other known topoisomerase II
inhibitors. Bellamy et al. (14) have studies the effects of the
candidate AMAPs on 8226/S human myeloma cells by alkaline elution
and found that each produced single- and double-strand breaks and
protein-DNA crosslinks. Furthermore, the amount of DNA damage
produced by the four AMAPs at their respective IC_{50}s (crisnatol
- 2.49 μM, 773U82 - 1.43 μM, 502U83 - 8.95 μM and 7U85 - 5.0 μM)
was the same.

We are currently examining the activity of a large number of
AMAPs (of general structure $ArCH_2NHC(CH_3)CH_2OH)_2$) in both the
cleavable complex assay and the unknotting assay. Preliminary
data show that the activity in these two assays and in vivo antitumor activity is related to the shape of the AMAP, not the actual
ring system.

The apparent low activity of 502U83 in cytotoxicity experiments and in a number of the cell-free assays has been puzzling
since its activity profile in all of the in vivo studies is similar to that of the other three candidate AMAPs.

CONCLUSIONS

This overview on AMAPs has only briefly discussed the extensive amount of work that has been accomplished over the last
decade. The selection of the clinical candidate AMAPs was difficult, and to a certain extent reflects the biases of the scientists performing the tests on this large group of congeners. As a
first effort in the development of a new class of antitumor drugs
we opted to select compounds with the basic AMAP structure that
showed the broadest spectrum of preclinical antitumor activity and
that represented the broadest range of physical properties possible. The fact that all of the clinical candidates have the same
side chain was a result of the need to use one side chain in the
examination of the effects of aromatic ring variation. Whether

the ring systems and side chain represented in the clinical candidate AMAPs are the correct ones will be determined as data from Phase II clinical trials becomes available.

ACKNOWLEDGEMENTS

I would like to acknowledge the efforts of the many scientists at Burroughs Wellcome Company and our collaborators at other institutions whose work has been presented in this AMAP overview. I especially would like to recognize Vincent C. Knick, Drs. Richard L. Tuttle and David J. Adams for their tireless work that has been instrumental in moving the AMAPs from the laboratory into the clinic.

REFERENCES

1. Gale EF, Cundliffe E, Reynolds PE et al: The Molecular Basis of Antibiotic Action, Second Edition, John Wiley and Sons, London pp 270-273, 1981.
2. Bair KW, Tuttle RL, Knick VC et al: (1-pyrenylmethyl)amino alcohols, a new class of antitumor DNA intercalators. Discovery and initial side chain structure-activity studies. J. Med. Chem. 33:2385-2393, 1990.
3. Bair KW, Andrews CW, Tuttle RL et al: 2-[(arylmethyl)amino]-2-methyl-1,3-propanediol DNA intercalators. An examination of the effects of aromatic ring variation on antitumor activity and DNA binding. J. Med. Chem. 34:0000, 1991.
4. Bair KW, Andrews CW, Tuttle RL et al: Biophysical studies and murine antitumor activity of arylmethylaminopropanediols (AMAPs), a new class of DNA binding drugs. Proc. Am. Assoc. Cancer Res. 27:424, 1986.
5. Cory M, Bair KW, McKee DD et al: DNA as a receptor for arylmethylaminopropanediols (AMAPs): Biophysical and molecular modeling studies. Proc. Am. Assoc. Cancer Res. 28:266, 1987.
6. Knick VC, Tuttle RL, Bair KW, Von Hoff, DD: Preclinical antitumor activity of BW A7U: A heterocyclic arylmethylaminopropanediol (AMAP). Sixth NCI-EORTC Symposium on New Drugs in Cancer Therapy 4:22, 1987.
7. Knick VC, Tuttle RL, Bair KW, Von Hoff DD: Arylmethylaminopropanediols (AMAPs); Discovery, antitumor activity and selection of clinical candidates. Fifth NCI-EORTC Symposium on new drugs. Cancer Therapy 4:32, 1986.
8. Knick VC, Tuttle RL, Bair KW, Von Hoff DD. Murine and human tumor stem cell activity of three candidate arylmethylaminopropanediols (AMAPs). Proc. Am. Assoc. Cancer Res. 27:424, 1986.

9. Everitt BJM, Grebe G, Mackars A et al: Comparative pharma-
    cology and toxicology of three arylmethylaminopropanediols
    (AMAPs): BW A770U, BW A773U and BW A502U. Proc. Am. Assoc.
    Cancer Res. 27:424, 1986.
10. Painter GR, Bair KW, Grunwald R et al: Interaction of aryl-
    methylaminopropanediols (AMAPs) with vesicle membranes: Rela-
    tionship of membrane binding to local anaesthetic activity.
    Proc. Am. Assoc. Cancer Res. 28:270, 1987.
11. Adams DJ. An _in_ _vitro_ pharmacodynamic assay for drug develop-
    ment. Application to Crisnatol, a new DNA intercalator.
    Cancer Res. 49:6615-6620, 1989.
12. Adams DJ, Watkins PJ, Knick VC et al: Evaluation of aryl-
    methylaminopropanediols by a novel _in_ _vitro_ pharmacodynamic
    assay: Correlation with antitumor activity _in_ _vivo_. Cancer
    Res. 50:3663-3669, 1990.
13. Carter CA, Bair KW: Effects of isomeric 2-(arylmethylamino)-
    1,3,-propanediols (AMAPs) and clinically established agents
    on macromolecular synthesis in P388 and MCF-7 cells. Investi-
    gational New Drugs 9:0000, 1991.
14. Bellamy WT, Dorr RT, Bair KW, Alberts DS: Cytotoxicity and
    mechanism of action of 3 arylmethylaminopropanediols (AMAPs).
    Proc. Am. Assoc. Cancer Res. 30:562, 1989.

7

MECHANISM-BASED APPROACHES TO CANCER DRUG DISCOVERY

Paul H. Fischer, Eric R. Larson, Robert L. Dow and Penny E. Miller

INTRODUCTION

Advances in our understanding of the molecular basis of cancer and tumor cell biology have suggested novel anticancer drug targets. Approaches directed toward the inhibition of tumor angiogenesis, invasion and metastasis are feasible (1-7). Numerous growth factors have now been implicated in a variety of human cancers (8,9) and a large body of data suggest that both oncogenes and tumor suppressor genes play important roles in the etiology of human cancer (10-12). In addition, we are gaining an improved understanding of the basic mechanisms underlying treatment failure with our current agents (13-16). Of particular relevance to drug discovery is the fact that specific targets, potentially amenable to mechanism-based discovery approaches, have been described for many of these advances. As with any rapidly developing area, it is not certain that interference with the function of these novel targets will yield useful therapeutic effects. Nonetheless, the possiblity of exploiting these targets and developing new classes of drugs with improved toleration and efficacy is both reasonable and exciting.

This discussion will briefly review some of the issues encountered in mechanism-based discovery approaches within the context of target selection, lead discovery and characterization, and compound development for potential new anticancer therapies. Detailed reviews of current approaches for the discovery new drugs in general are available (17-20).

TARGET SELECTION

Target selection can be viewed as an investment decision in which an attempt to balance risk and return is made in a rapidly changing market with insufficient information. In mechanism-based drug discovery programs which address novel targets, both risk and potential return appear to be relatively high. Since there are no clinically active prototypes, efficacy is not guaranteed even after sucessful discovery of new pharmacological entities. At times, a project's scientific rationale seems unrealistically sensitive to recently published data. On the other hand, potential pitfalls of the approach are only vaguely appreciated and the excitement of an entirely new class of drugs is contagious. An estimate of return depends on a reasonable assessment of medical need at the time the drug will actually be marketed. This is especially difficult when no clinical prototypes exist. Similarly, the lack of a precedent increases the problem of accurately assessing the technical feasibility of a particular strategy. Technically daunting programs should be aimed at large, unmet, medical needs. At the core of a mechanism-based approach is the scientific rationale. The success of the program is linked to validation of the hypothesis being challenged. Despite extensive experimental biological data, therapeutic validation of the strategy awaits the development of an adequate pharmacological tool. This often forces commitment to the entire discovery and developmental pathway at an early stage, before success can be guaranteed.

Protein tyrosine kinases are a newly identified family of proteins which appear to mediate the transduction of signals initiating cellular replication (21-23). They represent possible targets in a cancer drug discovery program (24,25). Many oncogene products, including several altered growth factor receptors, are protein tyrosine kinases (26). The activation of c-abl in chronic myelogenous leukemia (27), the expression of c-erb-B-2 in breast cancer (28,29), and the enhanced activity of c-src in colon carcinomas are protein tyrosine kinases which have been associated with human cancers (30-33). If, in comparison with other poten-

151

tial targets, tyrosine kinases are considered of interest, it is
still difficult to assess which of these many protein kinases is
best suited for pharmacological attack. This assessment requires
careful consideration of medical need, the strength of the data
supporting an important role in human cancer, the likelihood of
achieving therapeutic selectivity and the technical feasibility of
the appproach. Unfortunately, key pieces of information are
usually lacking, and if present, it is likely that the approach
is, in fact, not novel.

LEAD IDENTIFICATION

Lead identification and validation are key to drug discovery
programs and a variety of approaches should be considered for each
new target. A combination of factors, including resources, technical feasibility, and experience must be considered in choosing a
strategy. Depending on the target, the best approach to lead
identification could range from random screening to molecular
modeling (17-20).

In the case of tyrosine kinases, the design of reversible and
irreversible protein and nucleotide substrate-based inhibitors has
been considered (34). Multisubstrate inhibitors, combining ATP
and tyrosine, have also been synthesized (35,36), but target
specificity has been difficult to achieve and the large number of
protein kinases (37) compounds this problem. Nonetheless, a recently reported series of dicyanostyrenes appears to inhibit the
EGF receptor kinase much more effectively than the insulin receptor kinase (38). Importantly, inhibition of EGF-dependent, but
not EGF-independent, cell growth was shown. A priori, as has been
demonstrated for protease inhibitors, if the targets are structurally distinct, selective inhibitors can be developed (39).

Illustrative of the directed synthesis approach is a series
of benzyl phosphonic acids which we synthesized as tyrosine kinase
inhibitors (Figure 1). Several derivatives appeared to selectively inhibit the tyrosine kinase activity of v-src versus cAMP
protein kinase with IC50 values in the 20-30 uM range (Table 1).

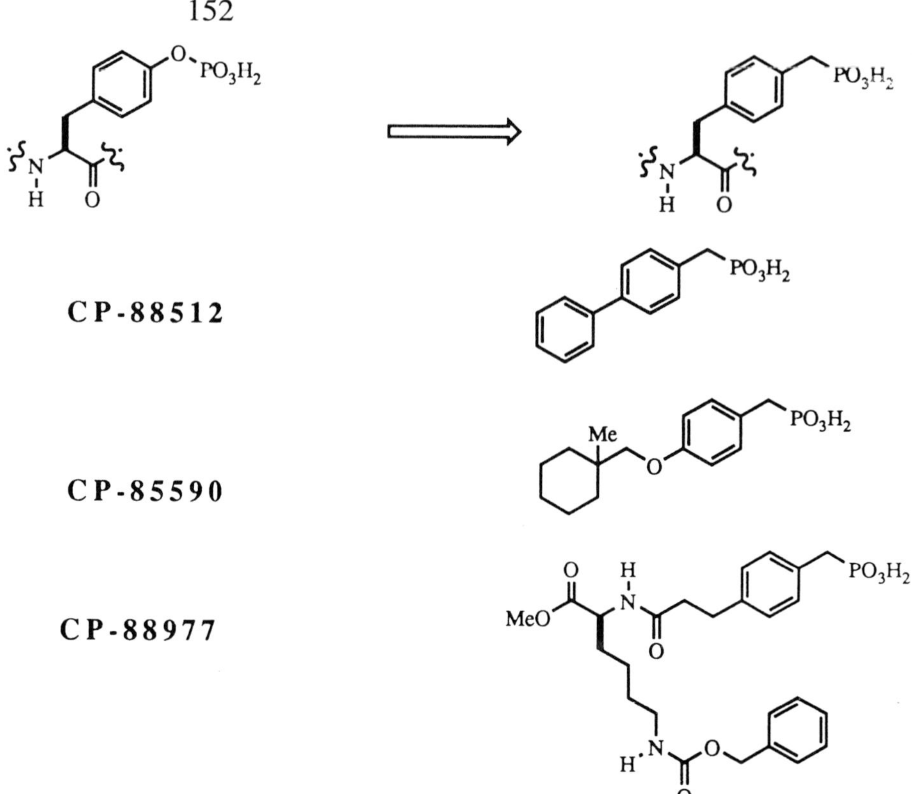

C P - 8 8 5 1 2

C P - 8 5 5 9 0

C P - 8 8 9 7 7

Figure 1. Protein kinase inhibitors.

Table 1
Protein Kinase Inhibition

	IC50 (uM)	
Compound	v-scr	cAMP
CP-85,590	20.5	580
CP-88,512	24	>1000
CP-88,977	31	>1000

Compounds were assayed for inhibition of peptide phosphoryla-
tion using a phosphocellulose paper binding assay. The peptide
substrates were val[5]-angiotensin II for the v-src kinase and
kemptide for cAMP-dependent protein kinase. The reactions were
initiated by the addition of substrate and [^{32}P]-ATP following
incubation with the test compounds for 10 min. The reactions were
run for 30 min at 30^{0} and terminated by the addition of acid.
Portions of the reaction mixture were spotted on phosphocellulose
paper, which was then washed, dried and counted by liquid scin-
tillation spectrometry.

Surprisingly, the inhibitory effects of these compounds on the
v-src kinase were strongly dependent on the presence of manganese
and the inclusion of magnesium markedly antagonized the activity
of these phosphonates (Figure 2).

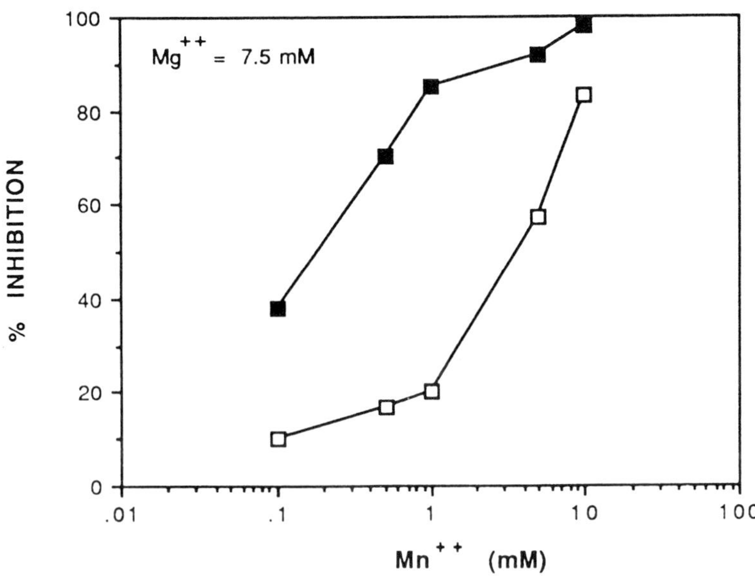

Figure 2. Effect of manganese on v-src inhibition. The assay for
v-src kinase was conducted as described in Table 1 with 7.5 mM
Mg^{++} in the incubation mixture. The effects of CP-85,590 at 20
uM (open squares) and 100 uM (closed squares) are shown.

The disappointing manganese-dependence of these compounds
emphasizes the key role that _in vitro_ assay conditions can play in
describing inhibitor specificity. Good cellular assays are
essential in the early follow-up of new inhibitors in order to
insure that the _in vitro_ effect can be translated to activity in
intact cells.

DEVELOPMENTAL PATHWAY

In a mechanism-based drug discovery approach, a relatively
high level of confidence in the mode of action of a compound is

desired. Ideally, in the cellular, animal and human testing of a candidate, data supporting the mechanism of action will be generated and, thereby, increase the probability that the hypothesis under study is actually being tested. In anticancer programs, non-specific cytotoxic effects can easily confound interpretation of the data. In the case of tyrosine kinase inhibitors, good cellular controls may be available. The EGF-dependent growth inhibition demonstated with the dicyanostyrenes certainly increases confidence in the mechanism of action of these compounds (37).

In the clinical evaluation of inhibitors directed toward novel targets, a thorough understanding of the biochemical pharmacology of the agent will aid in decision making. A determination as to whether toxicity is mechanism related is critical since the clinical rationale is linked to the target mechanism and not the phenomenology of the model. This is in contrast to many model-based approaches to the discovery of potential new cancer therapeutants.

SUMMARY

Mechanism-based drug discovery is an intellectually exciting endeavor in which newly discovered chemical entities provide the means of testing important clinical hypotheses. At the pre-clinical level this approach is scientifically satisfying and it solicits creative, target-based monitoring in clinical evaluation protocols. The strength of this approach, the rigorous testing of hypotheses, is, however, usually dependent on one or more key assumptions. Consequently, significant risk is associated with such novel programs. In addition, a certain degree of serendipity is lost when the discovery approach is focussed on a particular mechanism. As a consequence, compounds with new mechanisms of action may be missed or deliberately excluded. The rapidly expanding knowledge base in cancer biology, coupled with strikingly more powerful technical capabilities, presents an ever changing landscape of new therapeutic targets. Efficient and flexible mechanism-based discovery strategies should be part of our efforts to develop new cancer therapeutants.

REFERENCES

1. Folkman JJ: What is the evidence that tumors are angiogenesis Dependent? Natl. Cancer Inst. 82:4-6, 1990.
2. Liotta LA: Gene products which play a role in cancer invasion and metastasis. Breast Cancer Res. Treat. 11:113-124, 1988.
3. Liotta LA, Wewer U, Rao NC et al: Biochemical mechanisms of tumor invasion and metastases. Adv. Exp. Med. Biol. 233:161-169, 1988.
4. Fidler IJ: Origin of cancer metastases and its implications for therapy. Isr. J. Med. 24:456-463, 1988.
5. Nicolson GL: Cancer metastasis: Tumor cell and host organ properties important in metastasis to specific secondary sites. Biochim. Biophys. Acta 948:175-224, 1988.
6. Sobel ME: Metastasis suppressor genes. J. Natl. Cancer Inst. 82:267-276, 1990.
7. Zetter BR: The cellular basis of site-specific tumor metastasis. N. Engl. J. Med. 322:605-612, 1990.
8. Heldin C-H, Betsholtz C, Claesson-Welsh L, Westermark, B: Subversion of growth regulatory pathways in malignant transformation. Biochim. Biophys. Acta 907:219-244, 1987.
9. Moyer JD: Inhibition of growth factor action as an approach to cancer chemotherapy. In: Developments in Cancer Therapy II, RI Glazer (ed), CRC Press, Boca Raton, pp. 25-41, 1988.
10. Weinberg R: Oncogenes, antioncogenes, and the molecular bases of multistep carcinogenesis. Cancer Res. 49:3713-3721, 1989.
11. Spandidos DA, Anderson ML: Oncogenes and onco-supressor genes: Their involvement in cancer. J. Pathol. 157:1-10, 1989.
12. Sager R: Tumor suppressor genes: The puzzle and the promise. Science 246:1406-1411, 1989.
13. Goldstein LJ, Galski H, Fojo A et al: Expression of a multidrug resistance gene in human cancers. J. Natl. Cancer Inst. 91:116-124, 1989.
14. Bradley G, Juranka PF, Ling V: Mechanism of multidrug resistance. Biochim. Biophys. Acta 948:87-128, 1988.
15. Morrow CS, Cowan NH: Glutathione S-transferase and drug resistance. Cancer Cells 2:15-22, 1990.
16. Tew ND: Enzyme changes linked to anticancer drug resistance. Ann. Rep. Med. Chem. 23:265-274, 1988.
17. Williams M, Malick JB: Drug discovery and development reflections and projections. In: Drug Discovery and Development, M Williams and JB Malick (eds), Human Press, Clifton, pp. 3-29, 1987.

18. Baldwin JJ: Drug Design. In: Drug Discovery and Development, M Williams and JB Malick (eds), Human Press, Clifton, pp. 33-71, 1987.
19. Maxwell RA: The state of the art of the science of drug discovery-an opinion. Drug Devel. Res. 4:375-389, 1984.
20. Testa B: Drugs? Drug research? Advances in drug research? Musings of a medicinal chemist. Adv. Drug Res. 13:1-58, 1984.
21. Hunter T, Cooper JA: Protein-tyrosine kinases. Ann. Rev. Biochem. 54:897-930, 1985.
22. Foulkes JG, Rosner MR: Tyrosine-specific protein kinases as mediators of growth control. In: Molecular Mechanisms of Transmembrane Signalling, P Cohen and MD Houslay (eds), Elsevier, Amsterdam, pp. 217-252, 1985.
23. Yarden Y, Ullrich AA: Molecular analysis of signal transduction by growth factors. Biochemistry 27:3113-3119, 1988.
24. Brugge JS, Chinkers M: Tyrosine-specific protein kinases. Ann. Rep. Med. Chem. 18:213-224, 1983.
25. Larson ER, Fischer PH: New approaches to antitumor therapy. Ann. Rep. Med. Chem. 24:121-128, 1989.
26. Yarden Y, Ullrich A: Growth factor receptor tyrosine kinases. Ann. Rev. Biochem. 57:443-478, 1988.
27. Konaka JB, Watanabe S, Witte ON: An alteration of the human c-abl protein in K562 leukemia cells unmasks associated tyrosine kinase activity. Cell 37:1035-1042, 1984.
28. Slamon DJ, Clark GM, Wong SG: Human breast cancer: Correlation of relapse and survival with amplification of the HER-2/ neu oncogene. Science 235:177-182, 1987.
29. Guerin M, Barrois M, Terrier M-J et al: Overexpression of either c-myc or c-erbB-2/neu proto-oncogenes in human breast carcinomas: Correlation with poor prognosis. Oncogene Res. 3:21-31, 1988.
30. Bolen JB, Viellette A, Schwartz AM et al: Activation of pp60^{c-src} protein kinase activity in human colon carcinoma. Proc. Natl. Acad. Sci. USA 84:2251-2255, 1987.
31. Bolen JB, Viellette A, Schwartz AM et al: Analysis of pp60^{c-src} in human colon carcinoma and normal human colon mucosal cells. Oncogene Res. 1:149-168, 1987.
32. Cartwrignt CA, Namps MP, Meisler AI et al: pp60^{c-src} activation in human colon carcinoma. Clin. Invest. 83:2025-2033, 1989.
33. Cartwright CA, Meisler AI, Eckhart W: Activation of the pp60^{c-src} protein kinase is an early event in colonic carcinogenesis. Proc. Natl. Acad. Sci. USA 87:558-562, 1990.
34. Kenyon GL, Garcia GA: Design of kinase inhibitors. Med. Res. Rev. 7:389-416, 1987.
35. Kruse CH, Holden NG, Pritchard ML et al: Synthesis and evaluation of multisubstrate inhibitors of an oncogene-encoded tyrosine-specific protein kinase. Med. Chem. 31:1762-1767, 1988.

157

36. Kruse CH, Holden NG, Offen PH et al: Synthesis and evaluation of multisubstrate inhibitors of an oncogene-encoded tyrosine-specific protein kinase. 2. Med. Chem. 31:1768-1772, 1988.
37. Hunter T: A thousand and one protein kinases. Cell 50:823-829, 1987.
38. Yaish P, Gazit A, Gilon C, Levitski A: Blocking of EGF-dependent cell proliferation by EGF receptor kinase inhibitors. Science 242:933-935, 1988.
39. Ondetti MA, Ruin B, Cushman DW: Design of specific inhibitors of angiotensin-converting enzyme: New class of orally active antihypertensive agents. Science 196:441-444, 1977.

8

DISCOVERY AND BULK PRODUCTION OF NATURAL PRODUCTS WITH ANTICANCER
ACTIVITY: THE ROLE OF CHEMICAL ECOLOGY

Matthew Suffness

INTRODUCTION

There are many problems involved in screening natural products, especially those introduced by poor solubility, colored
materials, natural oxidants and reductants which interfere with
assay reading, reversal of antimetabolite assays, high salt
concentrations in marine samples, and residual solvent in extracts, to name but a few. While all of the above-cited problems
in getting reproducible data from natural products are important,
the overwhelming issue often is whether the desired bioactive
metabolite is present at anywhere near the concentration that it
was in previous samples. I therefore chose a topic which is even
more fundamental to drug discovery and development: "where do
natural products come from, and why are they produced?".

Two of the most serious problems with discovery and development of natural products are finding and reproducing the activity
of extracts in the discovery phase and being able to acquire
sufficient pure chemical to go on to toxicology and clinical
trials in the development phase. I wish to present examples which
demonstrate that the levels of natural products in particular
samples can often be a result of their interactions with their
environment and that the study of such interactions can be crucial
to assure production of the desired metabolite. First let us
define the term "natural product".

NATURAL PRODUCT - A SECONDARY METABOLITE PRODUCED BY A PLANT, ANIMAL OR MICROORGANISM

Thus, natural products are not involved in the primary metabolism of the organism, and the next logical question is "why are natural products produced?". What functions do they perform in the organism or indeed, do they have functions at all. In a recent review (1), Williams et al. discussed some of the many theories on why natural products are produced including the possibilities that:

1) they are end products of metabolism and serve no function other than a way to eliminate excess levels of primary metabolites; i.e. they are metabolic dead ends.

2) they are the result of a long series of neutral mutations in the organism, and can be regarded as evolutionary ballast.

3) they represent evolution in progress and are a pool of new possibilities for future changes. They have a role in further evolution of the organism and genetic diversity.

4) they are compounds which formerly had a role in the organism, but no longer do so; they are vestigial.

5) they have evolved as a part of the organism's strategy for survival. They have important functions in attracting, repelling, and otherwise interacting with other organisms, either within the species or with other species.

Current thinking now favors the last possibility, that these natural products do have functions important to the survival of the organism.

Before proceeding further, perhaps we should ask another very important question: "why should plants or marine organisms or microbes produce compounds effective against human cancer?". They shouldn't. The anticancer effects of natural products are quite probably incidental to the real functions of the compounds in the organism which might include antibiotic, anti-parasitic, antifeedant, attractant, repellent, or growth regulatory activities to name but a few possibilities. These kinds of biological activities form the basis for the science of CHEMICAL ECOLOGY, which can be defined as THE CHEMICAL BASIS FOR INTERACTIONS BETWEEN

161

ORGANISMS. Some of the well known classes of interactions between
organisms are listed in Table 1. It is apparent that production
of few of these chemical signals would need to be constantly

Table 1

Examples of Chemical Interactions between Organisms

Interaction	Type	Example
attractant	intraspecies	insect pheromone
repellent	interspecies	plant anti-feedant
alarm substance	intraspecies	fear odorant
defense substance	interspecies	skunk odorant
recognition	intraspecies	firefly glow mother and pup
reproductive regulator	interspecies	germination inhibitor
territorial marker	intraspecies	urinary odorant
living space protector	interspecies	antifoulant

occurring and that in some cases (e.g. alarm substances) their
value to the organism would be totally lost if they were to be
constantly produced. Substances such as specific anti-infectives
could be produced and sequestered in the organism against future
attack or could be present in negligible amounts and only produced
en masse when there was need. Thus we can conclude that, using
the terminology of classic enzymology, many of the "natural
products" produced are adaptive rather than constitutive and that
this will greatly affect both our ability to discover their
presence and bioactivities through screening as well as to produce
them on a mass scale as needed for development. This line of
reasoning can explain why seemingly equivalent biological samples
may show excellent activities in a screen one time and be almost

devoid of activity the next. In a similar way, many researchers in natural products drug development have had the nasty experience of making a large scale collection of organism to isolate bulk drug for advanced stages of preclinical development only to find that the yield of active drug is only 10% or 25% of what was expected based on previous collections. This can be true even if the collection locality, the season, and the climate have been much the same as previously. In the area of anticancer plants, for example _Catharanthus_ (=_Vinca_), the source of vinblastine and vincristine has not been a major problem and it is likely that these alkaloids are at least partly constitutive or that selective breeding has resulted in such strains. Perhaps the majority of plant toxins may be constitutive as they might possess a kind of permanent antifeedant role, but as the assays we use in cancer drug discovery are less directed towards cytotoxicity and are more directed towards enzyme and receptor based assays and phenomena such as metastasis, angiogenesis, cellular differentiation, growth factors, and inhibitors of gene expression, we must be fully aware of the possibility that many of the natural products active in these assays may be "adaptive" and consequently their production will be under regulation that has nothing whatsoever to do with cancer. As we encounter such cases the obvious question will be: "how can we control the production of these natural products?", and the answer will be that: "we must try to discover the reason for production of these compounds by the source organism and discover the stimuli that are involved. The discovery of the role of a natural product in its source organism is often a rather painstaking research project requiring observation of changes in the organism, analysis of levels of the substance in question in conjunction with different types of stress situations for the organism, and laboratory and field tests of the substance on organisms which interact with the source organism. The usual case is for ecologists or field biologists to observe an effect and then track down the chemical substances responsible for the effect by bioassay directed fractionation. Careful reading of the literature in chemical ecology can often give very interesting hints for drug discovery, although this literature has been largely ignored by people in the drug discovery field at least in part due to lack of knowledge of its existence. In the next section several examples are presented which may be instructive.

LEADS FOR DRUG DISCOVERY IN CHEMICAL ECOLOGY
<u>The Monarch and the Milkweed</u>

The monarch butterfly (<u>Danaus</u> <u>plexippus</u>) is a very beautiful and very obvious butterfly which has bright orange and black coloration and is found over most of the United States. Despite its bright coloration, it is largely avoided by birds and research into the reason for this has shown that the monarch sequesters high levels of cardenolides which result from its larvae feeding almost exclusively on the milkweed plant (<u>Asclepias</u> <u>species</u>) which in its turn is largely avoided as a food source because of the toxic nature of the cardenolides therein. A classical ecology study involved exposure of naive blue jays (raised from the egg without exposure to monarchs) to these butterflies. The naive jays attacked with gusto but immediately spat out the monarchs and when exposed to monarchs again, would not attack them, even if very hungry (2). This part of the story is an ecology classic demonstrating the ability of organisms to sequester toxins from their food and use them for protection. From a drug development viewpoint the really interesting question is why the monarch larvae and the monarchs themselves are immune to cardenolides. The fascinating answer is not that they can sequester the cardeno-lides in a compartment and keep them away from their cells but rather that the target of cardenolides, sodium-potassium dependent ATPase, is extremely resistant to inhibition by cardenolides such as ouabain and this is associated with lowered affinity for the enzyme (3). If one knew the changes in amino acid sequence which gave rise to this resistance and could model the binding site, it would be very helpful to design of better cardiotonic drugs.

164

The Indiana Cedar Barrens

The cedar barrens are an area of sandy poor soil where almost no flowering plants grow. The ecology is dominated by cedar trees and very large amounts of lichens on the ground. The chemical basis for the lack of flowering plants was not understood. The answer came during the course of an unrelated project on simple bioassays which might correlate with cytotoxicity. An assay was developed measuring inhibition of growth of duckweed (_Lemna species_). Duckweed is a very fast growing plant which is found in fresh water ponds and it grows not by increasing leaf (frond) size but by adding new fronds and elongating its stem. Thus growth inhibition can be measured by a simple counting of frond number in treated versus control plants. Those compounds or extracts active in the assay were then examined in the brine shrimp toxicity assay and in a series of human tumor cell lines to seek correlation levels (4). A series of blinded compounds were tested and one of them, usnic acid, was much more growth inhibitory to the _Lemna_ than to the brine shrimp or the human cell lines. The suspicion was that it was a new class of plant growth regulator, and subsequent studies found usnic acid to be growth inhibitory to a wide variety of plants. Since usnic acid is a lichen metabolite and is sometimes found in quite high concentrations in those groups of lichens which produce it, this gave a possible reason for the lack of flowering plants in the cedar barrens. Extraction of lichen samples from the cedar barrens showed that they had very high concentrations of usnic acid, in the range of 1.0-2.0% of dry weight and thus the hypothesis is confirmed. Although this result came somewhat serendipitously, it is clear that observation of the ecology of the cedar barrens and subsequent analysis of cedar trees and lichens for plant growth inhibitors would have led to both an understanding of the ecology on a chemical basis and the discovery of usnic acid as a plant growth inhibitor. This could be an interesting lead for agrichemical development.

The Giant Silk Moth and the Lytic Peptides

The giant silk moth (_Hyalophora cecropia_) which is native to Central America and Northern South America has been studied as a possible source of commercial silk. Part of that investigation looked at its resistance to infection and it was found that a series of specialized peptides, called cecropins, were produced in response to bacterial infection. The cecropins lysed bacteria by forming a pore in the membrane. Further studies showed that the cecropins consisted of about 35 amino acids and that the sequence of amino acid residues was such that when the molecule organized into a typical alpha helix, all the non-polar residues lined up on one side whereas all the polar side chains lined up on the other, giving the molecule an amphipathic nature. The individual alpha helices then self-assembled such that they formed a hollow tube in the cell membrane with the non-polar faces all directed into the lipid bilayer while the polar faces all directed inward forming a central pore which permitted leakage of intracellular contents and cell lysis (5). Follow-up studies have found that the cecropins can lyse mammalian cells as well as bacterial cells and that they may have some selectivity for lysing tumor cells in preference to normal cells. A series of analogs has been made in which certain of the amino acid residues are altered (being careful to sub-stitute polar for polar and non-polar for non-polar residues to retain the amphipathic nature) and a compound with enhanced potency named Shiva-1 (after the Hindu god of destruction) has been discovered. Another interesting observation is that the cytoskeleton seems to be a key mediator of resistance to the cecropins; antimitotic agents such as colchicine which block formation of the microtubules which form the essence of the cytoskeleton enhance the lytic abilities of the cecropins, sug-gesting possible use in combination chemotherapy (5). Thus ecological observations on the giant silk moth of Central America have given us a quite novel type of lead for cancer chemotherapy.

BULK PRODUCTION OF NATURAL PRODUCTS

Before any compound can become a candidate for development leading to clinical trials, a large and reproducible source of supply must be secured. There are many possible ways to approach the supply issue and most of these are noted in Figure 1.

- TOTAL SYNTHESIS

- SEMISYNTHESIS

- CULTIVATION
    - AGRICULTURE
    - AQUACULTURE
    - HYDROPONICS
    - TISSUE CULTURE
    - FERMENTATION

- DIRECTED BIOSYNTHESIS
    - PRECURSOR FEEDING
    - ANALOG PRODUCTION

- STRAIN SELECTION
    - NATURAL SELECTION
    - MUTATIONAL STUDIES

Figure 1. Approaches to bulk production of natural products.

Not listed in Figure 1 is the possibility of production by genetic engineering, but this is still rather distant for non-peptide derived molecules. Many of the bioactive secondary metabolites in plants are produced by complex biogenetic pathways involving as many as 10 to 20 enzyme catalyzed steps and production by genetic technology would involve isolation of these enzymes, finding the corresponding genes, sequencing them, and transferring all of them to a suitable host for expression. The amount of effort involved is huge; another factor to consider is that in the source plant, biosynthesis may involve compartmentalization and transfer of intermediates from leaves to roots to seeds, etc. Another problem at present is that the detailed biosynthetic pathways for most natural products of plant or marine animal origin are unknown and are very difficult to work out because of the low levels of potent metabolites produced and the consequent difficulties in getting adequate incorporations of labelled precursors.

Let us set aside for a moment the less understood production of secondary metabolites in plant and animals and reflect on the situation with microorganism produced compounds, in particular antibiotics. First, we know that these compounds are adaptive rather than constitutive since they are produced only under some specialized culture conditions and not others; second, we know that production of antibiotics is independent from growth since we can find many conditions under which the organisms grow luxuriantly, but produce no antibiotic. It is extremely likely that the antibiotics are in fact stress metabolites, produced in response to some specific chemical cue resulting from attack by other microbes. We produce these antibiotics on complex media often containing degraded proteins and complex mixtures of carbohydrates and all sorts of foreign secondary metabolites (see Figure 2) which may contain the stressors necessary to initiate the production of the desired antibiotic. It is no wonder that the selection of fermentation media is still considered to be somewhat of a "black art".

I would rather prefer to try an ecological approach to finding specific stressors to control the production of antibiotic in the fermentation. One could isolate a substantial number of cultures of other microorganisms from the same soil sample and test either the microbes themselves or extracts of these microbes on the producing organism to find one which stimulates production of the desired antibiotic; it would then be possible to use production of antibiotic as a bioassay to isolate the specific chemical substances or at least a key fraction which acts as a potent stimulus to antibiotic production. I am not aware of this approach having been tried, but it seems that it might be able to enhance production levels beyond those achievable by manipulation of media and physico-chemical conditions.

168

- YEAST EXTRACT

- PEPTONE BROTH

- CORN STEEP LIQUOR

- WHEY SOLIDS

- FISH MEAL

- COTTONSEED MEAL

- SEA WEED EXTRACT

- RAT CHOW

- POTATO DEXTROSE MEDIA

Figure 2. Examples of carbon/nitrogen sources in fermentation media.

For the case of higher plants, I can state that in the National Cancer Institute's (NCI) program we have had a number of cases where an initial collection showed quite good activity but one or two subsequent recollections of the same plant material, from the same general area, at about the same season, were inactive. In most of these cases we were fully confident of both the identity of the raw material and of the bioassay data; these remain as unsolved cases, but the suspicion is that the plants which gave rise to the active samples may have been under pressure from an ecological stressor which was absent in the inactive samples. Loss of production by plant cells in tissue culture, or by cultivated versus wild strains may likewise have roots in chemical ecology. A rather well studied example of a bioactive stress metabolite is that of ipomeanol (Figure 3), a simple furan isolated from moldy sweet potatoes (_Ipomea_ _batatas_) which is a powerful lung toxin (6). Ipomeanol is not produced by the sweet potato in the absence of infection and it is not produced by the infecting fungus, a _Fusarium_ species, under a variety of culture conditions; further, it has antibiotic activity against _Fusarium_.

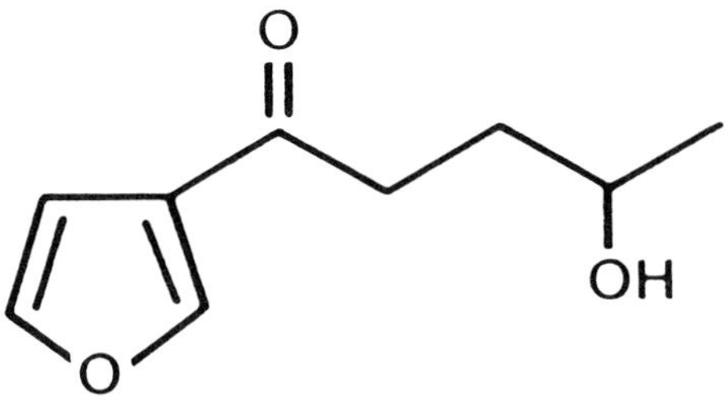

Figure 3.   Ipomeanol.

Although ipomeanol is readily synthesizable and would not be
produced for bulk use from the sweet potato, it is easy to imagine
that if it was a more complex metabolite and less amenable to
synthesis, significant difficulties would be encountered in its
production from the plant source unless the ecology was understood.

An interesting case of bulk production of a plant product is
that of maytansine, a macrolide isolated from a variety of plant
sources. Maytansine is a tubulin polymerization inhibitor and
antimitotic agent which showed good preclinical antitumor activity
in murine models and was selected for development to clinical
trials. The original isolation was by the Kupchan group in 1972
at a yield of only 0.00002% (0.2 ppm) based on weight of dried
plant (7). Isolations of maytansine from various natural sources
are summarized in Table 2. Judging from the relationship of the
chemical structure of maytansine (Figure 4) to that of ansamycins
and other macrolide antibiotics which were known at the time, and
given the extremely low yield of the drug, it seemed quite likely
that the actual source could be microbial.

The NCI sent a microbiologist to Kenya to collect samples
from on and in the vicinity of the _Maytenus_ plants but despite
intensive workup of more than 700 samples no producing cultures
were identified. Lacking a microbial source, the NCI, through
collaboration with the U.S.D.A., made a massive collection of the

Table 2. Selected Sources of Maytansinoids

Source Organism	Family	Type	Group	Year	Ref.
Maytenus serrata	Celastraceae	higher plant	Kupchan	1972	7
Maytenus buchananii	Celastraceae	higher plant	Kupchan	1977	8
Colubrina texensis	Rhamnaceae	higher plant	Wall	1973	9
Putterlickia verrucosa	Celastraceae	higher plant	Kupchan	1977	8
Nocardia sp. C-15003 (N-1)	Actinomycetaceae	actinomycete	Higashide Asai	1977 1979	10 11
Trewia nudiflora	Euphorbiaceae	higher plant	Powell	1981-2	12,13
Thamnobrynum sandei	Neckeraceae	moss	Sakai	1988	14
Isthecium subdiversiforme	Lembophyllaceae	moss	Sakai	1988	14
Claopodium crispifolium	Thuidaceae	moss	Cassady	1990	15
Anomodon attenuatus	Thuidaceae	moss	Cassady	1990	15

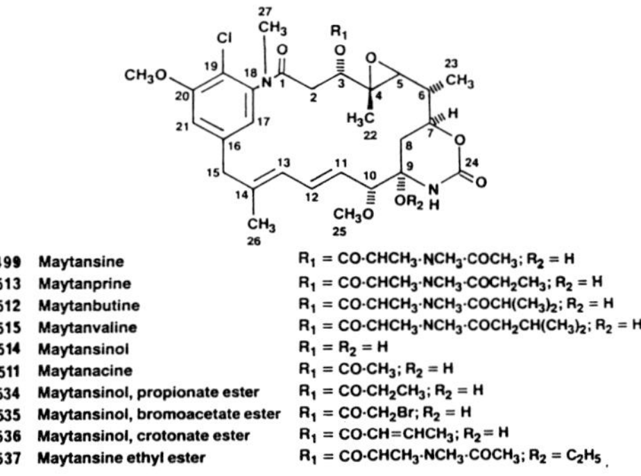

Figure 4. Maytansinoids from _Maytenus_ species.

source plant, _Maytenus buchananii,_ in Kenya in 1976. Over 30,000 pounds of dried leaves, twigs and bark were collected and processed to yield about 15 grams of pure maytansine at a cost of over $650,000 (16). In 1977, the Takeda Chemical Company found a microbial source of maytansinoids, a _Nocardia_ species (10,11), and assisted the subsequent NCI clinical trials by converting their maytansinoids to maytansine and donating 5 grams of maytansine to the NCI. Did the NCI miss the producing organism in the microbial collections in Kenya, or is maytansine really produced in the plant? We will come back to this in the next section but the point to be made now is that the ecology of higher plants and animals is very complex.

SOURCES OF NATURAL PRODUCTS

The idea that if a substance is isolated from a given organism, then that organism is the source, is quite unrealistic. Figure 5 lists some of the interactions between organisms that can result in the appearance of the end product in a particular species, and total biosynthesis in the observed source is only one of several possibilities. The cases for higher plants are complex enough, but when one studies marine organisms which acquire many compounds through their diet which can be sequestered, slightly modified, or used as starting materials for extensive modification, the issues of "true source" become even more complicated and the need for understanding the ecology of the organism becomes even more important.

We have seen above that the source from which maytansine was originally isolated, _Maytenus_ species, may or may not be a "true" source. There are interesting arguments to be made on both

- TOTAL BIOSYNTHESIS IN HOST

- MODIFICATION OF DIETARY
  PRECURSOR

- MODIFICATION OF PRECURSOR
  FROM MICROBIAL ASSOCIATE

- COOPERATIVE BIOSYNTHESIS WITH
  MICROBIAL ASSOCIATE

- TRANSFER (UNMODIFIED) FROM
  MICROBIAL ASSOCIATE

- ACCUMULATION FROM DIET

Figure 5. Possible sources of secondary metabolites.

sides. Arguments favoring <u>Nocardia</u> or other microbes as the true source of maytansinoids are that: 1) related compounds (ansamycins) are known to be of microbial origins; 2) the yields in higher plants are generally very low and may represent acquisition from microbial associates rather than innate biosynthesis; 3) the plant sources represent three families of higher plants and three families of mosses (Table 2) which are not closely related and wouldn't be expected to possess similar biosynthetic pathways for secondary metabolites. Counter arguments favoring biosynthesis in the plant sources as well as in <u>Nocardia</u> are that: 1) Most isolations from higher plants (i.e. not including mosses) have been from the genera <u>Maytenus</u> and <u>Putterlickia</u> in the family Celastraceae which either points to total biosynthesis in these genera or a close cooperative association with a particular microbial group; 2) Concentrations of maytansinoids in the seeds of <u>Maytenus</u> <u>rothiana</u> (=<u>Gymnosporia</u> <u>rothiana</u>) and in <u>Trewia</u> <u>nudiflora</u> are quite high and seem to represent a mechanism to protect seeds from infection or predation. The concentrations found seem too high to be a result of sequestration of microbially-derived compounds; 3) The <u>Trewia</u> compounds (Figure 6) have significant structural differences from other maytansinoids and appear to be species specific.

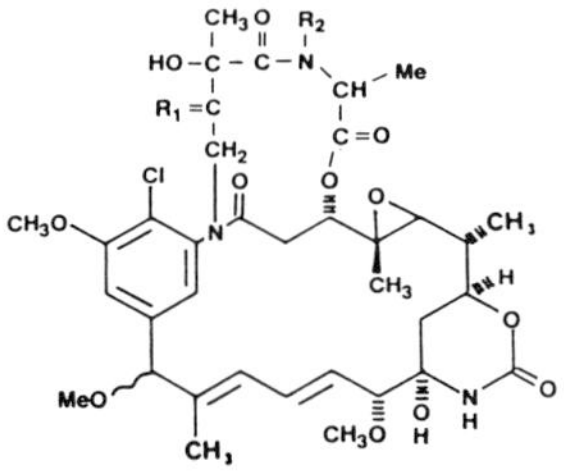

		R₁	R₂
516	N-Methyl trenudone	O	CH₃
521	Treflorine	H₂	H
522	Trenudine	H, OH	H

Figure 6. Modified maytansinoids from <u>Trewia</u> <u>nudiflora</u> (euphorbiaceae).

The question of origin of the maytansinoids remains unresolved, although it seems unlikely that all of them are of microbial origin. This could be a case of convergent evolution, or perhaps at some ancient point in evolution there was transfer of genetic material from microbes to at least some of the plants which are now producers.

A truly classic case which formerly seemed solved only to now be rather open is that of the origin of tetrodotoxin (TTX, Figure 7) the existence of which has been known since antiquity in China and Japan (17,18). Ancient documents from both of these countries

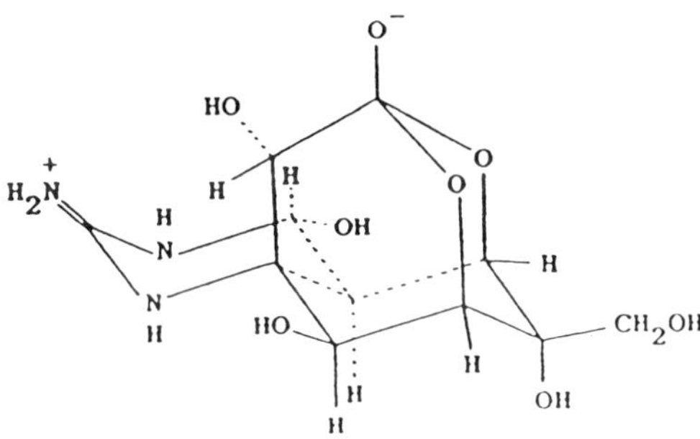

Figure 7. Tetrodotoxin.

describe the toxic effects of ingestion of puffer fish, with the same pattern of neurologic symptomology that we see today in cases of poisoning by toxic puffers and although the toxic component was not isolated in pure form and characterized until 1964 (19). The case for TTX being a product of total biosynthesis in the puffer and related fishes was very strong considering the taxonomic relatedness of the fish from which it was known, all of which are in the order Tetraodontiformes (Figure 8). This was the situation until the 1930s when a very similar toxicity was shown for a material from the California newt, _Taricha torosa_ (17,18). This newt was, until fairly recently, the only amphibian to have the

174

FISHES:

> CLASS: OSTEICHTHYES (BONY FISHES)
>
> ORDER: TETRAODONTIFORMES
>
> FAMILIES:
>
>> - TETRAODONTIDAE (PUFFERS)
>> - DIODONTIDAE (PORCUPINEFISH)
>> - CANTHIGASTERIDAE (SHARP-NOSED PUFFERS)
>> - MOLIDAE (OCEAN SUNFISH OR MOLAS)

Figure 8. Sources of tetrodotoxin fishes.

same type of mammalian toxicity as the puffer fish and this was
considered an anomaly. The structure elucidation of TTX and the
evidence that the same toxin came from such diverse species as a
puffer fish and a newt resulted in a more detailed look at the
evidence for origin of the toxin in puffer fish and certain pieces
of data which had long existed now raised meaningful questions
about the origin of TTX. For example: toxicity is seasonal in
puffers and the degree of toxicity can vary widely among the same
species even in the same waters; some species are quite toxic from
one location and not others; the pattern of toxic tissues (mainly
digestive and reproductive tracts, liver, and skin) is not incon-
sistent with an exogenous origin. When juvenile puffers were fed
on an artificial diet and kept separated from adults, they were
non-toxic but when they were exposed to adult puffers, they became
toxic suggesting some kind of transfer of toxic capability
(20-22). Work on tetrodotoxin itself had been very difficult
because of the extremely polar nature of the molecule and its lack
of easily detectable functional groups, and analysis of the
presence of TTX in samples of fish or tissues of poisoned animals
was a major challenge until the late 1970s. Once the analytical
methods were available, mainly reverse phase HPLC with paired ion
or fluorometric detectors (22-23), TTX began to be found in
herbivorous fish, crabs, the blue-ringed octopus, an annelid worm,
algae, a bacterium which is epiphyic on algae (an _Alteromonas_

species) and in a <u>Vibrio</u> <u>sp.</u> isolated from a crab (21,22,24). Yotsu and co-workers isolated a TTX producing <u>Pseudomonas</u> <u>sp.</u> from the skin of a puffer, <u>Fugu</u> <u>poecilonotus</u> (24), and also were able to produce TTX and anhydroTTX by fermentation of a <u>Psueudomonas</u> <u>sp.</u> This data together with the large variety of organisms recently shown to be TTX producers would seem to present a convincing case that the puffer fish is not a true biosynthetic source of TTX, but a recent report of production of the toxin from a gland in the skin of the puffer without microbial involvement seems to confound this (25). An excellent review of the role of chemical ecolgy in marine organisms has recently appeared (26). Certainly if one had to produce this toxin on a commercial scale, the microbial approach might be very attractive.

CONCLUSIONS

The examples cited in this paper are but a very few of many which could be cited and explained. Plants and marine organisms have become more important sources of materials for screening in recent years due to the advent of high capacity, inexpensive preliminary assays for many diseases, including cancer, and some special points about the ecology of these organisms need to be stressed.

First, many natural products are stress metabolites and as such their levels in the unstressed organism may frequently be below the level of detection in the assay used. Thus important leads can be missed through screening and the screening effort should be supplemented with observations from field biology and from the literature.

Second, the role of stressors must be considered whenever activity data is not reproduced as this may be one of the single most significant factors affecting levels of secondary metabolites. This is even more of a concern when making major changes in the ecology of the producing organism, as when attempting to put a wild species under cultivation.

Third, even though an organism is productive under cultivation, it may be even more productive if the organism's natural stressors are introduced. Thus ecological understanding may have great impact upon bulk drug supply.

Fourth, we must always be aware that the compound we are seeking may not be a product of biosynthesis in the source organism, but may depend heavily on the food chain of the organism or on microbial associates. There is an excellent possibility that new cancer drugs will be discovered from natural products, but to successfully develop these agents into marketable entities, a knowledge and understanding of the chemical ecology of the producing organisms is essential.

REFERENCES

1. Williams DH, Stone MJ, Hauck PR, Rahman SK: Why are secondary metabolites (natural products biosynthesized?) J. Nat. Prod. 52:1189-1208, 1989.
2. Brower LP: Ecological Chemistry. Scientific American 220(2):22-29, 1969.
3. Vaughan GJ, Jungreis AM: Insensitivity of lepidopteran tissues to ouabain: Physiological mechanisms for protection from cardiac glycosides. J. Insect Physiol. 23:585-589, 1977.
4. Anderson JE, Goetz CM, Suffness M, McLaughlin JL: A blind comparison of simple bench-top bioassays and human tumor cell cytotoxicities as antitumor prescreens. Phytochemical Analysis 2:107-111, 1991.
5. Jaynes J: Peptides to the rescue. New Scientist 124(1695): 42-44, 1989.
6. Christian MC, Wittes RE, Leyland-Jones B et al: 4-Ipomeanol: A novel investigational new drug for lung cancer. JNCI 81:1133-1143, 1989.
7. Kupchan SM, Komoda Y, Court WA et al: Maytansine: A novel antileukemic ansa macrolide from _Maytenus ovatus_. J. Amer. Chem. Soc. 94:1354-1356, 1972.
8. Kupchan SM, Komoda Y, Branfman AR et al: The maytansinoids. Isolation, structural elucidation, and chemical interrelation of novel ansa macrolides. J. Org. Chem. 42:2349-2357, 1977.
9. Wani NC, Taylor HL, Wall ME: Plant antitumor agents: Colubrinol acetate and colubrinol, antileukemic ansa macrolides from _colubrina texensis_. J. Chem. Soc. Chem. Commun. 1973:390, 1973.
10. Higashide E, Asia M, Ootsu K et al: Ansamitocin, a group of novel maytansinoid antibiotics with antitumor properties from _Nocardia_. Nature 270:721-722, 1977.
11. Asai M, Mizuta E, Izawa M et al: Isolation, chemical characterization and structure of ansamitocin, a new antitumor ansamycin antibiotic. Tetrahedron 35:1079-1085, 1979.

12. Powell RG, Weisleder D, Smith CR Jr: Novel maytansinoid tumor inhibitors from _Trewia_ _nudiflora_: Trewiasine, dehydro-trewiasine, and demethyltrewiasine. J. Org. Chem. 46:4398-4403, 1981.

13. Powell RG, Weisleder D, Smith CR Jr et al: Treflorine, trenu-dine, and N-methyltrenudone: Novel maytansinoid tumor inhibi-tors containing two fused macrocyclic rings. J. Amer. Chem. Soc. 104:4929-4935, 1982.

14. Sakai K, Ichikawa T, Yamada K et al: Antitumor principles in mosses. The first isolation and identification of maytan-sinoids including a novel 15-methoxyansamitocin P-3. J. Nat. Prod. 51:845-850, 1988.

15. Suwanborirux K, Chang C-J, Spjut RW, Cassady JM: Ansamitocin P-3, a maytansinoid, from _Claopodium_ _crispifolium_ and _Anomodon_ _attenuatus_ or associated actinomycetes. Experien-tia 46:117-119, 1990.

16. Suffness M, Douros J: Drugs of plant origin. In: Methods in Cancer Research, Vol. XVIa, VT DeVita and H Busch (eds), Academic Press, New York, pp. 73-126, 1979.

17. Halstead BW: Class Osteichthyes: Tetrodotoxic fishes. In: Poisonous and Venomous Marine Animals of the World, Vol. 2, U.S. Govt. Printing Office, Washington, D.C., pp. 679-903, 1967.

18. Fuhrman FA: Tetrodotoxin, tarichatoxin, and chiriquitoxin: Historical perspective. Annals N.Y. Acad. Sci. 479:1-13, 1986.

19. Mosher HS: The chemistry of tetrodotoxin. Annals N.Y. Acad. Sci. 479:32-43, 1986.

20. Matsui T, Hamada S, Konosu S: Difference in accumulation of puffer fish toxin and crystalline tetrodotoxin in the puffer fish, _Fugu_ _rubripes_ _rubripes_. Bull. Jpn. Soc. Scient. Fish. 47:535, 1981.

21. Noguchi T, Jeon JK, Arakawa O et al: Occurrence of tetrodo-toxin and anhydrotetrodotoxin in _Vibrio_ sp. isolated from the intestine of a xanthid crab, _Atergatis_ _floridus_. J. Biochem. (Tokyo) 99:311-314, 1986.

22. Yasumoto T, Nagai H, Yasumura D et al: Interspecies distri-bution and possible origin of tetrodotoxin. Annals N.Y. Acad. Sci. 479:44-51, 1986.

23. Onoue Y, Noguchi T, Hashimoto K. In: Seafood Toxins, EP Ragelis (ed), A.C.S. Symposium Series No. 262, American Chemical Society, Washington, D.C., pp. 345-355, 1984.

24. Yotsu M, Yamazaki T, Meguro Y et al: Production of tetrodo-toxin and its derivatives by _Pseudomonas_ sp. isolated from the skin of a pufferfish. Toxicon 25:225-228, 1987.

25. Kodama M, Shigeru S, Ogata T et al: Tetrodotoxin secreting glands in the skin of puffer fishes. Toxicon 24:819-829, 1986.

26. Scheuer P: Some marine ecological phenomena: Chemical basis and biomedical potential. Science 248:173-177, 1990.

9

CHEMICAL APPROACHES TO IMPROVED RADIOTHERAPY

W.R. Leopold and Judith S. Sebolt-Leopold

INTRODUCTION

Treatment with ionizing radiation is a major modality for the treatment of cancer. Between 50 and 60 percent of all cancer patients receive treatment with ionizing radiation at some time during the course of their disease (1). Thus, approximately 600,000 new patients will receive radiotherapy this year in the United States alone. Despite the proven efficacy of radiotherapy in the treatment of certain tumor types, nearly one half of the patients treated with radiotherapy will die with at least microscopic recurrence of tumor at the irradiated site (2).

In addition to the perhaps obvious difficulties associated with uniform and selective dosimetry of radiation to irregularly invasive tumor masses, a number of other properties of solid tumors are thought to limit the efficacy of radiotherapy. Included among these properties are the existence of hypoxic regions within the tumor mass and the enzymatic repair of x-ray induced DNA damage (3). Each of these limitations has stimulated research on potential methods of enhancing the efficiency of tumor cell killing with radiation. Approaches taken to overcome hypoxia related resistance to radiation have included the design of electron-affinic radiosensitizers (4), the use of hypoxia-selective and bioreductively activated cytotoxic agents (5), and more recently, the modification of tumor blood flow (6). The use of inhibitors of DNA repair (7), the design of elaborate dose-fractionation schemes (8, 9), and the variation in the quality of the radiation used (10) have been explored as methods to reduce the amount of damage repaired within the irradiated tumor.

Our efforts have concentrated on two different approaches to the development of radiosensitizers: the design of electron-affinic compounds that contain an alkylating moiety to increase the efficacy of x-irradiation in the hypoxic regions of tumors, and the development of inhibitors of the repair of x-ray induced DNA damage. Each approach requires the use of significantly different screening and evaluation strategies, and each type of compound carries with it significantly different implications for clinical use. Prototype compounds representative of each approach are depicted in Figure 1.

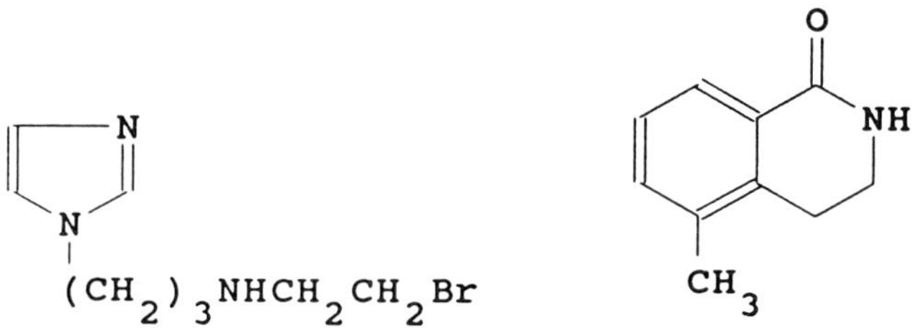

N
N
$(CH_2)_3NHCH_2CH_2Br$

PD 130908

O
NH
CH_3

PD 128763

Figure 1. Representative examples of electron affinic and DNA repair inhibiting radiosensitizers.

TUMOR HYPOXIA AS A TARGET FOR ELECTRON-AFFINIC SENSITIZERS

It is well established that solid tumor masses often either outgrow or even destroy their blood supplies. This leads to increased diffusion distances for oxygen and other nutrients between the capillary and various subpopulations of cells within the tumor. This effect, coupled with the metabolic consumption of oxygen along the diffusion path, results in a condition of relatively long term hypoxia within select areas of the tumor. In addition to the relatively chronic hypoxia produced by an inadequate vascular bed, intermittent occlusion of vessels within tumors has been demonstrated, leading to a more acute form of tumor hypoxia (11).

Both forms of hypoxia discussed above can reduce the cell killing potential of x-irradiation. Mammalian cells in culture are on average 2.5- to 3-fold more sensitive to x-irradiation under oxic conditions than when hypoxic (12). Although severe chronic hypoxia induces tumor cell death, moderate levels of hypoxia produce relatively quiescent tumor cell populations. In addition to being resistant to radiation therapy by virtue of an oxygen deficiency, these cells are also often resistant to many chemotherapeutic agents because of the quiescent nature of hypoxic subpopulations.

The reason for the relative lack of effect of ionizing radiation on hypoxic cells is shown in Figure 2. Oxygen is required

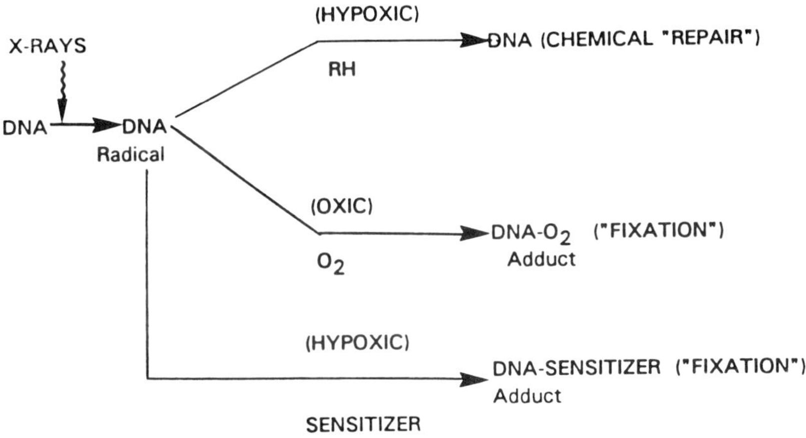

Figure 2. Schematic of the rationale for "electron-affinic" and "inhibition of repair" approaches to radiosensitization. Adapted from (13).

for the fixation of x-ray induced damage within the cell. A primary initial lesion produced by x-irradiation of a cell is thought to be the formation of free radical damage in the DNA. In normally oxygenated tissues these DNA radicals react with oxygen to produce DNA adducts which in general require "enzymatic repair," a relatively slow process (seconds to hours). In hypoxic tissues the concentration of oxygen is low enough to make the abstraction of protons from a variety of sources a major factor in the fate of the DNA radical damage. This "chemical repair" of the DNA occurs on a much faster time scale (msec), making the damage correspondingly less cytotoxic. Electron-affinic radiosensitizers are intended to be oxygen mimetic in that they take the place of oxygen in reaction with the DNA radical to "fix" the damage in a form requiring enzymatic repair (Figure 2). In order for a radiosensitizer to provide improved penetration into the tumor relative to oxygen, potential drug candidates should have appropriate log P values and should not be metabolized appreciably in oxic tissues (thus eliminating metabolic consumption as a negative factor with respect to diffusion distance from the capillary).

Our approach to the development and evaluation of an electron-affinic radiosensitizer is illustrated by PD 130908, a desoxy, ring-opened analog of RSU 1069 (Figure 1). RSU 1069 is a highly efficient electron-affinic radiosensitizer with high activity in both _in vitro_ and _in vivo_ model systems. In addition to its activity as an electron-affinic radiosensitizer mediated by the 2-nitroimidazole ring (14), RSU 1069 is also an efficient hypoxia-selective cytotoxin (15). This cytotoxicity in the absence of radiation is at least in part mediated by the reactive aziridine substitution on the side chain (16). Phase I clinical trials of RSU 1069 were terminated in part because of severe emesis at doses well below those predicted to produce a significant radiosensitizing effect (17), and partly because of the chemical instability and difficulty of synthesis of RSU 1069 that created a supply problem.

Analogs of RSU 1069 were synthesized in the hope of discovering compounds that maintained its highly efficient radiosensitizing activity and hypoxia-selective cytotoxicity, while also possessing lower emetic potential and improved chemical stability following a more facile synthesis. PD 130908 is representative of these compounds.

Initially, PD 130908 was evaluated for cytotoxicity to both hypoxic and oxic cultures of V79 cells. Exposure to PD 130908 was carried out at 37^0 C for three hr. PD 130908 proved to retain at least some of the hypoxia-selective cytotoxicity (15-fold) of the parent compound RSU 1069 (50- to 60-fold) (18,19). The IC_{50} values for oxic and hypoxic cultures treated with PD 130908 were 1.8 mM and 0.12 mM respectively.

PD 130908 was then tested for its radiosensitizing activity in vitro against V79 cells (18,19). PD 130908 proved to be an extremely efficient radiosensitizer (Table 1). The common measure of radiosensitizing efficiency is the $C_{1.6}$ value, the concentration of sensitizer that produces a sensitizer enhancement ratio (SER) of 1.6. The sensitizer enhancement ratio in turn may be thought of as the ratio of the x-ray doses for treatment with x-ray alone and for treatment with x-ray plus sensitizer that produce equal cell killing. (In practice, the SER is calculated as the ratio of the slopes of the exponential portions of the x-ray dose response curves.) Thus, for an SER of 1.6, the addition of a radiosensitizer allows an approximate 62.5% reduction of x-ray dose to produce the same cell kill as x-ray alone. PD 130908 produced a $C_{1.6}$ value of 0.48 mM. This value was essentially identical to that of RSU 1069 and considerably lower than those of misonidazole (3 mM) and SR 2508 (1.8 mM). Misonidazole was evaluated in the clinic where results were generally disappointing, although a small subset of the patient population was reported to benefit from its use (20). SR 2508 was developed as an improved analog of misonidazole (21) and is currently in clinical trial.

The reduced cytotoxicity of PD 130908 relative to that of RSU 1069 produced a strikingly superior sensitizer enhancement ratio at their maximum nontoxic concentrations of 3 mM and 0.8 mM, respectively (Table 1). The maximum achievable SERs under these conditions were 2.7 for PD 130908 and 2.0 for RSU 1069 compared to the theoretical maximum of about 3.0, based on the observed difference in radiosensitivity between oxic and totally hypoxic cultures (18,19).

The ability of PD 130908 to radiosensitize in vivo has been measured in several different tumor models (Figure 3). Initial studies employed in vivo treatment of subcutaneous KHT sarcomas followed by excision of the tumors and subsequent plating of sin-

Table 1

In <u>Vitro</u> Radiosensitizing Activity of PD 130908

Radiosensitizer	$C_{1.6}$ (mM)	Maximum Noncytotoxic Concentration (mM)	SER
PD 130908	0.48	3.0	2.7
RSU 1069	0.33	0.8	2.0
SR 2508	1.8	>3.0	1.9
Misonidazole	3.0	>3.0	1.7

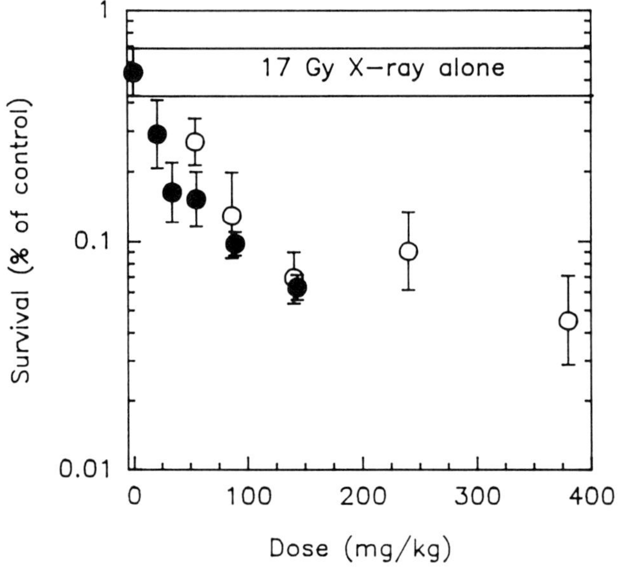

Figure 3. <u>In vivo</u> activity of PD 130908 against subcutaneous implants of the KHT sarcoma. Male $B6C3F_1$ mice bearing 100-200 mg KHT tumors were injected with a single dose of PD 130908 either IP (●) or PO (O) 30 min. before a 17 Gy x-ray treatment. Tumors were excised 18 hr later, dispersed into single cell suspensions, and plated for clonogenic survival. Results are presented as the mean (+/- std. error) for three mice.

gle cell suspensions for assessment of clonogenic survival. These
studies involved the determination of the optimal time for drug
administration relative to irradiation (30 min prior to irradiation), determination of drug dose response, and evaluation of the
effect of x-ray dose on sensitizing activity (18,19). For PD
130908 the _in vivo_ enhancement ratio at the maximum tolerated dose
was 1.9 compared to 2.1 and 1.5 for RSU 1069 and SR 2508, respectively (18,19). Qualitatively similar results were obtained for
the SCC7 sarcoma.

We also evaluated the efficacy of PD 130908 against the KHT
sarcoma when given orally (Figure 3). To our surprise, PD 130908
was just as efficient when given PO as when given IP or IV (IV
data not shown). In addition, it proved considerably less toxic
when given PO, with maximum tolerated single doses of 150 mg/kg
and 400 mg/kg for IP (or IV) and PO administration, respectively
(18,22). It is not yet clear whether significant additional cell
killing can be achieved or whether the ultimate effect of the lower toxicity on oral administration will only be an improved therapeutic index.

Finally, since the severe emesis observed in the clinical
trial of RSU 1069 contributed to a decision to discontinue development of the compound, we evaluated PD 130908 for its emetic activity (Figure 4). We tested equitoxic doses of RSU 1069 and PD
130908 based on the mouse equivalent LD_{10} ($MELD_{10}$) in groups
of 4 beagle dogs. Incidence, number of emetic episodes, and time
to onset of emesis were recorded. PD 130908 proved to be considerable less emetic than RSU 1069 with the threshold dose for a 50%
incidence of emesis of 16 umol/kg (1/4 of the $MELD_{10}$) for PD
130908. We also evaluated the ability of antiemetic therapy to reverse the emesis produced by PD 130908 and have found that ondansetron, and to a lesser extent, metoclopramide, are effective (18,
19,23).

MANIPULATION OF DNA REPAIR AS AN APPROACH TO RADIOSENSITIZATION

Treatment of most cell cultures with varied doses of x-irradiation produces a cell survival curve characterized by a shoulder

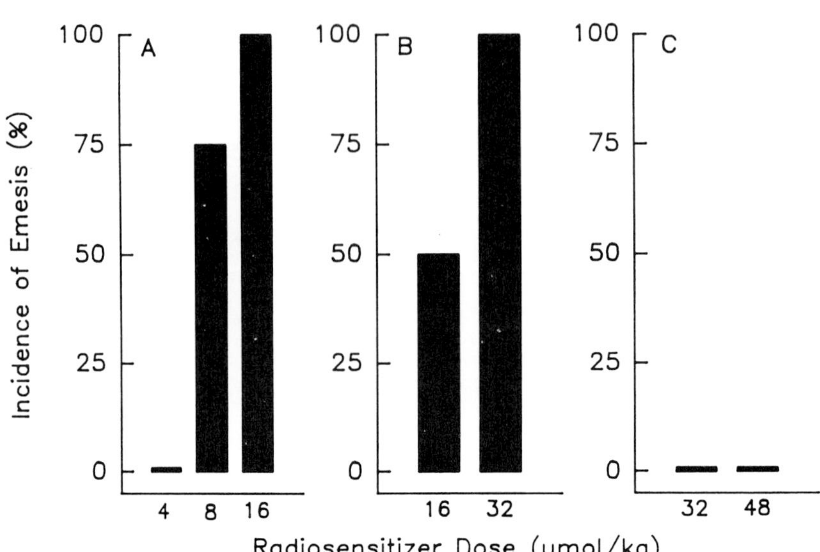

Figure 4.   Relative emetic potentials of PD 130908 and RSU 1069.
Groups of 4 beagle dogs received a 10 min. IV infusion of radiosensitizer at the indicated dosages.   The dogs were monitored for
up to 24 hr and the number of dogs with emesis, the number of emetic episodes for each animal, and the time of onset of emesis was
recorded.   Treatments were as follows: A, RSU 1069; B, PD 130908;
C, ondansetron (0.3 mg/kg) given 30 min. before the indicated dose
of PD 130908.

region at low doses and a region of exponential cell killing at
higher doses. The width of the shoulder region and the slope of
the exponential killing region vary with cell type. Electron-affinic sensitizers primarily affect the slope of the exponential
killing region of the survival curve and are hence expected to be
less effective at low x-ray doses than at high doses. Current
radiotherapy employs highly fractionated dosing to reduce normal
tissue damage and to allow for reoxygenation of the tumor between
treatments. The falling off of the cell killing potential of x-
irradiation at low x-ray doses (i.e., the shoulder of the survival
curve) is largely determined by the capacity of the cell to repair
and recover from x-ray induced damage. Clinically, the repair capacity of cells is inversely correlated with their radiosensitivity
(24). Given current radiotherapy practice employing multiple low
doses of x-rays and the domination of the response at low doses by

cellular repair processes, the modulation of the repair of x-ray induced DNA damage is a theoretically attractive target for radio-sensitization.

Our efforts in this area have been directed toward the enzyme poly(ADP-ribose) polymerase (ADPRP). This chromatin-associated nuclear enzyme is thought to be involved in several aspects of the repair of x-ray induced DNA damage (24-30). In addition, ADPRP levels are increased in response to DNA damage from x-irradiation. Finally, at the time we began our work, 3-aminobenzamide (3-AB) was the most potent known inhibitor of ADPRP, and it and structurally related compounds had been shown to be weak inhibitors of DNA repair and also had been shown to be weak radiosensitizers (31-33). These observations served as the basis of the rationale for our work.

PD 128763 is one of the compounds synthesized during the course of our studies (Figure 1). It arose from an attempt to determine the relationship between the position of the amide group relative to the rest of the molecule and inhibition of the enzyme (34). Several compounds were made with the amide group fixed in space via ring closure; these compounds were then modified with various substitutions on the rings.

PD 128763 was found to be about 60-fold more potent against the enzyme than the previous most potent inhibitor 3-aminobenza-mide (Figure 5). Its IC_{50} was 0.13 μM compared to 8 μM for 3-AB.

This improved activity relative to 3-AB was reflected in two of the most common assays of the ability of whole cells to recover from x-ray damage. In the first of these assays, the sublethal damage repair (SLDR) assay, exponentially growing V79 cells were exposed to two 5 Gy doses of x-ray separated by varied periods of time and the surviving fraction was measured by standard techniques (Table 2). The survival of cells treated only with x-ray improved about 3-fold (recovery ratio = 2.8) if the two x-ray doses were separated by at least 1 hr, reflecting repair of sublethal damage. Treatment with 3 mM 3-AB inhibited recovery completely. In contrast, treatment with 0.5 mM PD 128763 not only

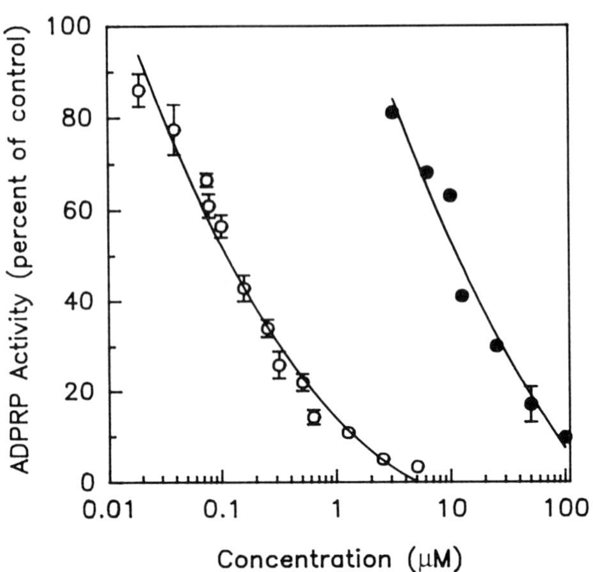

Figure 5. Inhibition of ADPRP by PD 128763 (O) and 3-AB (●). ADPRP was purified >800-fold from calf thymus (34) and assayed by measuring incorporation of [adenosine-2,8-^{3}H] into poly (ADP-ribose) (34,35). Results are presented as mean and standard error of at least 3 determinations.

Table 2

Inhibition of Cellular Recovery Processes by PD 128763

	Mean Recovery Ratio	
Treatment	SLDR	PLDR
Control	2.8	1.8
3-AB	1.0	1.0
PD 128763	0.6	0.4

completely inhibited the recovery process but also resulted in increased cell killing of approximately 2-fold (36-38).

In a similar assay, an assay for potentially lethal damage repair (PLDR), plateau phase V79 cells were exposed to a single dose of 10 Gy of x-irradiation and then held for varied lengths of

time in the presence or absence of inhibitor before plating in a
medium that allowed cell proliferation (Table 2). Once again, if
control cells were allowed a period of 1 hr for recovery prior to
plating in a growth conducive medium, survival improved roughly 2-
fold. At a concentration of 3 mM, 3-AB completely inhibited the
recovery process and 0.5 mM PD 128763 not only prevented recovery
but also increased the maximum cell killing, again by about 2-fold
over that obtained by x-ray alone with no recovery period (36,38).

These observations were extended by measurement of the repair
of DNA single and double strand breaks over time by alkaline and
neutral elution techniques. 3-aminobenzamide had little effect on
the repair of these lesions but PD 128763 reduced both the rate
and the ultimate degree of repair of these lesions (37,38).

PD 128763 is also a highly active radiosensitizer in vivo
(Figure 6). At the maximum tolerated dose of PD 128763 (100
mg/kg/injection), treatment with sensitizer plus x-ray produced

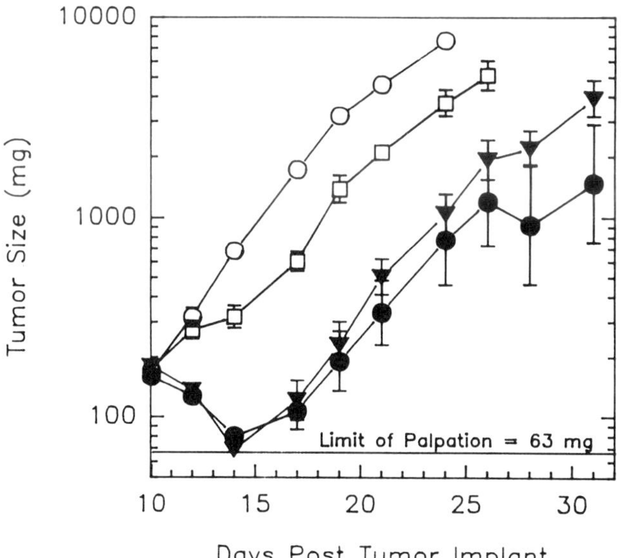

Figure 6. Radiosensitizing activity of PD 128763 against the SCC7
sarcoma. B6C3F$_1$ mice received 5x10^5 SCC7 sarcoma cells IM in
the right thigh on day 0. Treatment was given twice each day (12
hr apart) on days 10-13 as indicated: O, untreated controls; □,
2.5 Gy x-irradiation; ▼, 2.5 Gy x-irradiation + 62 mg/kg PD
128763; ●, 2.5 Gy x-irradiation + 100 mg/kg PD 128763. Data represent the mean and standard error from groups of 6 animals.

partial tumor regressions (>50% reduction in tumor burden) in 70% of the mice and a significant median tumor growth delay (20 days). Thus, the addition of PD 128763 to the x-ray regimen more than tripled the therapeutic effect of x-ray alone without an increase in host toxicity. In similar assays, the addition of PD 128763 to the treatment regimen has also produced enhanced tumor growth delays of 10 days or greater against the RIF-1 and KHT sarcomas suggesting the general utility of this approach to radiosensitization (39,40).

SUMMARY

We have explored two quite dissimilar chemical approaches to improved use of radiotherapy. In the first approach, we have attempted to take advantage of the potential tumor selectivity afforded by the development of hypoxic regions which are insensitive to x-irradiation. We targeted hypoxic cells by developing electron affinic or oxygen mimetic agents that are also hypoxia-selective cytotoxins. PD 130908 is one such compound. Its activity is characterized by: 1) high efficiency as a radiosensitizer, 2) high sensitizer enhancement ratios at maximum tolerated doses, 3) hypoxia-selective cytotoxicity (15-fold), 4) high activity on oral dosing, possibly resulting in either an improved therapeutic index and/or increased efficacy relative to parenteral dosing, 5) significant _in vivo_ activity in clinically relevant fractionated dosing regimens in several tumor models (data not shown), and 6) reduced emetic potential.

The hypoxia-selective cytotoxicity of compounds such as PD 130908 may prove to be highly significant. Brown and Koong have modeled the response of tumors to three different types of agents used with fractionated radiation regimens (41). These agents included a modulator of tumor oxygenation, an electron-affinic radiosensitizer, and a hypoxia-selective cytotoxin. Their study suggests that the use of a hypoxia-selective cytotoxin could produce a significantly superior reduction in tumor burden compared to other approaches if the hypoxia-selective cytotoxin could kill at least 50% of the hypoxic cell population at each treatment. This

approach takes full advantage of the potential selectivity afforded by the development of hypoxic regions within tumors. PD 130908
may be one such agent. Recent work by Cole et al. (22) confirmed
the ability of PD 130908 to kill hypoxic tumor cells _in vivo_, and
work from our laboratory (18) has demonstrated that significant
tumor growth delays can be produced by treatment of animals with
PD 130908 5 min after an x-ray dose. Under these conditions PD
130908 could not be acting as a classical electron-affinic radiosensitizer. These data are compatible with the idea that the
x-ray dose reduces the oxic fraction to a level at which the killing of hypoxic cells by PD 130908 can be measured.

In the second approach, we have attempted to reduce tumor
cell survival after irradiation by inhibition of cellular recovery
processes. PD 128763 is one of the most potent inhibitors known
of the enzyme ADPRP. We have been able to demonstrate its inhibition of whole cell recovery processes and even its potentiation
of radiation induced cell killing by several methods. Consistent
with those data, we have also shown that PD 128763 inhibits the
repair of DNA damage (both single and double strand breaks). The
observation of potentiated cell killing beyond the effects of
inhibition of recovery was unexpected and is as yet unexplained.
PD 128763 was also found to have significant activity on clinically relevant fractionated treatment regimens _in vivo_.

Although both of these approaches have resulted in compounds
with significant radiosensitizing activity _in vivo_, they differ
strongly in several ways with respect to their potential clinical
utility in conjunction with radiation therapy. The use of hypoxia-
selective electron-affinic agents carries with it a strong rationale for selectivity taking advantage of the development of hypoxia, both chronic and intermittent, within tumors. Normal, well
oxygenated tissues in theory would not be radiosensitized by such
an agent, nor would they be subject to a direct cytotoxicity if
the agent's degree of selectivity for hypoxic cells were high
enough. A key weakness of this approach is the theoretical loss
of efficacy of this approach at low x-ray doses such as those currently employed in the clinic. This is especially true for tumors

with large shoulders on the x-ray dose/survival curve. Hence, this approach appears poorly adapted to current radiotherapy practice. Nevertheless, studies in our laboratory have demonstrated the efficacy of PD 130908 on fractionated radiation regimens similar to those used in the clinic. A key factor in the potential utility of compounds like PD 130908 may be the combination of hypoxia-selective cytotoxicity with the conventional radiosensitizing activity.

The weakness of the inhibition of repair approach is its weak rationale for selectivity beyond that afforded by the local or regional aspect of radiotherapy itself. It is known that repair capacities vary widely among different cell types or lines, but little data exist to suggest that tumor cells have a uniformly higher or lower capacity for repair than normal tissues. We are currently evaluating the degree of tumor versus host cell selectivity of PD 128763 in combination with x-irradiation. The data presented here and elsewhere do suggest that for whatever the reason we achieve significant therapeutic benefit with little obvious toxicity. A major strength of this approach is that it is uniquely suited to the highly fractionated radiotherapy regimens currently in use. Current therapy involves radiation doses clearly within or very near the shoulder of the response curve for most cells. The key role of cellular recovery processes in this region of the x-ray dose response curve provides the rational for the approach. Our data clearly suggest that this approach has potential utility on clinically relevant therapeutic regimens.

It is perhaps noteworthy that these two approaches to improved radiotherapy have complimentary strengths and weaknesses. Given that both approaches have demonstrated significant activity in our experimental models, it seems reasonable to suggest that they might prove most efficacious when used in combination with one another. Clearly, the combination of dissimilar drugs has been the mainstay of chemotherapy for many years. The use of drugs, even as single agents, for the improvement of radiotherapy is still in its infancy. Nevertheless, given the heterogeneity of human tumor cell populations, the combination of dissimilar

193

"radiosensitizing" agents, once they are available, may prove a significant advance in radiotherapy just as it was for chemotherapeutics.

ACKNOWLEDGMENTS

The work reviewed here represents the combined efforts of a large number of investigators and their staffs. These include (Warner-Lambert) Drs. W.L. Elliott, C.M. Arundel-Suto, M. Suto, and H. Showalter; (MRC) Drs. G. Adams, M. Fielden, I. Stratford; and (U Rochester) Dr. D. Siemann.

REFERENCES

1.   Brady LW, Sheline GE, Suntharalingam N, Sutherland RM: The interdisciplinary program for radiation oncology research: Overview. Cancer Treat. Symp. 1:1-11, 1984.
2.   Diamond JJ, Hanks GH, Kramer S: The structure of radiation oncology practices in the continental United States. Int. J. Radiat. Oncol. Biol. Phys. 14:547-548, 1988.
3.   Russo A, Mitchell J, Kinsella T et al: Determinants of radiosensitivity. Sem. Oncol. 12:332-349, 1985.
4.   Adams GE Clarke ED, Flockhart IR et al: Structure-activity relationships in the development of hypoxic cell radiosensitizers. Int. J. Radiat. Biol. 35:133-150, 1979.
5.   Weissberg JB, Son YH, Papac RJ et al: Randomized clinical trial of mitomycin C as an adjunct to radiotherapy in head and neck cancer. Int. J. Radiat. Oncol. Biol Phys. 17:3-9, 1989.
6.   Chaplin DJ: Hydralazine-induced tumor hypoxia: A potential target for cancer chemotherapy. J. Natl. Cancer Inst. 81:618-622, 1989.
7.   Nakatsuguwa S: Potentially lethal damage repair and its implication in cancer treatment. In: Modification of Radiosensitivity in Cancer Treatment. T Sugahara (ed), Academic Press, Toyko, pp. 221-250, 1984.
8.   Thames HD, Peters LJ, Withers HR, Fletcher GH: Accelerated fractionation vs. hyper fractionation rationales for several treatments per day. Int. J. Radiat. Oncol. Biol. Phys. 9:127-138, 1983.
9.   Svoboda VHJ: Further experience with radiotherapy by multiple daily sessions. Br. J. Radiol. 51:363-369, 1978.
10. Glatstein E, Lichter AS, Fraass BA et al: The imaging revolution and radiation oncology: Use of CT, ultrasound, and NMR for localization, treatment planning and treatment delivery. Int. J. Radiat. Oncol. Biol. Phys. 11:299-314, 1985.
11. Brown JM: Evidence for acutely hypoxic cells in mouse tumours, and a possible mechanism of reoxygenation. Br. J. Radiol. 52:650-656, 1979.

12. Alper T: Cellular Radiobiology. Cambridge University Press, Cambridge, 1979.
13. Coleman CN, Bump EA, Kramer RA: Chemical modifiers of cancer treatment. J. Clin. Oncol. 6:709-733, 1988.
14. Adams GE, Ahmed I, Sheldon PW, Stratford IJ: Radiation sensitization and chemopotentiation: RSU 1069, a compound more efficient than misonidazole _in vitro_ and _in vivo_. Br. J. Cancer 49:571-577, 1984.
15. Chaplin DJ, Durand RE, Stratford IJ: The radiosensitizing and toxic effects of RSU-1069 on hypoxic cells in a murine tumor. Int. J. Radiat. Oncol. Biol. Phys. 12:1091-1095, 1986.
16. Silver ARJ, O'Neill P: Interaction of the aziridine moiety of RSU-1069 with nucleotides and inorganic phosphate. Implications for alkylation of DNA. Biochem. Pharmacol. 35:1107-1112, 1986.
17. Horwich A, Holliday SB, Deacon JM, Peckham MJ: A toxicity and pharmacokinetic study in man of the hypoxic cell radiosensitizer RSU-1069. Br. J. Radiol. 39:1238-1240, 1986.
18. Sebolt-Leopold JS, Arundel-Suto CM, Elliott WL et al: Preclinical evaluation of PD 130908, a desoxy analog of RSU 1069 with superior potency and reduced toxicities. Proc. 38th Annual Mtg. Radiat. Res. Soc. Abst. Cv 14, 1990.
19. Leopold WR, Arundel-Suto CM, Elliott WL et al: _In vitro_ and _in vivo_ evaluation of the radiosensitizer PD 130908, an analog of RSU 1069 with superior potency and reduced toxicity. Proc. Am. Assoc. Cancer Res. 31:393, 1990.
20. Overgaard J, Hansen HS, Jorgensen K, Hansen MH: Primary radiotherapy of larynx and pharynx carcinoma - an analysis of some factors influencing local control and survival. Int. J. Radiat. Oncol. Biol. Phys. 12:515-521, 1986.
21. Brown JM, Yu NY, Brown DM, Lee WW: SR-2508, a 2 nitro imidazole amide which should be superior to misonidazole as a radio sensitizer for clinical use. Int. J. Radiat. Oncol. Biol. Phys. 7:695-703, 1981.
22. Cole S, Stratford IJ, Fielden EM et al: Dual function nitroimidazoles less toxic than RSU1069: Selection of candidate drugs for clinical trial (RB 6145 and/or PD 130908). Int. J. Radiat. Oncol. Biol. Phys. In press.
23. Sebolt-Leopold JS, Vincent PW, Beningo KA et al: Pharmacologic/pharmacokinetic evaluation of emesis induced by analogs of RSU 1069 and its control by antiemetic agents. Int. J. Radiat. Oncol. Biol. Phys. In press.
24. Thraves PJ, Mossman KL, Brennan T, Dritschilo A: Differential radiosensitization of human tumor cells by 3-aminobenzamide and benzamide: Inhibitors of poly (ADP-ribosylation). Int. J. Radiat. Biol. 50:961-972, 1986.
25. Benjamin RC, Gill DM: Dependence of poly (ADP-ribose) synthesis on strand breakage in DNA. J. Biol. Chem. 255:10493-10501, 1980.
26. Oghushi H, Yoshihara K, Kaniya T: Bovine thymus poly (ADP-ribose) polymerase. Physical properties and binding to DNA. J. Biol. Chem. 255:6205-6211, 1980.

27. Durkacz BW, Omidiji O, Gray DA, Shall S: (ADP-ribose)$_n$
    participates in DNA excision repair. Nature (London)
    283:593-596, 1980.
28. Nduka N, Skidmore CJ, Shall S: The enhancement of cyto-
    toxicity of N-Methyl-N-Nitroso-Urea and of gamma-irradiation
    by inhibitors of poly (ADP-ribose) polymerase. Eur. J.
    Biochem. 105:525-530, 1980.
29. Ben-Hur E, Utsumi H, Elkind MM: Inhibitors of poly (ADP-
    ribose) synthesis enhance x-ray killing of log phase chinese
    hamster cells. Radiat. Res. 97:546-555, 1984.
30. Wasserman K, Newman RA, McLaughlin JD et al: A possible role
    for altered poly(Adenosine diphosphoribose)-synthesis in the
    sensitivity of human head and neck squamous carcinoma cells
    to ionizing radiation. Biochem. Biophys. Res. Commun.
    154:1041-1046, 1988.
31. Lunec J, George AM, Hedges M et al: Postirradiation sen-
    sitization with the ADP-ribosyltransferase inhibitor
    3-acetamidobenzamide. Br. J. Cancer Suppl. VI. 49:19-25,
    1984.
32. Huet J, Laval F: Influence of poly (ADP-ribose) synthesis
    inhibitors on the repair of sublethal and potentially lethal
    damage in -irradiated mammalian cells. Int. J. Radiat.
    Biol. 47:655-662, 1985.
33. Brown DM, Evans JW, Brown JM: The influence of inhibitors of
    poly (ADP-ribose) polymerase on x-ray induced potentially
    lethal damage repair. Br. J. Cancer Suppl. VI. 49:27-34,
    1984.
34. Suto MJ, Turner WR, Arundel-Suto CM et al: Dihydroisoquino-
    linones: The design and synthesis of a new series of potent
    inhibitors of poly (ADP-ribose) polymerase. Anticancer Drug
    Design 6:107-117, 1991.
35. Shizuta Y, Ito S, Nakata K, Hazaishi O: Poly (ADP-ribose)
    synthetase from calf thymus. Methods in Enzymology
    66:159-165, 1980.
36. Arundel-Suto, CM, Scavone SV, Turner WR et al: Effects of
    PD128763, a new potent inhibitor of poly (ADP-ribose) poly-
    merase, on x-ray induced cellular recovery processes in
    Chinese hamster V79 cells. Radiat. Res. 126:367-371, 1991.
37. Arundel-Suto CM, Sebolt-Leopold JS: Inhibition of DNA double
    strand break repair by inhibitors of poly (ADP-ribose) poly-
    merase and its relationship to inhibition of cellular re-
    covery in Chinese hamster V79 cells. Submitted for publica-
    tion.
38. Sebolt-Leopold JS, Arundel-Suto CM, Scavone SV et al:
    Development of a new series of potent ADP-ribosyltransferase
    inhibitors: The dihydro-isoquinolinones. Proc. Am. Assoc.
    Cancer Res. 31:418, 1990.
39. Elliott WL, Sebolt-Leopold JS, Leopold WR, Siemann DW: In
    vivo evaluation of a new potent inhibitor of ADP-ribosyltrans-
    ferase activity, PD128763. Proc. Am. Assoc. Cancer Res.
    31:418, 1990.

40. Siemann DW, Sebolt-Leopold JS, Leopold WR, Elliott WL:
     Effects of PD128763, a new potent inhibitor of ADP-ribosyl
     transferase, on radiation induced cellular recovery processes
     in solid tumors. Proc. 38th Annual Mtg. Radiat. Res. Soc.
41. Brown JM, Koong A: Therapeutic advantage of hypoxic cells in
     tumors: A theoretical study. JNCI 83:178-185, 1991.

10

LARGE SCALE ANTICANCER DRUG SCREENING AT STERLING DRUG INC.

Paul F. Cavanaugh, Jr. and Kenneth C. Mattes

Historically, large scale anticancer drug discovery screening programs have identified clinically useful antitumor agents
as evident from the high success rate in the chemotherapeutic
treatment of selected forms of cancer (primarily hematologic neoplasms). The relatively poor response rates for the treatment of
solid tumors most likely reflects the screening systems from which
most clinically used agents were discovered, namely leukemia based
screens. New assay systems, such as those developed by Dr. Thomas
Corbett and colleagues (1) are based on discovering those agents
with solid tumor activity and possibly selectivity. Because leukemia based screens often select various structural classes with
identical chemotypes, it is our opinion that screening systems
geared to select those agents demonstrating selective toxicity
versus solid tumors may identify new chemotypes.

The Eastman Kodak and Sterling Drug Chemical Inventories
offer a diverse new source of potential anticancer agents. Our
primary goal was to screen this inventory in the most expeditious
manner possible to discover new anticancer agents. As with any
screening program where very little bias is placed on compound selection, the number of useful leads discovered is directly related
to both the compound throughput and cut-off criteria utilized to
declare compounds either active or inactive at the _in vitro_ and _in
vivo_ levels. In addition, the types of compounds discovered will
no doubt reflect the type of screen chosen (e.g., solid tumor selective or leukemia selective).

198

To ensure an adequate compound throughput, not only is a good assay system required but a well characterized organization of one's chemical file and logistic support to handle compound collection, distribution, and data management is imperative. The purpose of this presentation is to review the results of the past two years of our large scale anticancer drug discovery program at Sterling Drug in collaboration with Dr. Tom Corbett and colleagues at Wayne State University.

The primary assay system chosen was the soft agar disk diffusion assay of Corbett, et. al., as described in more detail in other chapters of this book and in reference 1. As shown in Figure 1, this tumor stem cell assay involves plating of murine tumor cells which have been passaged _in vivo_ or human tumor cells which have been passaged continually in tissue culture. The assay system was purposely devised to accommodate very small amounts of sample (50-500 ug/disk) to be spotted on filter paper disks and placed on the edge of the petri dish containing a lawn of tumor cells. The cytotoxicity of a compound is measured by the zone of cytotoxicity (no cell growth) observed, similar to a Kirby-Bauer disk diffusion assay (Figure 1). This clonogenic assay has two main advantages, namely ease of the assay and the small amount of sample material which is needed. This second point is critical

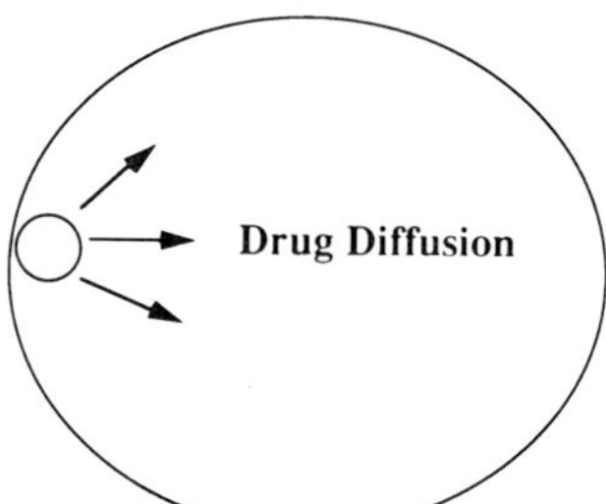

Figure 1. Schematic of the Disk Diffusion Soft Agar Assay with the four possible results indicated.

199

when screening a large compound inventory as often very little
sample is available for evaluation.

A flowchart of the screening operation is presented in Figure
2. The chemical file was initially split into distinct structural
classes by Dr. Bill Washburn and coworkers at the Kodak Research
Laboratories. Ten percent of the compounds from each structural
class were selected for primary evaluation. Samples chosen also

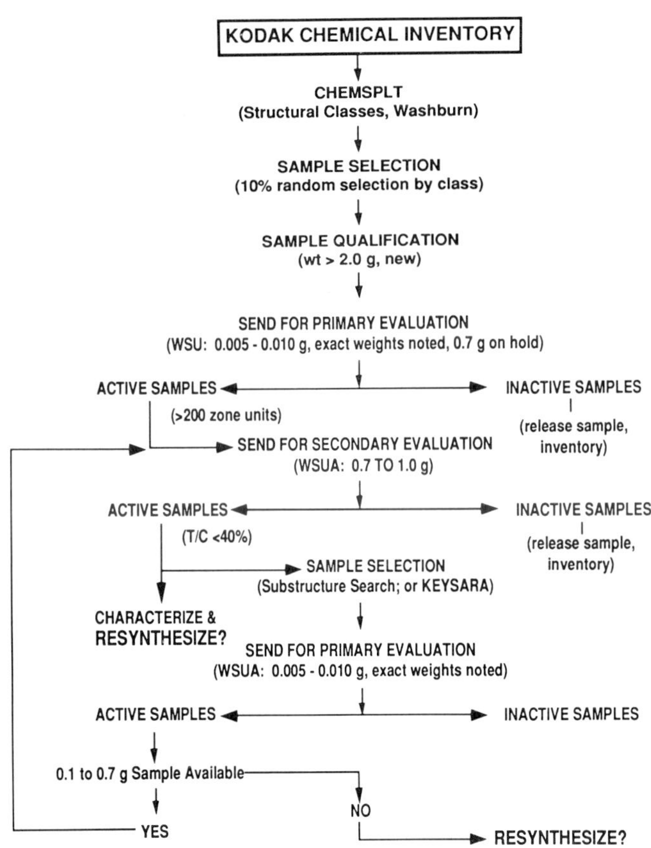

FIG. 2   ANTICANCER DRUG SCREENING FLOWCHART

Figure 2. Anticancer drug screening flowchart.

had an intitial qualification that at least 2 grams or more of sample be available for primary and secondary _in vitro_ screening, _in vivo_ screening, and analytical (purity and structure verification) analysis. Therefore, a known sample amount was reserved solely for this screening program until results indicated that it was of no utility and could be released for use in other testing programs. Approximately 5-10 mg of each sample chosen was sent for primary evaluation in the soft agar disk diffusion assay. Samples were declared to be active at this level if the difference of zone units of cytotoxicity in the solid tumor line(s) tested was greater than or equal to 200 zone units (200 zone units = 6 mm). At this point, 700-1000 mg of material were designated for evaluation in the murine solid tumor model where activity was seen _in vitro_.

For each compound, the dose, route, and schedule of administration was initially optimized to reach the maximally tolerated nonlethal total dose and schedule. Compounds displaying a percent Treated/Control (% T/C) value for tumor mass of less than 40% at the maximum nonlethal dose were considered active. The compound inventory was subsequently searched in a systematic manner for compounds containing related substructures. Analogs were sent for _in vitro_ analysis in the primary assay. In addition, at this point the structure of any _in vivo_ active was verified. Given the age of some of the materials tested and the fact that some structures had been assigned without the benefit of modern physicochemical techniques, the inclusion of structural verification at this stage was deemed to be extremely important. Compound resynthesis and retesting was initiated for two of the most active leads (% T/C <10%) at this point in addition to analog design and preparation.

As mentioned previously, compounds were chosen for _in vivo_ testing based on their different cytotoxicity in solid tumors versus leukemia. Figure 3 displays the number of compounds from a set of 3,120 unique samples which were run through the primary assay and displayed various differences in activity between the solid tumor lines indicated and L1210 leukemia. The relative sensitivity of each cell line is apparent. What is also apparent is

the fact that all the murine lines were much more sensitive than
the cultured human tumor lines used. Figure 4 compares the percent of compounds tested in each line which displayed various zone
unit differences versus L1210 leukemia. At a cut-off level of
>200 zone units using the murine lines colon 38, panc 03, or colon

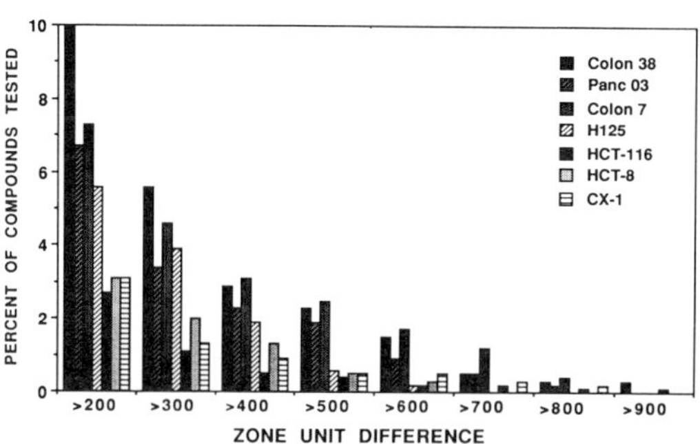

Figure 3. Solid tumor selectivity of compounds evaluated in the
soft agar disk diffusion assay. Results are expressed as the number of compounds which displayed the indicated zone unit differences in the cell lines used (One zone unit = 6.5 mm).

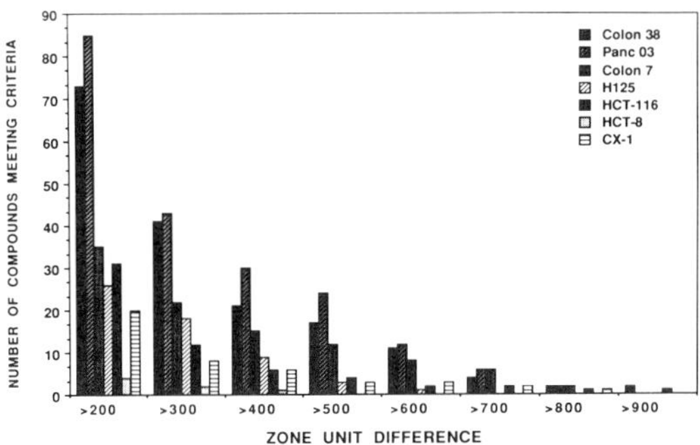

Figure 4. Solid tumor selectivity of compounds evaluated in the
soft agar disk diffusion assay. Results are expressed as the percent of compounds tested which displayed the indicated zone unit
differences in the cell lines used (One zone unit = 6.5 mm).

7, 6-10% of compounds tested met the criteria of >200 zone units difference compared to L1210 leukemia. The bargraphs also emphasize the relative insensitivity of human tumor cell lines passaged in culture versus the _in vivo_ passaged murine lines used. Whether this is a general phenomena to be expected with the use of murine solid tumors passaged _in vivo_ and cultured human lines or specific to the lines selected is not known.

Of the compounds screened to date, which represented over 13,000 at the _in vitro_ level and over 320 at the _in vivo_ level, one compound (Compound A), displayed promising _in vitro_ activity in the primary disk diffusion assay as displayed in Table 1.

Table 1

Disk Diffusion Soft Agar Assay Results for a Lead Compound (Compound A) Discovered by the Screening System Employed.

Agent	µg/Disk	Zone Units					
		L1210	Colon 38	Colon 7	HCT 116	HCT-8	LMC
Compound A	350	0-260	600-670		0-380		120-370
Compound A	125	100-150		500-600		0-150	0-150

Although active against L1210 leukemia, it was much more active against both the colon 38 and colon 7 tumors, whereas activity in the human lines and a low malignancy cell line (LMC) was very low. Had the criteria for choosing these compounds been based on activity against cultured human tumor cells, this compound would clearly not have been selected for _in vivo_ evaluation.

Initial _in vivo_ evaluation of Compound A in colon 38 resulted in % T/C values of 3% at the maximum nonlethal dose (Table 2). This compound has displayed potent activity in a number of murine tumor models. Most notably, it is curative in the highly metastatic murine tumor model colon 51 (Table 2). Resynthesis and retesting of this compound has reconfirmed this activity. Studies to determine breadth of activity and analog activity are in progress at this time.

Table 2

In <u>Vivo</u> Antitumor Activity of Compound A Administered s.c.

Tumor	Schedule	Total Dose (mg/kg)	Max.Wt. Loss	Drug Deaths	% T/C	Log Kill	Cures
Mamm16/C	QD1-4	800	-2.6	0/5	0	2.1	0/5
Colon 51	QD3-7	840	-4.2	0/5	0	> 4	4/5
Colon 51	QD3-7	505	-2.0	0/5	0	> 4	4/5
Panc 03	QD3-8	1580	-3.6	0/5	0	1.8	0/5
Panc 03	QD3-9	1190	-2.4	0/5	12	1.2	0/5
Panc 03	QD3-9	700	-1.0	0/5	7	1.8	0/5
Colon 38	QD5-12	2240	-3.4	2/5	0	NA	0/5
Colon 38	QD5-12	1344	-1.8	0/5	3	NA	0/5
Colon 38	QD5-12	808	-1.2	0/5	45	< 1	0/5

To-date, of the 7% of compounds tested at the <u>in vitro</u> level
which were sent for <u>in vivo</u> evaluation and which have been tested
(~320 compounds), approximately 7% met the activity criteria of
% T/C <40% (Table 3). However, only two compounds, (0.6%) tested
<u>in vivo</u> were active at a level of % T/C <10% in at least one

Table 3

Summary of <u>in vivo</u> screening data for compounds selected from the
soft agar disk diffusion assay across all tumor models used (primarily colon 38 and panc 03). The best results for each compound
in any tumor line was included.

% T/C[b]	Number of Compounds	% Compounds Tested
<40	24	7.1
<30	14	4.1
<20	7	2.1
<10	2	0.6

murine tumor model. This exemplifies the low percentage of compounds discovered in an assay such as this which can be expected and re-emphasizes that large scale drug screening is a 'numbers game'. Indeed, it is quite likely that one sampling of a chemical file, although a statistically significant representation of that compound file would miss a considerable number of active compounds. This point is most clear when one observes the complete inactivity of analogs of a given series from the same class of compounds from which the original active compound resided. It can be expected based on probability that a rescreening of a large chemical inventory (excluding previously screened material) should yield a roughly equal percentage of new lead compounds. This places importance on the throughput of one's screening assay. Based on our experience, we feel that the disk difussion soft agar assay linked to murine solid tumor model systems, such as those described, offers an efficient method of discovering active anti-tumor agents from a large, organized, and diverse chemical collection.

ACKNOWLEDGEMENTS

The authors would like to thank Drs. Thomas Corbett and Frederick Valeriote and their laboratories for the evaluation of compounds, Ms. Linda Longaker and her staff in the Kodak Chemical Library for sample preparation and handling, Dr. Jerome Verlin, Mr. Larry Beattie, and Mr. Albert Lazarovici for data management support, and also the support of the National Cancer Institute (NCI Grant CA-45962).

REFERENCE

1. Corbett TH, Wozniak A, Gerpheide S, Hanka L: A selective two-tumor soft agar assay for drug discovery. In: In Vitro and In Vivo Models for Detection of New Antitumor Drugs; 14th International Congress of Chemotherapy. LJ Hanka, T Kondo, RJ White (eds), University of Tokyo Press, pp. 5-14, 1986.

11

ARE ANTISENSE OLIGONUCLEOTIDES THERAPEUTIC AGENTS OF THE FUTURE?

George S. Johnson

The idea of using sequence-specific oligonucleotides to inhibit the expression of individual genes and thereby cure a disease is a topic of great interest in the scientific as well as the financial communities. Most major pharmaceutical companies have a strong interest if not an active research group working on the topic. Numerous small "start-up" biotechnology companies have been organized in the past two or three years whose major or sole reason for existence is the development of oligonucleotides as therapeutic agents. Is this so-called "antisense" approach non-sense or is it realistic? Can we expect that anti-sense reagents will be the drugs of the future? An answer to these questions is not possible at this time. However, anti-sense is a fertile area of investigation. Much research and development is underway on many fronts. Clearly, insight into the feasability of anti-sense agents as therapeutic drugs will be forthcoming. In this article I will highlight some recent developments as well as bring out some of the problems and pitfalls encountered and the pursuits researchers are taking to circumvent these problems. Readers are referred to the recent reviews (1-3) and volumes (4-6) on anti-sense research for more specific details.

Genes are expressed by transcription of the "information" strand of DNA into RNA in the nucleus. The resultant transcript is processed into mRNA, transported into the cytoplasm, and translated into protein (Figure 1). A disease state could result if this normal process is altered. In some diseases genetic control mechanisms may not function properly leading to an

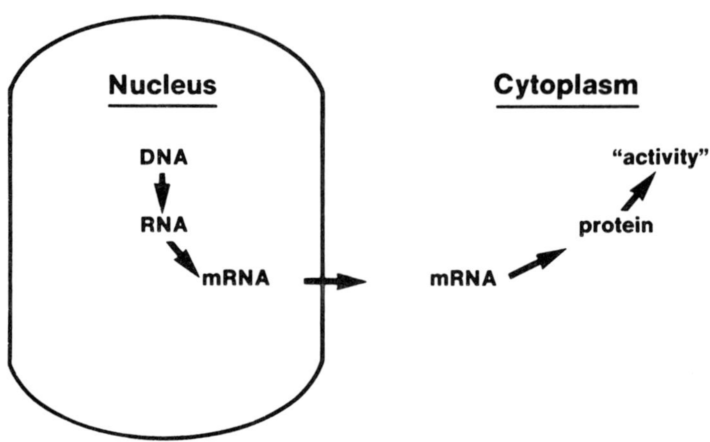

Figure 1.   Sequence of events in gene expression.

abnormal accumulation of a protein. If the DNA is mutated, an
abnormal protein may be produced. In other cases such as viral or
bacterial infection, proteins foreign to the cell are produced
causing the disease. In all situations to cure the disease it is
necessary to rid the organism of the abnormal protein or inhibit
its activity. Traditionally, drugs have been designed or selected
as enzyme inhibitors or as toxic agents to kill cells which
express the abnormal gene product. However, this approach suffers
from selectivity problems; i.e., identification of agents which
are target specific and do not act at other sites leading to
undesirable toxicity. A gene-based therapy to inhibit solely the
expression of the gene in question would eliminate the problem of
drug selectivity. Therein lies the strength and motivation for
the development of anti-sense technology.

The theoretical basis for anti-sense therapy is depicted in
Figure 2. The coding strand of the double stranded DNA is tran-
scribed into RNA. An added oligomer, the anti-sense molecule,
which is complimentary to the RNA, forms a duplex thereby "inactivating" the RNA and preventing its translation into protein.
Duplex DNA could also be a target of the anti-sense oligomer to

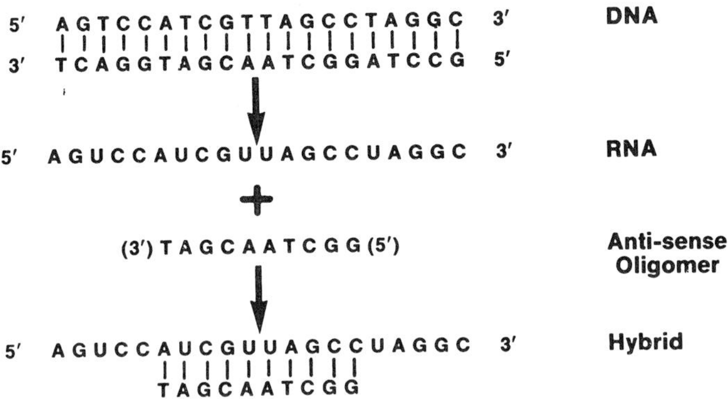

Figure 2. Theoretical basis of anti-sense therapy.

inhibit gene expression directly. More will be said about the
target nucleic acid later. Statistically an oligomer of about 15
bases should define a unique sequence and specifically inhibit the
gene. Anti-sense oligomers can be oligodeoxynucleotides chemically synthesized and added extracellularly, or alternatively RNA
produced from genetically engineered vectors. Each approach has
its own advantages and disadvantages and is under active investigation. This review will emphasize development of the oligodeoxynucleotides.

In designing a drug for therapeutic benefit several parameters have to be considered. First of all, the target must be
clear and optimally defined. For anti-sense development the gene
must be identified, isolated, and the base sequence determined.
Viruses provide a unique and well defined target, but most viruses
are genetically complex. Hence, it is not always apparent which
gene in the viral genome would serve as the most effective target.
For cancer therapy the situation may be even more complex. Oncogenes and growth factor/receptor genes are likely to be targets,
but in no case has it been established that suppression of any one
of them has therapeutic value in humans. In addition, once the

appropriate gene has been identified, the specific bases within
the gene to be targeted must be determined. It is impractical to
use an antisense molecule complementary to the entire gene or to
the complete mRNA since a polymer in the kilobase range would be
required. Moreover, in studies done to date not all 15-20 base
sequences complimentary to various regions of a given gene are
equally effective in inhibiting expression. In general, the 5′
regulatory region or splice junction sequences are more sensitive
than are coding sequences. Clearly, the most effective regions
will have to be defined for each gene.

Another critical question is whether RNA or DNA should be the
target of the anti-sense oligomer. In most studies published to
date RNA has been the object of investigation (1-6). The reasoning is that since it is found in the cytoplasm mRNA should be
readily accesible to the oligomer. In addition RNA-DNA base
pairing is well understood. However, there are serious theoretical drawbacks to RNA targeting. First of all, numerous, perhaps
thousands, of copies of a message exist in a cell. Secondly, it
would be expected that the anti-sense oligomers would have to be
applied for extended periods of time since mRNA is continuosly
being synthesized. These two problems raise the question of the
effectiveness of an oligomer to inhibit gene expression <u>in</u> <u>vivo</u>.
DNA may provide a more attractive target. In has been known for
many years that a third strand of DNA can form a triplex with
double stranded DNA (3). Such a complex would not likely be a
substrate for RNA polymerase, thereby preventing RNA synthesis.
Importantly, by targeting DNA it may be possible to cure some
genetic diseases or viral diseases where the viral genome is
stably integrated into the host chromsome such as is the case in
AIDS. The reasoning for this exciting possibility is that repair
of damaged DNA caused by a covalently attached third DNA strand
could cause a permanent inactivation of the genome. Such an inactivation would most likely occur if the coding sequence of the
gene were targeted so that the codons would be out of phase and
protein synthesis would not occur. Alternatively, if repair of
this abnormal complex is not possible or incomplete, cell death

may result. These scenarios are theoretical at the present time but they certainly merit serious consideration for exploitation. On the negative side, as a consequence of its nuclear location and the complex structure of chromatin, DNA may not be as accesible to exogenous oligomers as is RNA. Moreover, the physical-chemical parameters for triplex base pairing have not been clearly elucidated. More theoretical studies will have to be done to learn the third strand "binding code". Effective anti-sense drugs must be able to be administered to the patient, arrive at the diseased cell intact, enter the cell, and once inside the cell find and bind to the complimentary base sequences. At first thought meeting these requirements seems an impossible task. Nucleases in the blood or in the cell seem certain to at least partially degrade the oligomer. Also, conventional pharmacological principles would predict that such a highly charged molecule would enter the cell very slowly if at all. As an attempt to remedy these problems chemists have synthesized various DNA analogs. All published analogs to date have modifications in the phosphate backbone since alterations in the bases would likely interfere with base pairing (1-6). Phosphorothioates, in which one nonbridging oxygen is replaced with sulfur, are nuclease resistant and also have the advantage of maintaining the original charge of the DNA. Neutral analogs such as the methylphosphonates, phosphotriesters, and phosphoramidates have been synthesized and also found to be nuclease resistant. Each derivative has its own advantages and disadvantages, and none has emerged as superior enough over the others to be a clear candidate for therapeutic development. It should be noted that all of these synthetic compounds are a mixture of stereoisomers. As each monomeric unit is added during synthesis two stereoisomers are possible at the chiral phosphorus resulting in a oligomer of 2^{n-1} stereoisomers where n is the number of bases in the oligomer. A completely different and achiral analog based on formacetal linkages instead of the phosphate-oxygen structure has recently been synthesized, but biological activity with this analog has not yet been established (7).

Antisense oligonucleotides of various structural classes have been shown to have biological activity in model systems, but concentrations in the range of 10-100 μM are often required. However, it may not be feasible to achieve these concentrations _in vivo_. Hence, analogs by themselves may not be sufficient. Functional groups are being covalently added to oligomers to increase their potency. Examples include alkylating agents, intercalators, photoactivating agents, and chemical cleavage reagents such as Fe-EDTA. Another interesting concept is the use of tandem sequences (8). The idea is that two smaller sequences such as 15-mers in tandem may be almost as effective as the corresponding 30-mer, but much more practical to synthesize and administer. Certainly many more innovations will be forthcoming.

Do the oligomers actually enter the cell? Studies on the transport of the oligonucleotide analogs have been done, and uptake has been demonstrated. Neutral oligomers apparently enter by passive diffusion; whereas, charged species enter via a facilitated uptake system (1,3,4). The involvement of an 80 kilodalton protein has been suggested (9).

Obviously the most important result is the actual demonstration of biological activity in intact cells and in live animals. In tissue culture systems numerous base sequence specific effects have been reported. Examples include inhibition of expression of VSV, HSV, HIV, various oncogenes, retinol-binding protein, SV40 T-antigen, the mdr p-glycoprotein, and cyclic AMP-dependent protein kinase (1-6, 10-12). Examples of _in vivo_ activity have been reported only at conferences, and the results have not been published to the best of my knowledge. Topical administration in an ointment form of a methylphosphonate oligomer whose base sequence overlaps a splice junction of the Herpes simplex virus has been shown to attenuate HSV-induced lesions on mouse skin. This study is awaiting confirmation when more material becomes available (Paul Miller, Johns Hopkins University, personal communications). In another presentation it was reported that systemic administration of oligomers was effective in treatment of mice infected with tick-born encephalitis virus (Valentin

Vlassov, Novosibirsk, USSR) (3). As research progresses it is
expected that more _in vivo_ studies will be undertaken. A demonstration that a gene product can be diminished significantly in
the complex environment of an entire animal would greatly stimulate development of anti-sense technology.

The use of anti-sense oligonucleotides in human treatment is
the goal of this research; however, theoretical and practical
obstacles must be overcome before such therapy can be attempted.
Pharmacuetical considerations for anti-sense development have
recently been reviewed by Zon in (4). By making a few simple
assumptions several problems become apparent. Consider treatment
of a 70 kg human with a 15 base oligomer (molecular weight of
approximately 5,000 kilodaltons) which is active in _in vitro_ model
systems at 10 µM. At first approximation one would like to bring
the concentration of oligomer in the extracellular fluid (assume
14 liters) to this level. The minimal amount of material required
for this (assuming complete bioavailablity) would be 700 mg. At a
cost of $5 per mg (probably a minimum value for GMP produced
material with the chemical technology available today) it would
cost $3,500 per treatment. To make this estimate even approach
reality delivery mechanisms and schedules would have to be carefully delineated, and techniques would have to be developed to
sustain the peak concentration for longer periods of time. To
date only a few basic pharmacokinetic analyses have been done.
Following iv. bolus injection the oligomers are rapidly excreted
in the urine with a plasma half-life of 5-15 minutes depending
upon the conditions and the oligomer tested (3). Full scale
toxicology to determine safety remains to be done, and the
potential antigenicity of the oligomers must be carefully
evaluated.

It seems safe to conclude that for oligodeoxynucleotides to
become effective and realistic therapeutic agents, much development is necessary. The cost of the material will almost certainly
decrease when chemical engineers develop technology for production
of material on a kilogram scale. This will happen when, but probably not before, it becomes apparent that there is a need, i.e.,

convincing _in vivo_ efficacy of the agents is demonstrated. The
situation of anti-sense agents today is in some ways analagous to
the early days in the development of penicillin. At first the
antibiotic was scarce and expensive. But when it was clear that
penicillin would be a worthwhile drug, technology was developed to
produce it cheaply. It should be noted that the cost of synthetic
DNA (in mg amounts) has decreased by several orders of magnitude
in the thirty years since DNA was first synthesized by Khorana and
colleagues. Other means should be considered to optimize therapy
and decrease treatment cost. It seems doubtful that oligomers
could be considered for widespread use until potency is increased
at least 10-100 fold. To meet this need more potent derivatives
or oligomers with covalent adducts must be discovered. Perhaps
the most important but least studied area is drug delivery. Not
only must methods be worked out to deliver the oligomers to the
extracellular fluid at an effective dose, but the oligomers must
remain there for a sufficient length of time to be able to enter
the cells. Techniques should be developed to target cells which
express the abnormal gene product, a possibility in some diseases,
such that the entire organism need not be "bathed" in the oligomer. Some studies designed to augment delivery and uptake have
been undertaken. For example, covalent attachment of cholesterol
to oligomers has been found to increase the retention time in the
plasma several fold as well as facilitate uptake into the cell
(13). Also, attachment of poly-lysine as a carrier increases the
cellular uptake and potency (14).

One last point should be considered. Would a cost of up to
several thousand dollars per treatment allow widespread use of
anti-sense reagents as therapeutic agents? If the agents are
designed so that prolonged treatment, perhaps several times a
month for the rest of the patients's life, is necessary to control
the disease, the answer is probably, no. However, if only a few
treatments would cure the disease the answer would have to be,
yes. Even a total cost for the drug of $50,000 could be con-
sidered cheap if the treatment actually cures a disease for which
there is no better treatment and lifelong hospitalization is not

required. These concepts should be kept in mind when anti-sense
drugs are being contemplated and designed.

Are anti-sense agents drugs of the future? Today we cannot
be sure. The power of the concept is today's motivation. With a
few convincing demonstrations of _in vivo_ efficacy the theoretical
concept could quickly become a reality.

REFERENCES

1. Stein CA, Cohen JS: Oligodeoxynucleotides as inhibitors of
    gene expression: A review. Cancer Res. 48:2659-2668, 1988.
2. Zon G: Oligonucleotide analogues as potential chemothera-
    peutic agents. Pharm. Res. 5:539-549, 1988.
3. Rothenberg M, Johnson G, Laughlin C et al:
    Oligodeoxynucleotides as anti-sense inhibitors of gene ex-
    pression: Therapeutic implications. JNCI 81:1539-1544,
    1989.
4. In: Oligodeoxynucleotides: Antisense Inhibitors of Gene
    Expression, JS Cohen, (ed), CRC Press, Inc., Boca Raton, FL,
    1989.
5. In: Antisense RNA and DNA, DA Melton (ed), Cold Spring
    Harbor Laboratory, Cold Spring Harbor, NY, 1988.
6. In: Advances in Applied Biotechnology, Vol. 2, Discoveries
    in Antisense Nucleic Acids, CL Brakel (ed), Gulf Publishing
    Co., Houston, TX, 1989.
7. Matteucci M: Deoxyoligonucleotide analogs on formacetal
    linkages. Tetrahedron Lett. 31:2385-2388, 1990.
8. Maher L, Dolnick B: Specific hybridization arrest of dihydro-
    folate reductase mRNA _in vitro_ using anti-sense RNA or anti-
    sense oligodeoxynucleotides. Arch. Biochem. Biophys.
    253:214-220, 1987.
9. Loke SL, Stein CA, Zhang XH et al: Characterization of oligo-
    nucleotide transport into living cells. Proc. Natl. Acad.
    Sci. USA 86:3474-3478, 1989.
10. Vasanthakumar G, Ahmend NK: Modulation of drug resistance in
    a daunorubicin resistant subline with oligonucleoside methyl-
    phosphonates. Cancer Communications 1:225-232, 1989.
11. Cope FO, Wille JJ: Reteniod receptor antisense DNAs inhibit
    alkaline phosphatase induction and clonogenicity in malignant
    keratinocytes. Proc. Natl. Acad. Sci. USA 86:5590-5594,
    1989.
12. Tortora G, Clair T, Cho-Chung YS: An antisense oligodeoxy-
    nucleotide targeted against the Type II beta regulatory
    subunit mRNA of protein kinase inhibits cAMP-induced differ-
    entiation in HL-60 leukemia cell without affecting phorbol
    ester effects. Proc. Natl. Acad. Sci. USA 87:705-708, 1990.

13. Letsinger RL, Zhang G, Sun DK et al: Cholesteryl-conjugated oligonucleotides: Synthesis, properties, and activity as inhibitors of replication of human immunodeficiency virus in cell culture. Proc. Natl. Acad. Sci. USA 86:6553-6556, 1989.

14. Lemaitre M, Bayard B, LeBleu B: Specific antiviral activity of a poly(L-lysine)-conjugated oligodeoxynucleotide sequence complementary to vesicular stomatitis virus N protein mRNA initiation site. Proc. Natl. Acad. Sci. USA 84:648-652, 1987.

12

SUPERCOMPUTER AIDED DRUG DESIGN: APPLICATION IN ONCOLOGY AND
AIDS

Frederick H. Hausheer, U. Chandra Singh, Jeffrey D. Saxe,
Alexander L. Weis

Significant advancements in the treatment of cancer have developed during the last four decades as a result of dedicated clinical and experimental efforts. Many of the therapeutic gains are
related to discovery and development of more effective medicinal
agents, technologic advancements, and an enhanced understanding of
the fundamental chemical and biologic interactions involving the
pathogenesis and pathophysiology of these heterogenous diseases.
It is now possible to cure several types of malignancy and to
achieve significant palliation in a variety of other tumors. Unfortunately, many of the more common types of neoplasms (e.g. carcinomas of the lung, breast, GI tract, and melanoma) are refractory to therapy with currently available agents. A most significant obstacle to address in the coming years is multiple drug resistance in which the cytotoxic action of pharmacologic agents is
rendered ineffectual by a transmembrane pump in tumor cells
(1-3). Early in this past decade, infection with the human immunodeficiency virus (HIV) has presented a major health problem because of the lethal nature of the disease, significant latent interval between infection and disease manifestation, fluctuating/
evolving epidemiologic patterns, and the lack of effective therapy. An important complication of pharmacologic agents that must
be considered in the development of new therapeutic agents for the
AIDS and neoplastic disorders are the immediate and long term clinical toxicities that frequently affect the quality of life (4).
Because of the immediate and life-threatening nature of these diseases the untoward effects of these agents have been monitored

and managed expectantly, since some toxicities can be lethal to the patient. Our primary research is directed towards generating new classes of pharmacologic agents possessing highly specific cytotoxicity for neoplastic cells, and cells that have incorporated the HIV genome. The major goals of developing such agents will be to cure these diseases which are currently refractory to therapy with minimal patient toxicity.

The discovery that carcinogen and viral alterations in DNA play a central role in the pathogenesis and pathophysiology of malignancy and AIDS has been a significant accomplishment (1). There is increasing evidence of the existence of critical molecular targets in neoplastic cells and cells with incorporation of the HIV genome that distinctly differ from normal host cells. The partially redundant nature of DNA and the pattern of DNA sequence comprises a regulatory molecule that could be selectively inactivated by pharmacologic agents. Other molecular targets for therapy include various functional proteins and polysaccharides that are accessible to inactivation by pharmacophores and monoclonal antibodies. The most important marker of cytotoxicity is the loss of the cell's capacity to undergo replication. There are many independent cellular processes that are subject to pharmacologic modulation. The identification and characterization of molecular targets such as DNA and cellular proteins are increasing through state of the art applications of molecular biology, NMR, pharmacology, cytogenetics, and x-ray crystallography.

Biomedical research is entering an exciting new era with the advent of advanced molecular computational methods and supercomputers. The study of complex molecular processes can be more productively addressed by the combined efforts of a team of researchers composed of medicinal chemists, NMR spectroscopists, molecular biologists, bio-organic chemists, physical chemists, and x-ray crystallographers. The multidisciplinary efforts of these teams will be tightly coupled to computational analysis which will identify and permit greater understanding of key molecular interactions of interest, and will diminish the trial and error approach. Supercomputers are a critical component of this approach, since rapid feedback and design considerations must guide and complement experimental efforts to enhance productivity. The operating environment of these machines must be adaptable to many different algorithms and permit program enhancements on a frequent basis to simulate specific drug design problems of varying magnitude (5-11).

The interactions between drug and target molecules producing therapeutic effects are of an exceedingly complex nature. In nearly all instances the breadth of scientific questions dealing with understanding of these mechanisms far surpass the descriptive capacity of any single experimental discipline. For example, to describe the mechanisms of cytotoxicity of an agent related to methotrexate would involve conformational aspects of drug binding (x-ray crystallography), affinity of drug binding (protein chemistry), effects of DNA/RNA synthesis, functional effects of DNA/RNA-protein interactions (molecular biology, sequence analysis), and identification of transport and metabolism (cellular physiology, pharmacokinetics, and pharmacology). Clearly, the strength among individual experimental disciplines needs to be integrated into concisely identifying these processes through a common model and language. In the next decade researchers from different backrounds will rely heavily on graphically projected simulations made by supercomputer that will provide quantitative and qualitative predictions to guide and complement experimental efforts and drug design (15,18).

It is exciting to consider the prospective capacity to rationally design more effective agents useful in treating cancer and AIDS by optimally integrating the efforts and results of experimental disciplines with molecular computational methods and supercomputers. We believe that the speed and capacity of the developing generation of supercomputers can establish a tightly coupled theoretical and experimental effort to supplant traditional approaches to drug discovery and development. Supercomputers and numerical experimentation can provide rapid feedback between various laboratory experimental disciplines and focus the research effort (11,12). In a collaborative effort between Sterling Drug and the Drug Development Section of Medical Oncology at The University of

Texas Health Science Center at San Antonio, we are developing a multidisciplinary approach to enhance research productivity by numerical simulation of molecules involved in the treatment cancer and AIDS. These coupled theoretical/experimental efforts are beginning to provide qualitative and quantitative progress in understanding critical molecular interactions of interest. The results of such computations are applied to test ongoing hypotheses and to enhance considerations in experimental design by reducing (focusing) the number of possible considerations to more relevant elements. Use of these computational approaches will increasingly depend on supercomputers to provide rapid feedback to experimental research teams and provide an environment for the rapid development and enhancement of molecular computational algorithms.

Clinical experience has identified certain drug classes and individual agents which have significant intrinsic antitumor activity. The spectrum of malignancies for which these agents are active can vary considerably between individual agents, but there are certain consistent pharmacologic and clinical features that we consider significant. Our approach to developing new agents using molecular computational methods and Cray supercomputers (X-MP and Y-MP series) is based on the premise that these agents with significant clinical activity act via fundamentally important molecular interactions. If these molecular determinants were fully understood, this information could help to understand the mechanism(s) involved and the beneficial and untoward effects in both normal and neoplastic cells and to apply this information in rational drug design. Thus, our efforts involve studying agents with established curative potential and identifying molecular events that interact to produce clinical effects. In addition, by monitoring progress at all levels of drug testing and development we can identify newer agents with desirable chemical/biologic/pharmacologic features and subject these to similar analysis at an early stage.

One area of effort involves the use of _ab initio_ quantum mechanical and molecular mechanics methods to study chemical, conformational, electronic, and energetic properties of various

clinically active drug molecules which have been difficult to
study experimentally. One area pertains to cyclophosphamide, one
of the most widely used and effective anticancer and immunosuppressive agents. The activity profile of cyclophosphamide is broad
(solid tumors, leukemias, and lymphomas), and the recent capacity
to synthesize activated metabolites of this drug (e.g. 4-hydro-
peroxy-cyclophosphamide) has facilitated _ex_ _vivo_ purging of auto-
logous bone marrow for transplantation. With the supercomputer
and a hierarchy of advanced molecular computational methods
coupled to experimental efforts, a novel series of local chemical
determinants of DNA binding for this class of agent have been
identified (14). Certain metabolites of cyclophosphamide interact
with DNA and proteins of cells producing covalent crosslinks. The
major target of this class of drugs mediating cytotoxic events is
believed to be DNA, and most of the laboratory approaches in this
area dictate the use of highly complex experimental methods, which
in most instances can only partially characterize the interactions
at each step. _Ab_ _initio_ quantum mechanical calculations have provided structural, stereochemical, and chemical data for active
metabolites of the parent compound and prompted several previously
unconsidered experimental efforts that are yielding greater insight into the chemical properties of the drug. Using molecular
mechanics and molecular dynamics we have simulated the conformational and energetic interactions of six different crosslink complex ensemble trajectories in water at 300 K each for 50 psec.
These calculations helped to identify several previously unrecog-
nized molecular interactions that could significantly affect the
antitumor activity of this drug, and has given new leads for the
design of agents that bind efficiently to specific regions of DNA
(14). In the past, numerous attempts to describe specific struc-
tural/stereochemical relationships have eluded formidable efforts
by NMR or x-ray crystallography for several molecular species of
this class of antitumor agents. For example, _ab_ _initio_ calculations of several electronic states of one metabolic (phosphoramide
mustard) led us to design and use several previously unconsidered
and feasible experimental approaches, such as solid state NMR, and

additionally has provided new approaches, structural/chemical/ stereochemical data that is being used to design more effective agents. Based on computer simulations carried out over the past year and a half there is new evidence that agents in this class consistently bind DNA selectively, which is largely determined by specific factors including nucleotide sequence, conformation of the drug and DNA helix, electrostatic attraction and repulsion, and electron interactions involved in covalent adducts (14). During this time we have used these data to design prospectively a new series of multidisciplinary experimental approaches that delineate the magnitude of the effects projected by these calculations, and are devoting a strong effort to design more effective cytotoxic agents.

A significant advantage from computational analysis of molecular structure by supercomputer includes the capacity to interactively consider and test hypotheses prior to chemical synthesis and experimentation. Several anticancer drugs directly interact with DNA (e.g. mitomycin-C, doxirubicin, and DTIC), resulting in the formation of stable (covalent) nucleic acid adducts, or base intercalation. Other drugs such as methotrexate, VP-16 (and congeners) exert cytotoxic effects by binding to cellular proteins (dihydrofolate reductase and topoisomerase II, respectively). By simulating these interactions on the supercomputer we hope to identify molecular mechanisms of synergistic cell kill with combinations of agents in current use. There are several instances where multiple drug exposure exhibits cytotoxic effects by lethal inhibition of various cellular processes such as protein-DNA interactions, DNA replication, synthesis, and conformation. From such simulations, we have learned that interatomic distances between certain reactive sites under consideration in DNA vary as a function of the DNA sequence (and base composition). These are important developments since these interactions are considered to directly influence the ability of the drug to maximally exert its cytotoxic effects in the cancer cell. Other new findings from numerical simulation include the role of electrostatic interactions on the regional attraction or repulsion of a drug which regulate

initial binding of antitumor agents (19). The electrostatic potential surface of DNA varies significantly as a function of nucleotide sequence, making this project useful in identifying regions
in DNA where drugs can selectively interact. Since our goal is to
reduce the number of experimental considerations, we are attempting to define these interactions prospectively, and to develop a
systematic approach of predictive value.

The rational a priori design of molecules that bind specifically to certain regions of DNA involving regulation of gene expression or to the mRNA product of such genes is an exciting area of
investigation, and will enable the development of effective tumor-
specific therapy with minimal toxicity to the patient (13). This
area is being competitively pursued by many academic groups and
pharmaceutical companies. Introduction of specific chemical alterations in the base, sugar, and phosphate groups of DNA-like molecules can introduce a series of biochemical effects. In this way,
certain desirable chemical and biologic properties are retained
(e.g. regional mRNA sequence binding with a high degree of specificity, capacity to assume a similar conformation with native mRNA
and DNA, and resistance to cleavage by cellular enzymes) in a
"homing" molecule that inactivates specific cellular targets unique to tumor or AIDS infected cells. When these molecules are in
proximity to their target reversible binding is initially favored,
followed by irreversible covalent modification which inactivates
DNA and mRNA targets. These synthetic oligomers could be targeted
to a variety of mRNA or DNA targets involved in the pathogenesis
of malignancy. The use of similar agents in AIDS is likely to be
of potential benefit, since the pathogenesis of this disease involves alterations in the genome of host cells and is accompanied by
abnormal protein production (13).

A most challenging problem in this area involves chemical
modification of the phosphate backbone. Chemical modifications
(e.g. by sulfur, methyl, or ethyl groups) of the phosphorus atom
result in two diastereomers. It is important to identify whether
one type of chemical modification can enhance or inhibit the
binding of the parent molecule to the target. When there are 15

diastereomeric phosphorus atom centers in an oligomer (such as methylphosphonate or phosphorothioates) there are 2^{15} (32,768) different products from chemical synthesis. To reduce the number of experimental considerations we are using the supercomputer and theoretical methods to identify these relationships for a given molecular sequence. Computational methods have identified a significant chemical interaction which could decrease the binding affinity by interactions between the backbone and methyl groups on the modified base (16,17).

Advancement in molecular computational methods coupled with the power and flexible environment of general purpose supercomputers provides a new approach to the development of more effective pharmacologic therapy for malignancy and AIDS. By integrating this modern approach with the strengths of a coupled multidisciplinary experimental effort it will be possible to understand the pathogenesis and pathophysiology of these diseases and to develop new agents inactivating certain specific molecular targets that possess greater clinical efficacy. This is a field in its infancy, and although some limitations now exist, the dramatic progress in computational algorithms and hardware will continually reduce these problems commensurate with that of new approaches in the experimental scientific disciplines. The integration of theoretical and experimental efforts will be essential in expeditiously identifying and resolving scientific problems in the future. The major result of these developments will dramatically reduce mortality, morbidity, time and resource losses. The future of this field will have significant impact not only in cancer and AIDS, but in all areas of medicine involving the pharmacologic management of disease.

ACKNOWLEDGEMENTS

The authors gratefully acknowledge the research support of Sterling Drug, Inc., Gray Research, Inc., and the National Cancer Institute.

REFERENCES

1. In: Cancer: The Principles and Practice of Oncology. VT DeVita, S Hellman, SA Rosenberg (eds), Saunders, 1985.
2. Wittes RE: Current emphasis in the clinical drug development program of the National Cancer Institute. In: Cancer: The Principles and Practices of Oncology Supplement, Vol. I. VT DeVita, S Hellman, SA Rosenberg (eds), Saunders, 1987.
3. The Pharmacologic Basis of Cancer Treatment. BA Chabner (ed), Saunders, 1982.
4. Perry MC, Yarbro JW: Toxicity of Chemotherapy. Grune and Stratton, 1982.
5. Singh UC: QUEST (version 1.1), Scripps Clinic and Research Foundation,1987.
6. Singh UC, Kollrnan PA: An approach to computing electrostatic charges for molecules. J. Comput. Chem. 5:129-145, 1984.
7. Frisch MJ, Binlley JS et al: Gaussain 86. Carnegie-Mellon Quantum Chemistry Publishing Unit, Pittsburgh, PA, 1984.
8. Hehre WJ, Radom L, v.R.Schleyer P, Pople: Ab Initio Molecular Orbital Theory. Wiley Publishing Co., 1986.
9. Singh UC, Weiner PK, Caldwell JW, Kollman PA: AMBER VERSION 3.0 (University of California - San Francisco), 1986.
10. Weiner SJ, Kollman PA, Case DA et al: A new force field for molecular mechanical simulation of nucleic acids and proteins. J. Amer. Chem. Soc. 106:765-784, 1984.
11. Singh UC, Brown FK, Bash P, Kollman PA: An approach to the application of free energy perturbation methods using molecular dynamics. J. Amer. Chem. Soc. 109:1607-1614, 1987.
12. Singh UC: Probing the salt bridge in the dihydrofolate reductase-methotrexate coordinate complex by using the coordinate coupled free energy perturbation method. Proc. Nat. Acad. Sci. 85:4280-4284, 1988.
13. Miller P, T'so POP: A new approach to chemotherapy based on molecular and nucleic acid chemistry: MATAGEN. Anti-Cancer Drug Design 2:117-128, 1987.
14. Hausheer FH, Singh UC, Colvin OM: Identification of local determinants of DNA interstrand crosslink formation by cyclophosphamide metabolites. Anti-Cancer Drug Design 4:281-294, 1989.
15. Palmer TC, Hausheer FH, Saxe JD: Applications of ray tracing in molecular graphics. J. Mol. Graphics 7:160-164, 1989.
16. Hausheer FH, Singh UC, Saxe JD et al: Enhanced binding of methylphosphonate modified oligodeoxynucleotides in triple-stranded poly [dT] [dA] [dT] demonstrated by molecular dynamics. Proc. AACR 30:629, 1989.
17. Hausheer FH, Singh UC, Saxe JD et al: Can oligonucleotide methyphosphonates form a stable triplet with a DNA duplex? Anti-Cancer Drug Design 5:159-167, 1990.
18. Palmer TC, Hausheer FH, Saxe JD: Context-free spheres: A new method for rapid CPK image generation. J. Mol. Graphics 6:149-154, 1988.

19. Hausheer FH, Singh UC, Palmer TC, Saxe JD: Dynamic proper-
     ties and electrostatic potential surface of neutral DNA
     heteropolymers. Journal of American Chemical Society (in
     press) 1990.

13

EXTRACHROMOSOMAL DNA AS A TARGET FOR DRUG DEVELOPMENT

Daniel D. Von Hoff, M.D.

INTRODUCTION

Two of the greatest problems in clinical oncology today are
resistance of patients' tumors to chemotherapeutic agents and progression of patients' tumors with invasion and metastases. New approaches to both of these problems are certainly needed.

It has been known for some time that bacteria possess small
extrachromosomal circular DNA molecules (plasmids) which contain
drug resistance genes. These plasmids are anywhere from 2-4 kbp
in size. Because these plasmids are located in an extrachromosomal site rather than on the main chromosome, the plasmids can
replicate and make many copies of the drug resistance gene. This
increase in gene copy number is referred to as gene amplification
(1).

Plasmids have also been implicated in causing the crown gall
tumor in plants. These crown gall tumors are formed by the Ti
plasmid found in the <u>Agrobacterium</u> <u>Tumefaciens</u>. Thus, extrachromosomal DNA has been found in a very diverse group of organisms (2).

As will be seen below, there is increasing evidence that
animal and human tumor cell lines which are resistant to conventional antineoplastic agents or which possess oncogenes have those
amplified resistance genes or amplified oncogenes located on supercoiled extrachromosomal circular DNA called episomes (transposable
elements - elements which can move from an extrachromosomal site
to an intrachromosomal site). There is also increasing evidence
that one might be able to manipulate these episomes to modulate

the tumor cells' resistance to antineoplastic agents as well as modulate tumor cell progression.

GENE AMPLIFICATION IN CLINICAL ONCOLOGY

There are over 20 known examples of continuous cell lines in which amplification of a specific gene is known to be responsible for resistance to a specific drug (3). In addition, there are many examples of tumor cell lines with amplified oncogenes (4). There is also some evidence that amplifications are responsible for drug resistance in patients' tumors. For example, amplification of the dihydrofolate reductase gene (coding for the target enzyme dihydrofolate reductase which results in resistance to methotrexate) has been noted in patients with acute leukemia, ovarian cancer, and small-cell lung cancer (5-8). Amplification of the thymidylate synthase gene coding for resistance to 5FU has been also described in a patient's rectal cancer specimen (9). Also, over the last few years, amplification of the MDR-1 gene coding for multidrug resistance to vinblastine, doxorubicin, and other agents has also been described in a number of patients' tumors (10,11).

Amplification of oncogenes is becoming more important in clinical oncology. The presence of amplified oncogenes in patients' tumors may be an important prognostic factor. High levels of amplification of the N-myc oncogene have been correlated with a poor prognosis for patients with neuroblastoma (12). Amplification of the HER-2neu gene has been associated with a poor prognosis for patients with lymph node positive breast cancer and ovarian cancer (13,14). Amplification of c-myc has been associated with a poor prognosis for patients with small-cell lung cancer. This list of amplified oncogenes which seem to be associated with a poor prognosis for the patient is definitely increasing in size. It is clear that gene amplification has some importance in the progression of human tumors.

GENE TRANSFER METHODS YIELD EPISOMES

Investigators at the Salk Institute have been working for some time trying to understand the mechanism of gene amplification (15). Wahl and colleagues have been studying gene amplification mechanisms by introducing genes into random genomic locations using gene transfer methods. They inserted a Syrian hamster CAD gene (CAD is an acronym for the multifunctional protein containing carbamylphosphate synthetase, aspartate transcarbamylase, and di-hydroorotase - a gene that codes for resistance to PALA), into a CAD-deficient Chinese hamster ovary cell line. In performing this procedure they noticed that most of the clones that had survived treatment with PALA (the gene had been transferred successfully) actually possessed a chromosomal localization for the gene on a homogeneous staining region (HSR). However, they noted that one clone derived from the study was still resistant to PALA (so it did carry the CAD gene in an amplified form) but there was no chro-mosomal localization of the CAD gene by in situ hybridization. Carroll and colleagues from the same Salk Institute group noticed that there were actually copies of the amplified CAD gene located on submicroscopic circular supercoiled pieces of extrachromosomal DNA, which were approximately 250 kbp in size, which they called episomes (16). The size of these episomes was such that they would have been missed by light microscopy. As these cells were cultured in PALA containing media, these episomes seemed to in-crease in size (? multimerize) to form microscopically visible double minutes (17). This was the first clue as to the real origin of double minutes (submicroscopic episomes being their pre-cursors). Carroll et al. also observed that these episomes could integrate into chromosomal locations for amplification at those sites (an abnormal banding region or homogeneously staining region) (17). There was some criticism of the above model since it was a gene transfer model and not a spontaneously occurring model.

EPISOMES IN HUMAN TUMOR CELL LINES

One of the first tumor model systems in which a drug resistance gene was located on a circular chromosomal DNA element (episome) was the human squamous cell tumor line KBV1 which is resistant to vinblastine and doxorubicin based on the presence of amplification of the MDR-1 (P170 glycoprotein coding) multidrug resistance gene. Ruiz and colleagues noted that KBV1 cells contained an episome approximately 750 kbp in size. The episomes in that model replicated (just like the Chinese hamster ovary model above) in a semi-conservative manner (18).

Mauer and colleagues also described a HeLa BU25 subclone which was methotrexate resistant which contained amplified dihydrofolate reductase genes on submicroscopic episomes (19). VanDevanter et al. also described a methotrexate resistant squamous cell human tumor line which contained dihydrofolate reductase genes on submicroscopic episomes approximately 350 kbp in size (20). These latter two findings are particularly of interest since Garvey and Santi reported methotrexate resistant mutants of the protozoa <u>Leishmania</u> <u>major</u> have amplification of the dihydrofolate reductase gene with those amplified dehydrofolate reductase genes located on episomes (21).

More recently, Von Hoff and colleagues have documented that HL60 promyelocytic leukemia cells with amplification of the c-myc oncogene (early passages of the cells) have the copies of that amplified oncogene located on episomes approximately 230-250 kbp in size (22). They also found the neuroendocrine tumor Colo 320 DM cell line also had episomes containing the c-myc gene. They were supercoiled extrachromosomal DNA molecules of approximately 160 kbp in size (22). The great interest is that with additional work the same group has documented that as HL60 cells are carried in passage, the episomes multimerize to form double minutes. These double minutes are eventually incorporated into an intrachromosomal site (23). Thus, this is additional evidence that double minutes probably arise from episome precursors.

SPECIAL METHODS FOR ISOLATION OF EPISOMES

One of the major difficulties and probable reasons for not having noted episomes in human tumor cells before is that they are very large supercoiled molecules. They probably are quite fragile in terms of being easily nicked (Figure 1). In addition, having

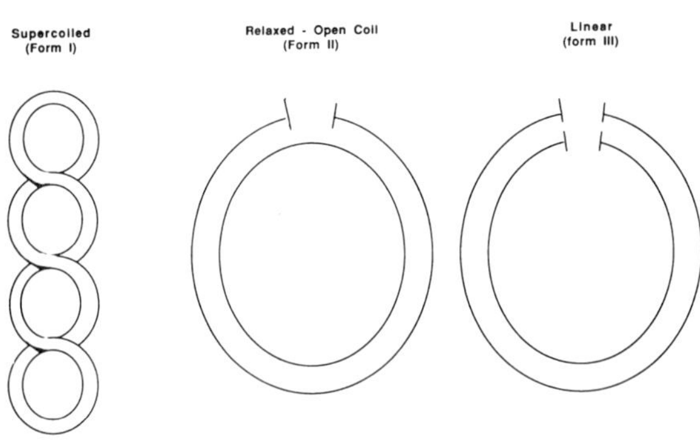

Figure 1. Three possible forms for episomes in tumor cell.

these molecules migrate in the usual agarose gel would be quite difficult since their topology would make most of them hang up on the agarose polymer as they attempted to percolate through the agarose gel.

Two methods have been developed for detecting episomes from tumor samples. The first method is the alkaline lysate method which is utilized to detect large herpes virus DNA molecules such as the Epstein Barr virus in mammalian cells (24,25). With the alkaline lysate technique cells are lysed at high pH (12.45). High pH, in addition to lysing the cells, actually denatures the linear duplex DNA while strands of covalently closed circular material (episomes) remain intertwined (17,22). Alkaline neutralization and extraction with phenol concentrates single strand DNA at the interphase while all covalently closed circular DNA (episomal

DNA) remains in the aqueous phase. The alkaline lysate material
is further analyzed by agarose gel electrophoresis. This is best
accomplished with very low voltage gel electrophoresis (loVE gel)
(26). Figure 2 graphically demonstrates the alkaline lysate technique. Figure 3 demonstrates a typical gel with isolation of
c-myc containing episomes in early passage HL60 cells using the
alkaline lysate and loVE gel technique. One of the major problems

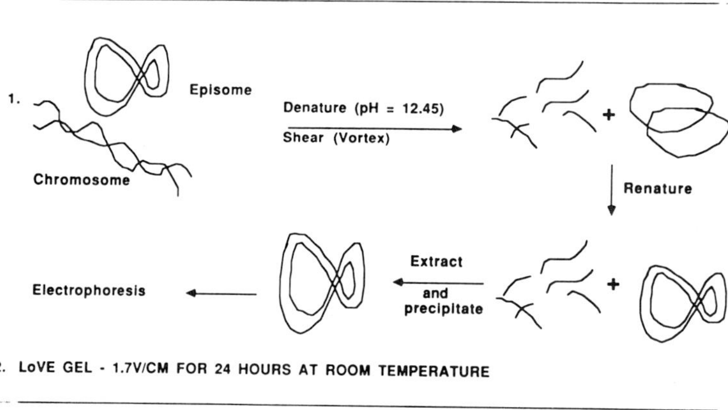

Figure 2. Graphic representation of the alkaline lysate technique
for isolation of episomes from tumor cells.

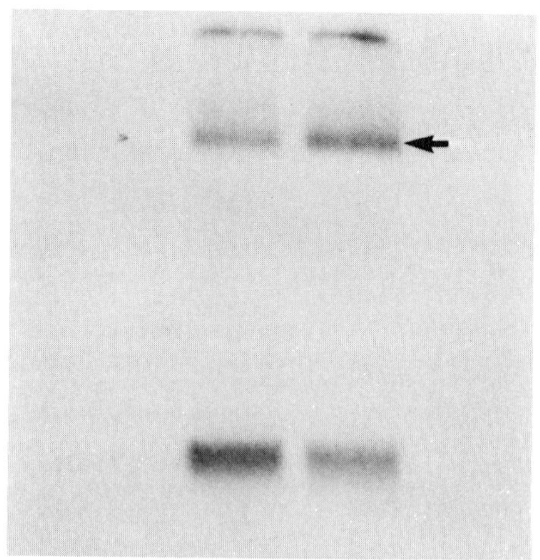

Figure 3. Gel demon-
strating isolation of
c-myc-containing episomes
in early passage HL60
cells. Technique used
was the alkaline lysis
technique with low
voltage electrophoresis
(LoVE gel). Arrow
designates episome.

with the alkaline lysate technique is major loss of episome
material because of the rather stringent conditions (high pH and a
large number of manipulations) which causes single strand and
finally double strand nicking which linearizes the molecules. A
more useful mechanism for isolation has been the use of an agarose
embedding technique whereby the cells are embedded in agarose
blocks (27) followed by a contour clamped homogenous electric
field (CHEF) electrophoresis. This is a form of field inversion
gel electrophoresis where the circular elements are coaxed along
through the agarose matrix by reversing directions of the field
and making the fields run at angles (28,29,26). To compliment
this technique, after the cells are embedded in agarose blocks and
lysed, they are gamma irradiated with ^{137}Cs. The ^{137}Cs causes
linearization of episomal molecules which show as a band on CHEF
gel electrophoresis. Figure 4 is a schematic representation of
the technique used to isolate episomes by the CHEF gel apparatus.
This technique has been successfully utilized to isolate episomes
from primary human neuroblastoma specimens (30).

1. CELLS ARE EMBEDDED AND LYSED IN AGAROSE BLOCKS

2. GAMMA IRRADIATION WITH ^{137}Cs

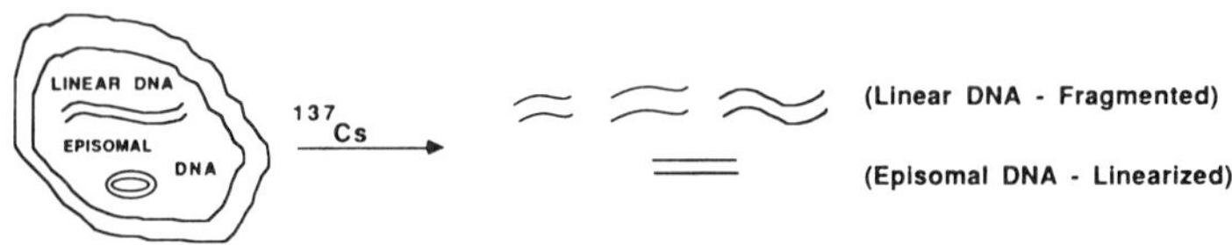

3. ELECTROPHORESIS USING CONTOUR CLAMPED HOMOGENEOUS ELECTRIC FIELD
   (CHEF) IN 0.6% AGAROSE GEL AT 14 DEGREES C WITH 60 MINUTE PULSES AT 50
   VOLTS FOR 158 HOURS

Figure 4. CHEF gel technique utilized to isolate episomes from
human tumor cells.

POSSIBLE WAYS TO ELIMINATE DRUG RESISTANCE GENE CONTAINING AND ONCOGENE CONTAINING EPISOMES FROM TUMOR CELLS

With the extrachromosomal localization of either oncogenes or drug-resistance genes on episomes, they are vulnerable to elimination from the cell. Once the episomes are incorporated into an intrachromosomal site they are no longer vulnerable to that elimination from the cell.

Snapka and Varshavsky have demonstrated that hydroxyurea at non-cytotoxic concentrations could eliminate double minutes containing the dihydrofolate reductase gene from methotrexate resistant mouse cells (31). We have used a similar strategy and have documented that both drug-resistance genes and oncogenes can be eliminated from human tumor cells (32,33). More work is needed in this area but this does appear to be a promising area.

POSSIBLE MODEL FOR GENE AMPLIFICATION

One very exciting possibility is that there may be a model for gene amplification which includes the deletion event. As can be seen in Figure 5, the deletion could occur secondary to a stress such as hypoxia or ultraviolet light. This could cause a deletion which circularizes and generates extrachromosomal elements (episomes). If the extrachromosomal element is lost from a cell that could mean there is a loss of the suppressor gene, which leads to tumorigenesis with more aggressive behavior. In a selective environment such as when drug is added, episomes can replicate and gene amplification takes place with development of double minutes and eventually incorporation into the chromosome. This is a very attractive theory which could explain oncogenesis, drug resistance, and amplification of oncogenes.

POSSIBLE TARGETS FOR DRUG DEVELOPMENT AREA

As outlined by other speakers in this conference, it is clear that new targets are needed for drug development. Figure 6 outlines possible targets for drug development using the episome models. The first possible target would be agents to prevent the deletion event. These agents could be used to decrease genome

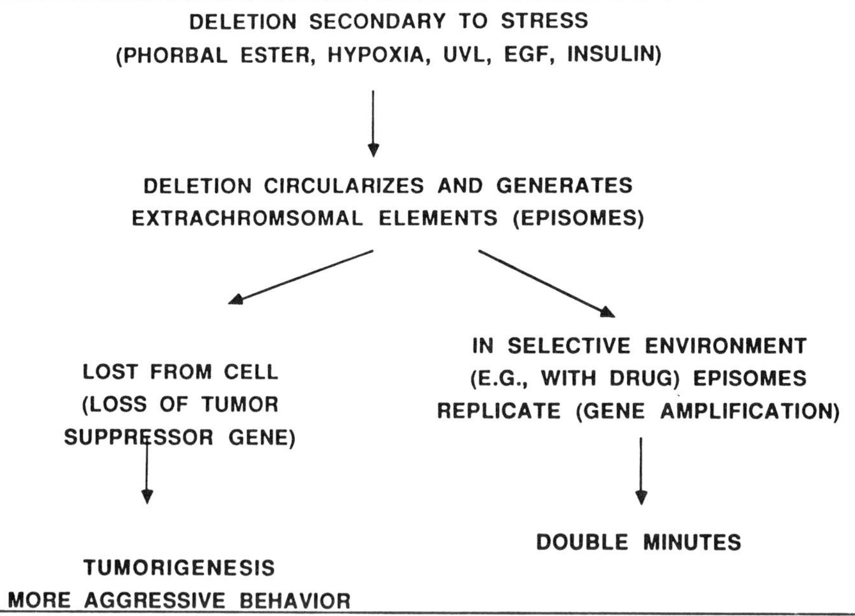

Figure 5. Possible deletion model for gene amplification.

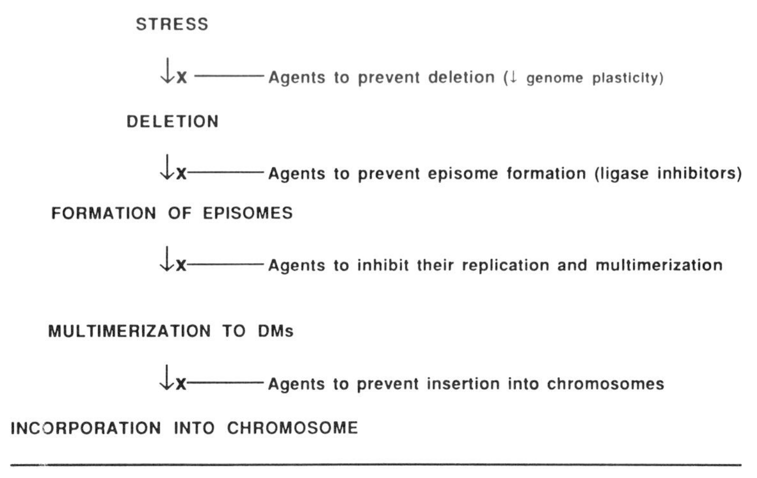

Figure 6. Possible targets for drug development involving the episome model.

234

plasticity. Undoubtedly there will be new agents in that area.
Even the retinoids could be considered a first step in the development of agents which might prevent deletion events.

A second area for development is agents to prevent episomal
formation. These could include ligase inhibitors. This is a very
understudied area.

A third area for possible drug development is agents to inhibit the replication of episomes and their multimerization. This
might include agents such as hydroxyurea discussed above.

One final target would be agents to prevent insertion into
chromosomes. As noted above, if one could prevent insertion of
amplified genes into chromosomes one might keep them extrachromosomal and make them vulnerable to loss from the cell.

SUMMARY

There is no doubt that episomes have now been documented to
occur in tumor cell lines as well as in primary human tumors.
This work has led to a model for gene amplification with episomes
as an intermediate. This model presents drug developers with a
variety of new targets. Promising results with elimination of extrachromosomal oncogene sequences as well as drug resistant gene
sequences located on these episomes have proved interesting. Whether or not the _in vitro_ results can be translated into _in vivo_ clinical and clinical trials only remains to be tested.

ACKNOWLEDGEMENTS

The author acknowledges the grant support of the National
Foundation for Cancer Research and of the Bristol Myers Company
Drug Resistance Grant Program.

REFERENCES

1. Watanable T: Infectious heredity of multiple drug resistance
    in bacteria. Bact Rev. 27:87-115, 1963.
2. Thomashow MF, Nutler R, Postle K et al: Recombination bet-
    ween higher plant DNA and the ti plasmid of agarobriterim
    tunefaciens. Proc. Nat. Acad. Sci. USA. 77:6448-6452, 1980.

3. Stark GR: DNA amplification in drug resistant cells and in tumors. Cancer Survey 5:1-23, 1986.

4. Alitalo K, Schwab M: Oncogenes amplification in tumor cells. Adv. Cancer Res. 47:235-281, 1985.

5. Carman MD, Schornagel IH, Ribert RS et al: Resistance to methotrexate due to gene amplification in a patient with acute leukemia. J. Clin. Oncol. 2:16-26, 1984.

6. Horns RC, Dower WI, Schimke RT: Gene amplification in a leukemia patient treated with methotrexate. J. Clin. Oncol. 2:2-7, 1984.

7. Trent I, Buick RN, Olson, S et al: Cytologic evidence for gene amplification in methotrexate resistant cells obtained from patients with ovarian adenocarcinomas. J. Clin. Oncol. 2:8-15, 1984.

8. Curt GA, Carney DN, Cowan KH et al: Unstable methotrexate resistance in human small cell carcinomas associated with double minute chromosomes. N. Engl. J. Med. 208:199-202, 1983.

9. Clark JL, Reizer SH, Mittelman A, Berger FG: Thymidylates synthase gene amplification in a color tumor resistant to fluoropyrimidine chemotherapy. Cancer Treat. Rep. 71:261-265, 1987.

10. Gerlach JH, Bell DR, KaraKonsis C et al: P-glycoprotein in human carcinomas: evidence for multidrug resistance. J. Clin. Oncol. 5:1452-1460, 1987.

11. Bell DR, Gerlach JH, Kartner N et al: Detection of P-glycoprotein in ovarian cancer: A molecular marker associated with multidrug resistance. J. Clin. Oncol. 3:311-315, 1985.

12. Seeger RC, Brodeur GM, Sather H et al: Association of multiple copies of the N-myc oncogene with rapid regression of neuroblastomas. N. Engl. J. Med. 313:1111-1116, 1985.

13. Slamon DJ, Clark GM, Wong FS et al: Human breast cancer: Correlation of relapse and survival with amplification of the HER-2/neu- oncogene. Science 235:177-180, 1987.

14. Johnson BE, Batley J, Linnoila I et al: Changes in the phenotype of human small cell lung cancer cell lines alter transection and expression of the c-myc proto-oncogene. J. Clin. Invest. 78:525-532, 1986.

15. Wahl GM, de Saint Vincent R, De Rose ML: Effect of chromosomal position on amplification of transfected genes in animal cells. Nature 307:516-520, 1984.

16. Carroll SM, Gaudray P, De Rose ML et al: Characterization of an episome produced in hamster cells that amplify a transfected CAD gene at high frequency: Functional evidence for a mammalian replication origin. Mol. Cell Biol. 7:1740-1750, 1987.

17. Carroll GM, De Rose ML, Gaudray P et al: Early events in gene amplification: A chromosomal deletion produces submicroscopic precursors of double minutes. Mol. Cell Biol. 8:1525-1533, 1988.

18. Ruiz JC, Choi K, Von Hoff DD et al: Autonomously replicating episome-containing mdr-1 gene in a multidrug resistant human cell line. Mol. Cell. Biol. 9:109-115, 1989.

19. Mauer BJ, Lai E, Hamkalo BA et al: Novel submicroscopic ex-
     trachromosomal elements containing genes in human cells.
     Nature 327:434-437, 1987.
20. VanDevanter DR, Von Hoff DD: Episomal DNA formation during
     hydroxyureaphorbal ester mediated dhfr gene amplification.
     Submitted, 1990.
21. Garvey EP, Santi DV: Stable amplified DNA in drug-resistance
     Leisnmania exists as extrachromosomal circles. Science
     253:535-540, 1986.
22. Von Hoff DD, Needham-VanDevanter DC, Yucel J et al: Ampli-
     fied oncogenes are contained in replicating submicroscopic
     circular DNA molecules in human tumor cells. Proc. Natl.
     Acad. Sci. USA 85:4804-4808, 1988.
23. Von Hoff DD, Forseth BJ, Clare N et al: Double minutes arise
     from extrachromosomal DNA intermediates which integrate into
     chromosomal sites in HL60 leukemia cells. J. Clin. Invest.
     In press, 1990.
24. Gardella T, Medveczky P, Sairenji T, Mulder C: Detection of
     circular and linear herpes virus DNA molecules in mammalian
     cells by gel electrophoresis. J. Virol. 50:248-254, 1984.
25. Cosse F, Boucher C, Julliot JS et al: Identification and
     characterization of large plasmids in rhizobium meliloti
     using gel agarose electrophoresis. J. Gen. Microbiol.
     113:229-242, 1979.
26. VanDevanter DR, Forseth BJ, Von Hoff DD: Optimal detection
     and further characterization of submicroscopic c-myc episomal
     DNA is HL60 cell. Submitted, 1990.
27. VanDevanter DR, Trammell HM, Von Hoff DD: Simple construc-
     tion of rubber-based agarose block molds for pulsed-field
     electrophoresis. BioTechniques 7:143-144, 1989.
28. Carle GE, Frank M, Olson MV: Electrophoretic separations of
     large DNA molecules by periodic inversion of the electric
     field. Science 232:65-68, 1986.
29. Van der Bliek AM, Lincke CR, Borst P: Circular DNA of 3T6R50
     double minute chromosomes. Nucleic Acids Res. 16:4841-4851,
     1988.
30. VanDevanter DR, Piaskowski VD, Casper JT, Von Hoff DD: Ampli-
     fied N-myc sequences can be located on circular extrachromo-
     somal DNA molecules in primary and metastatic neuroblastomas.
     J. Nat. Cancer Inst. (in press) 1990.
31. Snapka RM, Varshavsky A: Loss of unstably amplified dihydro-
     folate reductase gene from mouse cells is greatly accelerated
     by hydroxyurea. Proc. Natl. Acad. Sci. USA 80:7533-7537,
     1983.
32. Von Hoff DD, Eorseth B, Bradley T, Wahl G: Hydroxyurea can
     decrease oncogene copy number in human tumor cell lines.
     Proc. Am. Soc. Clin. Oncol. 9:55, 1990.
33. Von Hoff DD, VanDevanter D, Eorseth B et al: Hydroxyurea can
     decrease drug resistance gene copy numbers in tumor cell
     line. Proc. Am. Assoc. Cancer Res. In press, 1990.

14

PROSPECTIVE EVALUATION OF A PREDICTIVE MODEL FOR PLASMA CON-
CENTRATION-VERSUS-TIME PROFILES OF INVESTIGATIONAL ANTICANCER
DRUGS IN PATIENTS

David S. Alberts, Denise J. Roe, Patricia M. Plezia, John G. Kuhn
and Lisa E. Davis

INTRODUCTION

Several models have been proposed to predict target plasma
concentrations for new anticancer drugs in humans. Collins et al.
(1) have suggested a dose-escalation scheme based on the optimally
determined plasma concentration-versus-time (CXT) product in mouse
models. Phase I human studies are initiated at a dose of one-
tenth the LD_{10} in mice. Then, human pharmacology studies are
conducted to determine plasma CXT data in patients. The dose is
then escalated to approach a plasma CXT equal to that achieved in
the mouse model.

Scheithauer et al. (2) also have examined the relationship
between mouse LD_{50} values and human peak plasma concentrations
(PPCs) for 28 anticancer drugs. The rationale for such a comparison is based on the presumed relationship between toxicologic
end points in animal systems and the MTD in humans. A statistical
regression analysis between intraperitoneal mouse LD_{50} values
and PPCs in patients revealed a reasonable correlation (r^2=.501;
p<.001). These authors suggested that by using this regression
model, log (PPC)=-0.788+[0.755xlog(LD_{50})], a rational starting
point can be selected for <u>in vitro</u> screening of new agents for
which human PCC data are not yet available.

Davis et al. (3) have proposed a similar predictive model
using mouse intraperitoneal LD_{10} values and available human
plasma CXT data associated with standard anticancer drug MTDs for
22 commonly used anticancer drugs. Mouse toxicity data (LD_{10})
from two dosing schedules, daily times one and daily times seven,

were evaluated for BDF/1 mice. Strong correlations were found between LD_{10} and human plasma CXT data for both daily times one and daily times seven dosing schedules -- $\ln(CXT)=-1.6504+[0.8408 \times \ln(LD_{10})]$, r=.84, p<.0001, and $\ln(CXT)=-0.0754+[0.8954 \times \ln(LD_{10})]$, r=.90, p<.0001, respectively. It was concluded that these correlations may serve as useful models to predict the maximally tolerated dose of an investigational anticancer agent prior to entry into clinical trials and to assist in the selection of clinically relevant _in_ _vitro_ CXT's for new-agent screening against human tumors. In the present report we have attempted to apply this mouse LD_{10} versus human plasma CXT model to a group of recently studied experimental anticancer agents.

MATERIALS AND METHODS

Pharmacologic data for a clinically active anticancer drug were included in the model of Davis et al. (3) if two criteria were met. The first criterion was that an intraperitoneal LD_{10} value be available for BDF/1 or CDF/1 strain mice. The second criterion was that the human area under the CXT data curve be available for each standard and experimental anticancer drug included in the analysis. Human plasma CXT data were derived from published reports (4-6) and recent experimental data from our research laboratories concerning maximally tolerated, standard, single-dose drug regimens.

A linear regression analysis was performed to determine the correlation between the mouse toxicity data, i.e., LD_{10} for a single mouse species and the clinically achievable plasma CXT in humans (7). A logarithmic transformation of both LD_{10} and CXT was utilized to normalize the data. The mean plasma CXTs at the doses to be used in Phase II trials for three new experimental agents were used in an attempt to prospectively validate this LD_{10} versus plasma CXT model.

These experimental agents were recently studied in Phase I and pharmacokinetic trials (8-10). The mouse LD_{10} values for these agents were kindly provided from the manufacturer's pre-clinical toxicologic studies (11,12).

RESULTS

LD_{10} data for mice dosed with both a single ip injection or a daily times seven regimen along with the corresponding human plasma CXT data for each standard anticancer drug and the three experimental agents are shown in Table 1. The results of the linear regression analyses for the BDF/1 mice are shown in Table 2.

The regression lines of the logarithm of the mouse LD_{10} values versus the logarithm of the human CXT values are plotted in

Table 1

Usual Human CXT (ug x hr/ml) versus LD_{10} (mg/kg per dose), BDF/1 (or related species) Mice

Drug	Human dose	CXT (μg X hr/ml)	LD_{10} (mg/kg per dose) q day X 1	LD_{10} (mg/kg per dose) q day X 7†	Reference No.
5-Azacitidine*	150 mg/m² iv	1.56	42	NA	4
Bleomycin*	15 U/m² iv	4.99	42	NA	4
Brequinar	250 mg/m² iv	216.10	155	64	8
BW502U83	11,000 mg/m² iv. 72 hour infusion	121.50	81	47	9
Carmustine	95 mg/m² iv	1.02	31	5.2	4
Chlorambucil	0.60 mg/kg orally	2.38	15	12	4
Crisnatol	388 mg/m² iv, 6 hour infusion	63.31	65	60	10
Cisplatin	100 mg/m² iv	1.94	14	3.7	4
Cyclophosphamide	10 mg/kg iv	109.29	253	45	4
Cytarabine*	10 mg/kg iv	15.23	2,049	79	4
Dacarbazine	250 mg/m² iv	30.72	519	35	4
Dactinomycin	0.015 mg/kg iv	0.182	0.6	0.07	4
Daunorubicin	100 mg/m² iv	7.32	3.4	2.1	4
Doxorubicin	60 mg/m² iv	3.84	11	2.2	4
5-Fluorouracil*	15 mg/kg iv	16.33	193	33	4
Floxuridine*	2,000 mg/m² iv	44.88	445	73	5
Hexamethylmelamine	200 mg/m² orally	30	330	62	4
Hydroxyurea*	1,000 mg/m² orally	431.57	5,514	159	4
Melphalan	0.60 mg/kg iv	2.47	14	4.2	4
6-Mercaptopurine*	500 mg/m² iv	11.5	180	29	4
Methotrexate*	30 mg/m² iv	5.34	78	3.8	4
Mitoguazone	700 mg/m² iv	93.17	104	62	6
Mitomycin	20 mg iv	0.36	6.5	1.9	4
Vinblastine*	0.20 mg/kg iv	0.174	6.2	0.8	4
Vincristine*	0.025 mg/kg iv	0.064	3.1	0.02	4

*Cell cycle specific   †NA = not available

Table 2

Correlation between ln CXT (ug x hr/ml) in Humans and ln LD_{10} (mg/kg per dose) in Mice

Strain	Toxicity Dosing Schedule	No. of Drugs Tested	Slope*	Intercept*	Correlation Coefficient r	P value
BDF/1	ip q day X 7	20	0.8954 (0.69, 1.11)	-0.0754 (-0.72, 0.57)	.90	<.0001
BDF/1	ip q day X 1	22	0.8408 (0.59, 1.09)	-1.6504 (-2.78, -0.52)	.84	<.0001

*Values in parentheses = 95% confidence limits.

Figures 1 and 2 (daily x 7 and daily x 1 dosing schedules, respectively). The observed LD_{10} versus plasma CXT values of the three new agents were compared with the 95% confidence limits for a future agent from the original model, as shown.

There was no evidence that multiple-dose LD_{10} data were more predictive of the human plasma CXT data than the single-dose LD_{10} data for the 22 standard agents; however, data for the three experimental drugs appear to fit better in the multiple-dose LD_{10} model. Careful comparison of the regression analyses indicates that although neither dosing schedule provided a superior relationship, there was a difference between the intercepts of the regression lines between single-bolus and multiple-dose schedules, i.e., -1.6504 (SE = 0.5437) versus -0.0754 (SE = 0.3055). This difference in intercepts was due to the significantly higher LD_{10} values (mg/kg per dose) observed with single- versus multiple-dose schedules (p<.0001, paired t-test).

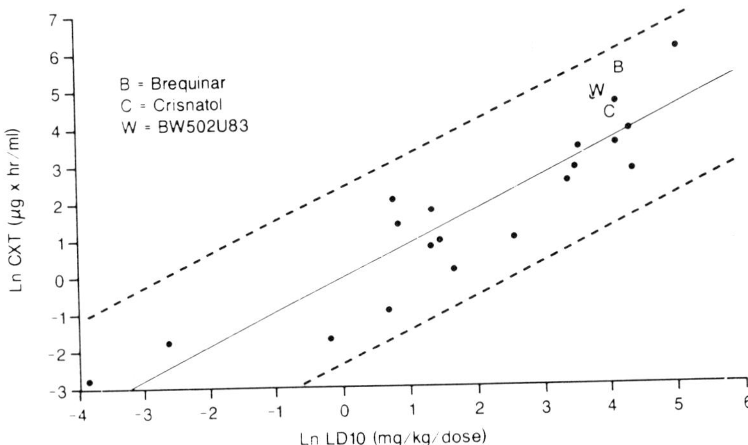

Figure 1. Human ln CXT (ug x hr/ml) vs. ln LD_{10} (mg/kg per dose). BDF/1 mice: ip q day x 7. ln (CXT) = -0.0754 + [0.8954 x ln (LD_{10})]. Solid line is the best fit by linear regression of ln transformed values; dashed lines are 95% confidence limits.

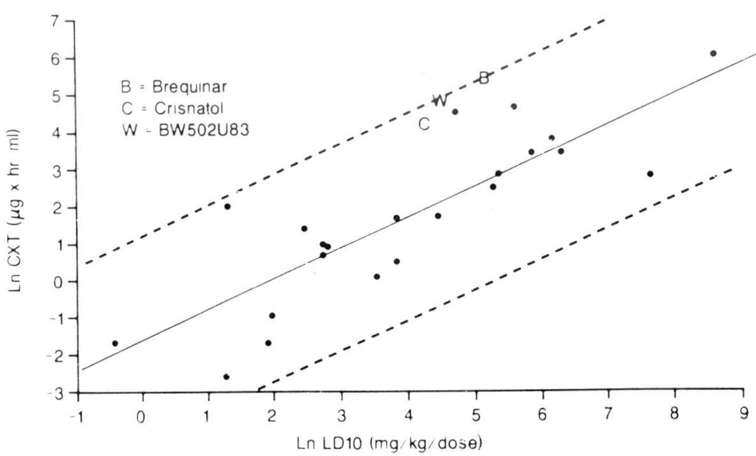

Figure 2. Human ln CXT (ug x hr/ml) vs. LD_{10} (mg/kg per dose). BDF/1 mice: ip q day x 1. ln (CXT) = -1.6504 + [0.8408 x ln (LD_{10})]. Solid line is the best fit by linear regression of transformed values; dashed lines are 95% confidence limits.

DISCUSSION

Commonly, the starting dose in a Phase I clinical trial of a new agent is based on 10% of the LD_{10} in mouse models, adjusted to the body surface area of an average-size adult male patient. Critical to the understanding of our approach is the assumption that the mouse LD_{10} bears a toxicological relationship to the MTD of an investigational or standard cytotoxic agent in humans. This has been demonstrated by numerous investigators and forms the basis of our current approach to the more efficient determination of the MTD dose in Phase I clinical trials (13,14). Since the MTD of a cytotoxic drug is reflected pharmacologically by its plasma CXT, we believe that the mouse LD_{10} can be rationally related to the plasma CXT of a cytotoxic agent following MTD doses in patients. Commonly administered anticancer drug doses are just below the MTD to achieve maximum dose intensity. From a pharmacokinetic viewpoint, our approach is based on the following relationships:

$$AUC_{mouse} = LD_{10\ mouse}/Cl_{T\ mouse} \quad \text{and}$$

$$AUC_{human} = \text{standard dose}_{human}/Cl_{T\ human}$$

From these relationships, it is obvious that if a relationship exists between total-body clearance (Cl_T) in the mouse and total-body clearance of the drug in humans, then there should be a relationship between area under the CXT curve (AUC) in the mouse and in humans. By extrapolation, then, one would expect there to be a relationship between $LD_{10\ mouse}$ and AUC_{human}.

The ability to predict the human plasma CXT associated with an MTD of an investigational agent prior to its entry into clinical trials could provide a powerful new tool in anticancer drug development. Preliminary estimates of the achievable plasma CXT could be used in the planning of <u>in vitro</u> Phase II drug trials against fresh human tumors and human tumor cell lines with clonogenic assays. Such plasma CXT data can maximize the clinical

243

applicability of the resulting dose-response data. Of even greater clinical significance, the early prediction of a maximal plasma CXT could serve as a benchmark for the potential therapeutic success of the new agent. For example, if the actual plasma human CXT associated with a toxic dose level of a new agent is significantly below that which was predicted by the mouse LD_{10}, then one might conclude that the new agent was unlikely to prove clinically useful and vice versa. This may occur, for example, when a species-specific toxicity is identified in humans at a relatively low dose, which would preclude using the drug at therapeutic concentrations. Finally, if an _in vitro_ assay predicts low antitumor activity at the achievable CXT, then one would not expect clinical usefulness for the agent.

Data currently available do not allow for analyses of populations with known differences in pharmacokinetic processes, i.e., sex, age, and weight. Very little, if any, such information is available for most antineoplastic agents. In addition, the CXT values reported here were based on total (i.e., free and protein-bound) concentration values. It is commonly assumed in the pharmacokinetic literature that free or unbound drug concentrations represent the active pharmacologic moiety. Although the predictive value of free concentrations of most antitumor agents has not yet been established, it is assumed that the predictive power of our model may be improved if CXT data were corrected for protein binding. The difference in the y-axis intercepts for the single-bolus and daily times seven dosing schedules should be kept in mind when making predictions with the LD_{10} versus plasma CXT relationship. It is empirically suggested that the LD_{10} data derived from the dosing schedule most analogous to the clinically proposed regimen be used to predict achievable human plasma CXT (3); however, as seen in Figures 1 and 2, the plasma CXT data for brequinar and crisnatol, which were administered by short-term iv infusion appear to fit better in the Q 1 day times 7 model. Obviously, it will require many more experimental drug LD_{10} vs. plasma CXT data sets before these models can adequately be validated.

ACKNOWLEDGEMENTS

We would like to acknowledge the assistance of Dr. Daniel Griswold who provided the "LD_{10} Summary Total Experience, May 16, 1960 - August 25, 1983, Southern Research Institute".

Supported by Public Health Service grants CA-17094 and CA-23024 from the National Cancer Institute, National Institutes of Health, Department of Health and Human Services; by the American Society of Hospital Pharmacists Research and Education Foundation; and by a donation from the Phi Beta Psi National Sorority.

REFERENCES

1. Collins JM, Zaharko DS, Dedrick RL et al: Potential roles for preclinical pharmacology in Phase I clinical trials. Cancer Treat. Rep. 70:73-80, 1986.
2. Scheithauer W, Clark GM, Salmon SE et al: Model for estimation of clinically achievable plasma concentrations for investigational anti-cancer drugs in man. Cancer Treat. Rep. 70:1379-1382, 1986.
3. Davis LE, Alberts DS, Plezia PM et al: Predictive model for plasma concentration versus time profiles of investigational anticancer drugs in patients. JNCI 80:815-819, 1988.
4. Alberts DS, Chen HS: Tabular summary of pharmacokinetic parameters relevant to _in vitro_ drug assay. In: Cloning of Human Tumor Cells, SE Salmon (ed), Liss, New York, pp. 351-359, 1980.
5. Sommadossi JP, Aubaert C, Cano JP et al: Kinetics and metabolism of a new fluoropyrimidine, 5'-deoxy-5-fluorouridine, in humans. Cancer Res. 43:930-933, 1981.
6. Marsh KC, Liesmann J, Patton TF et al: Plasma levels and urinary excretion of methyl-GAG following iv infusion in man. Cancer Tret. Rep. 65:253-257, 1981.
7. Snedecor GW, Cochran WG: Statistical methods. Ames, IA: The Iowa State University Press, 1967.
8. Arteaga CL, Brown TD, Kuhn JG et al: Phase I clinical and pharmacokinetic trial of brequinar sodium (DUP 785; NSC 368390). Cancer Res. 49:4648-4653, 1989.
9. Harman GS, Craig JB, Kuhn JG et al: Phase I and clinical pharmacology trial of crisnatol (BWA770U mesylate) using a monthly single-dose schedule. Cancer Res. 48:4706-4710, 1988.
10. Lam K, Alberts DS, Peng YM et al: Phase I and pharmacokinetic study of BW502U83 (an arylmethylaminopropanediol) in cancer patients. Proc. Amer. Soc. Clin. Onc. 9:68, 1990.
11. Data on file, Burroughs Wellcome Co., Research Triangle Park, NC, 1990.

12. Data on file, Dupont Co., Wilmington, DE, 1989.
13. Freireich EJ, Gehan EA, Rall DP et al: Quantitative com-
    parison of toxicity of anticancer agents in mouse, rat,
    hamster, dog, monkey, and man. Cancer Chemother. Rep.
    50:219-245, 1966.
14. Goldsmith MA, Slavik M, Carter SK: Quantitative prediction
    of drug toxicity in humans in small and large animals.
    Cancer Res. 35:1354-1364, 1975.

15

AGENT-DIRECTED PRECLINICAL TOXICOLOGY FOR NEW ANTINFOPLASTIC DRUGS

Charles K. Grieshaber

INTRODUCTION

Over the past forty to fifty years, toxicology has played a pivotal role in the later preclinical stages of drug development. The types of toxicology studies performed and their complexity have varied considerably over the interceding years but the reasons for carrying out such studies have remained essentially unchanged. The goals and objectives of preclinical toxicology studies, to estalish a safe drug dose for initiating Phase I clinical trials (quantitative toxicology), to predict the likely adverse effects in human trials (qualitative toxicology) and to describe the normalization of the acute adverse effects are as sound today as they were almost a half-century ago. There has been considerable debate, however, over whether these goals and objectives have been satisfactorily met in the past and are being met today. The main features of the debate and the outcomes impacting on present day drug development have been extensively documented over the past 25 years (1-10).

The design of studies for preclinical toxicology of anticancer drugs was more or less standardized in 1973 following the publication of the protocols by Prieur and co-workers (11). In order to understand the potential human risks of new chemotherapeutic drugs, lethal doses (LD) were established in dogs and monkeys from which nonlethal, progressively less toxic doses were derived. These protocols were designed to demonstrate the acute toxic effects of new agents in multiple biologic systems. Chronic effects and effects of repeated administration were assessed in dogs. Starting doses for clinical trials were calculated using one-third the dose with mild toxicity if the long-term and schedule-dependency studies established that serious toxicity was not present at these dose levels.

In 1981, the toxicology protocols were revised based on the finding that the entry level dose for clinical trial with new anticancer agents could be estimated from one-tenth the LD_{10} in mice (8). The streamlined protocols replaced the defined dose regimens in dogs and monkeys for clinical starting dose estimation with acute lethalily studies in mice using the clinically compatible single dose and five daily dose schedules (12,13). The qualitative toxicities of new drugs are determined by studies in dogs and rodents on the same schedules (12,13). These protocols have served as the standard studies for new cytotoxic agents prior to initiation of Phase I clinical trials.

Over their course of evolution, toxicology studies on new cytotoxic anticancer agents were initiated with the established hypothesis that all such drugs, regardless of cytotoxic mechanism, should be toxic to organs with dividing cell types such as the stem cells of the gastrointestinal tract, bone marrow, lymphoid organs and hair follicles. Today, we recognize that the types of studies performed should be modified and be based on the pharmacodynamic and pharmacokinetic characteristics of the individual agents to more closely associate dose levels and toxicity. This is described as the agent-directed approach. Not one single set of protocols is capable of serving as a blueprint to describe the toxicity and pharmacology for all conceivable kinds of new drug classes.

The astute and increasingly frequent use of screening procedures to identify new anticancer agents which demonstrate _in vitro_ activity versus solid tumors exemplified by the human tumor colony forming assay (14,15), the disk diffusion assay of Corbett, et al 16) as well as the advent of a large-scale, high capacity disease oriented new drug screen currently under validation at the National Cancer Institute (17-20) will, in all likelihood, select for new agents with specific, tumor cell oriented mechanisms of pharmacodynamic action in addition to unpredictable and/or unusual toxic effects. Toxicology studies like those characteristically employed in the past will presumably be of little utility in drug development of agents discovered by these screening methods necessitating a rethinking and modification of the methods used for contemporary toxicology studies in order to make the data meet the long-sought objectives.

In the mid-1980's, concern for the length of time taken to escalate doses to the maximally tolerated dose (MTD) in Phase I trials of anticancer drugs reached its zenith. In 1986, Collins and co-workers (21) made a major contribution to the preclinical-clinical interface in the early development of chemotherapeutic agents by proposing the escalation schemes in clinical trials be based on plasma drug concentration and duration of exposure. Building on the pharmacodynamic hypothesis that toxicity is a predictable, constant finding with cytotoxic agents in all species, and that similar biological effects, including toxicity, would likely occur at similar plasma drug exposure levels in both experimental animals and humans, these authors recognized the interspecies differences continually observed between the MTD in humans and the LD_{10} in mice must be due to pharmacodynamic and pharmacokinetic differences. To test the role of pharmacokinetics, the authors compared the area under the concentration versus time curve (AUC) values in mice at the LD_{10} with those in humans at the MTD. Table 1 illustrates the comparisons of these ratios for 13 investigational anti-cancer agents with the dose ratio of human MTD to murine LD_{10}. The data presented comprise a part of the recent and more comprehensive review (22) which updates the 1986 (21) information. For five of the drugs wherein the dose ratios are substantially greater or less than unity, Azacytidine, Doxorubicin, Teroxirone, PALA and Thiotepa, the concentration versus time ratios range between 0.8 and 1.0 indicating the pharmacodynamic hypothesis would have served as better predictor for dose escalation and human toxicity. In a second list of five drugs, Diaziquone, Indicine-N-oxide, AMSA, Tiazofurin and Pentostatin, the dose ratios and the CxT ratios were relatively similar affording

250

Table 1

Comparison of dose ratio and CxT ratio for human
MTD to murine LD_{10}

DRUG	MTD/LD_{10}	$\dfrac{\text{CxT at MTD}}{\text{CxT at } LD_{10}}$
Azacitidine	6.0	1.1
Doxorubicin	5.0	0.8
Teroxirone	4.3	0.8
Pirozantrone	2.1	0.8
Diaziquone	1.0	1.0
Indicine N-oxide	0.9	0.6
AMSA	0.8	1.3
Tiazofurin	0.7	0.9
Pentostatin	0.7	1.1
Thiotepa	0.4	1.0
PALA	2.8	3.3
Dihydroazacytidine	1.2	0.3
F-ara-AMP	0.1	0.1

Data Adapted From Collins et al (21,22)

no advantage to either method of interspecies toxicity correlation. It is noteworthy that with PALA the high AUC ratio (3.3)
offers no benefit to the description of toxicity over the interspecies dose ratio (2.8), with dihydroazacytidine the dose ratio
provides better insight into the interspecies toxicity relationships, and with Fludarabine (fluoro-ara-AMP) neither ratio provides insight into interspeces relationships. Each of these three
agents functions as an antimetabolite, thus cytotoxicity is not
necessarily a function of plasma drug exposure as much as a pharmacodynamic effect associated wth intracellular metabolism. The differences in cytotoxic action should remind us that the agent-directed approach to toxicity testing is vitally important. Nevertheless, the plasma AUC can be a helpful, prospective interspecies
predictor for the appearance of serious toxicity. This unique
comparative concept, coupled with the utilization of plasma drug

AUC to guide dose escalations in Phase I trials (21,22), provides an additional stimulus for the re-design of preclinical pharmaco-kinetically based, agent-directed toxicology studies for new anti-neoplastic agents.

We have limited experience with agent-directed preclinical pharmacology and toxicology studies over the past few years as "specialized studies" were added to the traditional protocols on an _ad_ _hoc_ basis to several new drugs developed by the National Cancer Institute. These special studies were based on known bio-logical and biochemical properties of each new drug at the time of initiation of toxicology studies and included measurement of plasma drug levels in mice and dogs to relate the observed toxic effect to a measure of plasma drug concentration. Furthermore, schedule dependency of toxicity was considered in order to design experiments wherein the least amount of toxicity could be induced at the maximum levels of drug (23).

Deoxyspergualin is a drug on which special studies were per-formed to determine the effect of administration schedule on toxi-city. This intriguing agent is the synthetic 15-deoxy analog of spergualin, a novel antibiotic isolated from culture broths of _Bacillus_ _Laterosporous_. Although the drug is a polyamine, mechan-istically it does not affect the polyamine pathways. Moreover, neither spermidine nor spermine inhibit its antiproliferative ef-fects. Maximal antitumor activity versus L1210 leukemia is sche-dule dependent in that the more freqently the drug is administer-ed, the better the antitumor activity. The log-cell kill of L1210 cells was enhanced approximately 4-fold following administration of deoxyspergualin via continuous infusion (24). In traditional Dx1 and Dx5 toxicology studies, the major adverse effects in rats and dogs were ataxia and bradypnea. Moderate myelosuppression was also noted as a consistent finding. Consideration of the schedule-dependency of L1210 activity prompted the use of a continuous in-travenous infusion schedule in toxicity studies in dogs. The toxicity pattern was altered from that seen with the bolus sche-dule. Neurologic and myelosuppressive effects observed with bolus dosing were alleviated by the infusion schedule and hemorrhagic

cystitis and subsequent anemia became the limiting toxicity. Moreover, the plasma drug concentrations at steady state ranged between 7-10 ug/ml (Table 2) with dose levels (2 mg/kg/hr) which produced little serious toxicity. These concentrations are in the

Table 2

Pharmacokinetic Parameters of 15-Deoxyspergualin
Following Continuous Infusion for 120 Hours

R_0 (mg/kg/hr)	N^b	Cp_{ss} (mg/l)	Clp^a (ml/hr/kg)	AUC (mg/l x hr)
2.0	1	7.2	279.2	859.5
6.0	3	21.9	279.7	2631.3
10.0	2	35.7	280.6	3866.6

[a] Total Body Plasma Clearance at Steady State
[b] Data Averaged from N Dogs

range of extrapolated levels in L1210 bearing mice whose tumor burden decreased significantly on the continuous administration schedule, thus canine toxicity was observed to be minimal at target
plasma levels. In fact, dose levels of 6 mg/kg/hr (2.9 gm/m^2/day)
could be administered via infusion in dogs producing a steady
state blood level of approximately 22 ug/ml. The design and results of the Phase I trials are outlined in Table 3. Plasma samples collected from patients on the highest dose levels during the
Phase I trials (>2100 mg/m^2/day) demonstrated drug concentrations
of 6-8 ug/ml (25,26), levels approximating those in effective antitumor preclinical studies. At doses greater than 2100 mg/m^2/day,
hypotension is the dose limiting toxicity, with other toxicities
including mild myelosuppression and mild diarrhea. Importantly,
qualitative studies in dogs producing hemorrhagic cystitis were
not predictive for humans.

In summary, the special study involving continuous intravenous infusion in beagle dogs permitted a higher entry dose for

Table 3

Summary of Phase I Clinical Trial Experiences
with Deoxyspergualin (NSC-356894)

SCHEDULE: CIV Infusion for 5 Days, Q4W

ENTRY DOSE: 80 $mg/m^2/day$

MTD: 2160 - 2792 $mg/m^2/day$

DLT: Hypotension

Other
Toxicities: Mild to moderate myelosuppression,
                 paresthesias agitation, slurred speech
                 gastrointestinal bleeding

ESCALATIONS: 8 - 11

PLASMA LEVEL: 5 - 7.5 ug/ml at the MTD

clinical trial because the drug load administered over 120 hours
was remarkably greater than that produced by five consecutive daily
bolus doses. The LD_{10} in mice on a daily x 5 schedule was 10 mg/
kg/day, suggesting a clinical entry dose of 1 mg/kg/day (3.2 $mg/m^2/$
day). Infusion studies in dogs indicated a dose of 2 mg/kg/hr
(960 $mg/m^2/day$) was tolerated, yielding a recommended clinical
starting dose of 320 $mg/m^2/day$ (calculated as 1/3 the lowest
dose administered in dogs). The actual starting dose for human
trials was 80 $mg/m^2/day$, although lower than projected was still
25 times higher than the traditional 1/10 mouse LD_{10}. As a result of using infusion schedules in preclinical toxicology (23),
there was a significant increase in the entry dose for phase I
clinical testing, with a consequential decrease in the time and
numbers of patients required to complete the human study.

A second category of special study used to enhance preclinical toxicology investigations centered on targeting specific efficacious drug exposure intensities (a plasma concentration for a
specific duration) in different animal species based on the pharma-
codynamically active _in vitro_ exposure intensities and identifying
drug exposure intensities which produce dose-limiting toxicity.

Such a pharmacologically guided toxicity study was conceived for the differentiation inducing agent, Hexamethylene Bisacetamide (HMBA).

HMBA is a polar-planar compound which induces terminal differentiation in murine erythroleukemia cells (27) and human promyelocytic leukemia cells (28) _in vitro_ when incubated at 2 to 5 mM for three to five days. The drug is essentially inactive in conventional _in vivo_ murine tumor models. Repeated drug administration at freguent intervals in rats or continuous intravenous infusions in dogs were employed in preclinical toxicology studies to target plasma drug concentrations in the effective _in vitro_ concentration range of 2-5 mM. Rats received intraperitoneal injections every four hours for twelve injections and dogs were continuously infused for 120 hours (29). HMBA administration produced CNS toxicity in both species. Convulsions were induced in dogs at doses of 60 mg/kg/hour yielding plasma steady state concentrations of 1 to 2 mM HMBA over the 120 hour infusion period.

In the Phase I trials (summarized in Table 4), clinical pharmacology studies revealed that plasma steady state HMBA concentra-

Table 4

Summary of Phase I Clinical Trial Experiences
with HMBA (NSC 095580)

SCHEDULE:	CIV Infusion for 5 Days, Q4W
ENTRY DOSE:	4.8 gm/m^2/day
MTD:	33.6 gm/m^2/day
DLT:	Neurotoxicity
Other Toxicities:	Thrombocytopenia, leukopenia nausea, vomiting, diarrhea
ESCALATIONS:	3 - 4
PLASMA LEVEL:	2 mM at the MTD

tions were dose dependent and that 1-2 mM could be achieved in patients with acceptable toxicity (30, 31). The MTD was reached in four dose escalations using plasma steady state drug level as the guide with the dose limiting toxicity consisting of agitation, confusion and occasional hallucinations. Importantly, administration of sodium bicarbonate to overcome metabolic acidosis due to metabolism of HMBA ameliorated the CNS toxicity and led to plasma HMBA concentrations of 2 mM with thrombocytopenia as dose limiting.

From the foregoing, a guideline for preclinical pharmacology and toxicology studies with new individual antineoplastic agents can be created in which interspecies pharmacokinetic similarities or differences are described along with the traditional toxicity parameters. The design of preclinical toxicology studies should revolve around the intended use of the drug in human studies, including route, schedule of administration and plasma concentrations of the drug.

CONCLUSION

A suggested compendium of agent-directed studies which constitutes a conscientious preclinical toxicology/pharmacology program for new anticancer drugs is illustrated in Table 5. These studies effectively re-define and slightly revise the objectives of preclinical toxicology studies to provide a framework for integrating pharmacokinetics into preclinical drug development. The first studies in each species provide a minimal plasma pharmacokinetic model from which intraspecies and interspecies predictions can be initialized. For instance, the plasma linearity of elimination, clearance, half-life and volume of distribution determined from two species will forecast, to a certain extent, the pharmacokinetic parameters in humans. The second set of studies describes the toxicity and the MTD in traditional terms to guide the design and analysis of the third series of studies.

The third, and final, series of studies are straightforwardly designed to correlate the administered dose with plasma concentrations (AUC, Cpss, etc.) of the parent drug (and metabolites, if necessary) with observable, acute toxic effects in the species of

Table 5

Agent-Directed, Pharmacologically Guided Preclinical Toxicology Studies for New Antineoplastic Agents

Rodents

Determine plasma pharmacokinetics on two schedules - single bolus and continuous infusion.

Determine the maximally tolerated dose (MTD) on the anticipated clinical schedules.

Determine the toxicity profile correlating toxicity to plasma concentration using the anticipated clinical schedule of administration.

Second Species

Determine pharmacokinetics on single bolus and the anticipated clinical schedule of administration.

Determine the toxicity profile at the proposed clinical trial entry dose and the expected MTD using the anticipated clinical schedule of administration.

choice. It is important to note that these studies can be accomplished with fewer rodents and dogs than called for by the traditional toxicology protocols. Furthermore, lethality studies in mice are eliminated and emphasis placed on clinical observations, clinical chemistry, hematology and histopathology as determinants of toxicity.

Over the recent past, it has been demonstrated that a mathematical relationship exists between peak plasma concentration of anticancer drugs in humans and the LD50 in mice (32) or between the AUC in humans at the MTD and the LD_{10} in mice (33). Collins (34) has correctly pointed out, however, that these models can only predict accurately for drugs with average clearance since plasma clearance values are not known for mice in either of the foregoing analyses. The presently proposed pharmacologically guided toxicology studies will provide these data and much more.

REFERENCES

1. Freireich EJ, Gehan EA, Rall DP et al: Quantitative comparison of toxicity of anticancer agents in mouse, rat, hamster, dog, monkey, and man. Cancer Chemother. Rep. 50:219-244, 1966.
2. Goldsmith MA, Slavik M, Carter SK: Quantitative prediction of drug toxicity in humans from toxicology in small and large animals. Cancer Res. 35:1354-1364, 1975.
3. Grieshaber CK, Marsoni S: Relation of preclinical toxicology to findings in early clinical trials. Cancer Treat. Rep. 70:65-72, 1986.
4. Guarino AM: Pharmacologic and toxicologic studies of anticancer drugs: of sharks, mice, and men. In: Methods in Cancer Research, VT DeVita Jr., H Busch (eds), Vol 15, Academic Press, Inc., New York, pp. 91-174, 1979.
5. Guarino AM, Rozencweig M, Kline I et al: Adequacies and inadequacies in assessing murine toxicity data with antineoplastic agents. Cancer Res. 39:2204-2210, 1979.
6. Homan ER: Quantitative relationships between toxic doses of antitumor chemotherapeutic agents in animals and man. Cancer Chemother. Rep. 3:13-19, 1972.
7. Penta JS, Rozencweig M, Guarino AM, Muggia FM: Mouse and large-animal toxicology studies of twelve antitumor agents: Relevance to starting dose for Phase I clinical trials. Cancer Chemother. Pharmacol. 3:97-101, 1979.
8. Rozencweig M, Von Hoff DD, Staquet MJ et al: Animal toxicology for early clinical trials with anticancer agents. Cancer Clin. Trials 4:21-28, 1981.
9. Schein PS, Davis RD, Carter S et al: The evaluation of anticancer drugs in dogs and monkeys for the prediction of qualitative toxicities in man. Clin. Pharmacol. Ther. 11:3-40, 1970.
10. Schein PS: Preclinical toxicology of anticancer agents. Cancer Res. 6:1934-1937, 1977.
11. Prieur DJ, Young DM, Davis RD: Procedures for the preclinical toxicologic evaluation of cancer chemotherapeutic agents: Protocols of the laboratory of toxicology. Cancer Chemother. Rep. 4:1-30, 1973.
12. Lowe MC: Large animal toxicological studies of anticancer drugs. In: Fundamentals of Cancer Chemotherapy, K Hellmann, SK Carter (eds), McGraw-Hill, New York, pp. 236-247, 1987.
13. Lowe MC, Davis RD: The current toxicology protocol of the National Cancer Institute. In: Fundamentals of Cancer Chemotherapy, K Hellmann, SK Carter (eds), McGraw-Hill, New York, pp. 228-235, 1987.
14. Hamberger AW, Salmon SE: Primary bioassay of human tumor stem cells. Science 197:461-463, 1977.
15. Shoemaker RH, Wolpert-DeFillippes M, Kern D et al: Application of a human tumor colony-forming assay to new drug screening. Cancer Res. 45:2145-2153, 1985.
16. Corbett TH, Wozniak A, Gerpheide S, Hanka L: A selective two-tumor soft agar assay for drug discovery. In: In Vitro and In Vivo Models for Detection of New Antitumor Drugs, LJ

Hanka, T Kondo, RJ White (eds), University of Tokyo Press, Tokyo, pp. 5-14, 1986.
17. Alley MC, Scudiero DA, Monks A et al: Feasibility of drug screening with panels of human tumor cell lines using a microculture tetrazolium assay. Cancer Res. 48:589-601, 1988.
18. Scudiero DA, Shoemaker RH, Paull KD et al: Evaluation of a soluble tetrazolium/formazan assay for cell growth and drug sensitivity in culture using human and other tumor cell lines. Cancer Res. 48:4827-4833, 1988.
19. Shoemaker RH, Monks A, Alley MC, et al: Development of human tumor cell line panels for use in disease-oriented drug screening. In: Prediction of Response to Cancer Chemotherapy. T Hall (ed), Alan R. Liss Inc., New York, pp. 265-286, 1988.
20. Boyd MR: Status of the NCI preclinical antitumor drug discovery screen. Prin. Prac. Oncol. Updates 3:1-12, 1989.
21. Collins JM, Zaharko DS, Dedrick R, Chabner B: Potential roles for preclinical pharmacology in Phase I clinical trials. Cancer Treat. Rep. 70:73-80, 1986.
22. Collins JM, Grieshaber CK, Chabner BA: Pharmacologically guided Phase I clinical trials based upon preclinical drug development. J. Natl. Cancer Inst. 82:1321-1326, 1990.
23. Collins JM, Leyland-Jones B, Grieshaber CK: Role of preclinical pharmacology in Phase I clinical trials: Considerations of schedule-dependence. In: Concepts in Cancer Chemotherapy. FM Muggia (ed), Martinus Nijhoff, Boston, pp. 129-140, 1987.
24. Plowman J, Harrison SD, Trader MW et al: Preclinical antitumor activity and pharmacologic properties of deoxyspergualin. Cancer Res. 47:685-689, 1987.
25. Havlin K, Koeller J, Craig J et al: Phase I clinical and pharmacokinetic study of deoxyspergualin. Proc. Am. Soc. Clin. Oncol. 7:59, 1988.
26. Jakubowski A, Scher H, Muindi J et al: Phase I and pharmacokinetic assessment of deoxyspergualin (DSG). Proc. Am. Assoc. Cancer Res. 29:191, 1988.
27. Fibach E, Reuben RC, Rifkind RA, Marks PA: Effect of hexamethylene bisacetamide on the commitment to differentiation of murine erythroleukemia cells. Cancer Res. 37:440-444, 1977.
28. Collins SJ, Bodner A, Ting R, Gallo RC: Induction of morphological and functional differentiation on human promyelocytic leukemia cells (HL-60) by compounds which induce differentiation of murine leukemia cells. Int. J. Cancer 25:213-218, 1980.
29. Chun HG, Leyland-Jones B, Hoth D et al: Hexamethylene bisacetamide: A polar-planar compound entering clinical trials as a differentiating agent. Cancer Treat. Rep. 70:991-996, 1986.
30. Egorin MJ, Sigman LM, Van Echo D et al: Phase I clinical and pharmacokinetic study of hexamethylene bisacetamide (NSC-95880) administered as a five-day continuous infusion. Cancer Res. 47:617-623, 1987.

31. Egorin MJ, Zuhowski EG, Cohen AS et al: Plasma pharmacokine-
    tics and urinary excretion of hexamethylene bisacetamide meta-
    bolites. Cancer Res. 47:6142-6146, 1987.
32. Scheithauer W, Clark GM, Salmon SE et al: Model for estima-
    tion of clinically achievable plasma concentrations for in-
    vestigational anticancer drugs in man. Cancer Treat. Rep.
    70:1379-1382, 1986.
33. Davis LE, Alberts DS, Plezia PM et al: Predictive model for
    plasma concentration-versus-time profiles of investigational
    anticancer drugs in patients. JNCI 80:815-819, 1988.
34. Collins JM: Pharmacology and drug development. JNCI 80:790-
    792, 1988.

16

PRECLINICAL STUDIES WITH BREQUINAR SODIUM: A NOVEL ANTICANCER AGENT

Shih-Fong Chen, Ph.D. and Daniel L. Dexter, Ph.D.

INTRODUCTION

A novel, substituted 4-quinolinecarboxylic acid, 2-(4-cyclo-hexylphenyl)-6-fluoro-3-methyl-4-quinolinecarboxylic acid, NSC 339768, was submitted to, and was found active in the National Cancer Institute's Developmental Therapeutics Program. Based on this finding, an analog synthesis program was initiated in our program; over 200 derivatives of NSC 339768 were prepared (1). One of these analogs, 6-fluoro-2-(2'-fluoro-1,1'-biphenyl-4-yl)-3-methyl-4-quinolinecarboxylic acid sodium salt, (NSC 368390, DuP 785, brequinar sodium, Figure 1), was selected for further study because of its antitumor activity and water solubility. This paper reviews the preclinical antitumor activity of brequinar sodium against murine tumors and human carcinomas xenografted in nude mice, the mechanism of action of the agent, and the structure activity relationship of this class of 4-quinolinecarboxylic acids.

ANTITUMOR ACTIVITY

Brequinar sodium was initially tested against L1210 leukemia; the compound caused an increase in life span of >80%. The acti-vity against L1210 was schedule dependent, and the compound was equally efficacious when administered i.p., i.v., s.c., or p.o. The agent was most active when administered on a daily x 9 sche-dule; intermittent dosing was less effective even when individual doses were increased to produce a cumulative total dose equal to that given on the daily x 9 schedule. Brequinar sodium also inhi-

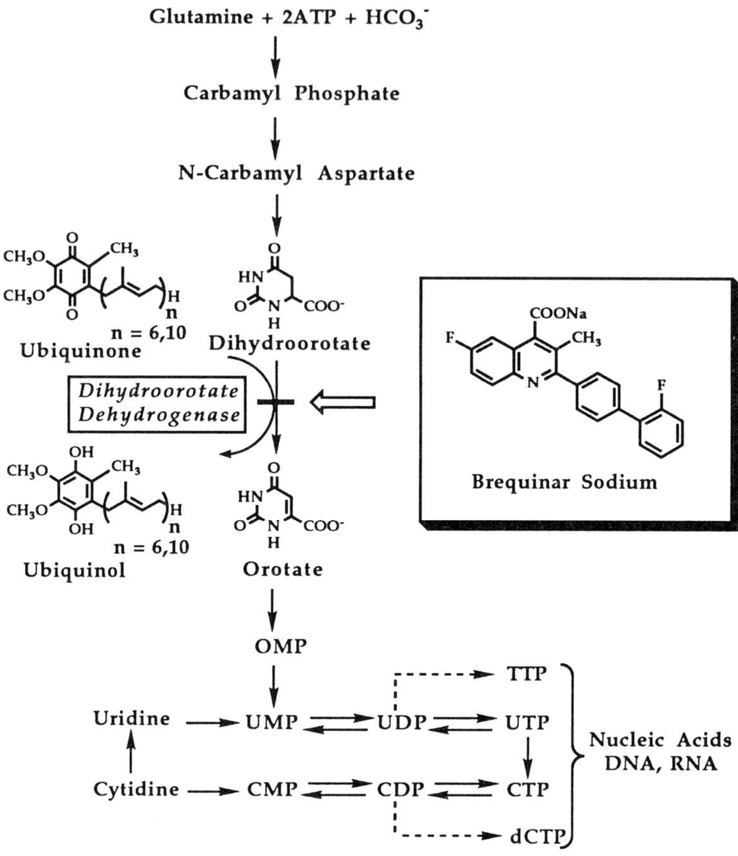

Figure 1. The chemical structure of brequinar sodium and its site of action on the pyrimidine _de novo_ biosynthetic pathway.

ited the growth of several human tumors xenografted in nude mice (Table 1); these human tumors included the DLD-2, clone A, HCT-15, and CX-1 colon tumors, the MX-1 mammary tumor and the LX-1 lung carcinoma (2).

Growth inhibition values in the range of 70-90% were generally obtained, identifying brequinar sodium as one of the more active agents reported versus human tumor xenografts (3). Braakhuis et al. also reported that the growth of an established line (HNX-LP) of human head and neck squamous cell carcinoma xenografted in nude mice was totally inhibited by brequinar sodium for a 17-day period (4). Loveless and Neubauer reported that brequinar sodium inhibited metastasis of B16 F10 melanoma in mice (5).

Table 1

Summary of Antitumor Activity of Brequinar Sodium
Against Human Tumor Xenografts in Nude Mice[a]

Nude mice with human tumors implanted subcutaneously or under the
subrenal capsule were treated with brequinar sodium on a daily X 9
schedule.

Human Tumor Type	Tumor Site	Dose (mg/kg/day)	Treatment Route	Growth Inhibition (%)
DLD-2 (colon)	s.c.	25	i.p.	>90
HCT-15 (colon)	s.c.	25-50	i.p.	58-89
Clone A (colon)	s.c.	12-50	i.p.	58-89
CX-1 (colon)	SRC[b]	10-32	i.p.	>90
MX-1 (mammary)	SRC	11-32	i.p.	>90
LX-1 (lung)	SRC	11-32	i.p.	80-89
BL/STX-1 (stomach)	SRC	20	i.p.	80-89
BL/STX-1	SRC	25	p.o.	80-89

[a]Data adapted from Ref. 2.
[b]Subrenal capsule

Combination chemotherapy experiments were conducted with
brequinar sodium and each of a series of marketed anticancer
drugs. Improved efficacies that were at least additive were
obtained when brequinar sodium was given i.p. with adriamycin,
melphalan, cytoxan or cisplatin to mice bearing L1210 leukemia.
Figure 2 shows the effect of brequinar sodium and adriamycin on
the survival of mice with L1210 leukemia. At a sub-optimal dose,
brequinar sodium (6.25 mg/kg) or adriamycin (2 mg/kg) alone,
caused only a slight increase in the life span of mice bearing
L1210 leukemia. However, when used in combination, more than
additive antitumor activity was seen; 20% of the mice survived for
30 or more days (6).

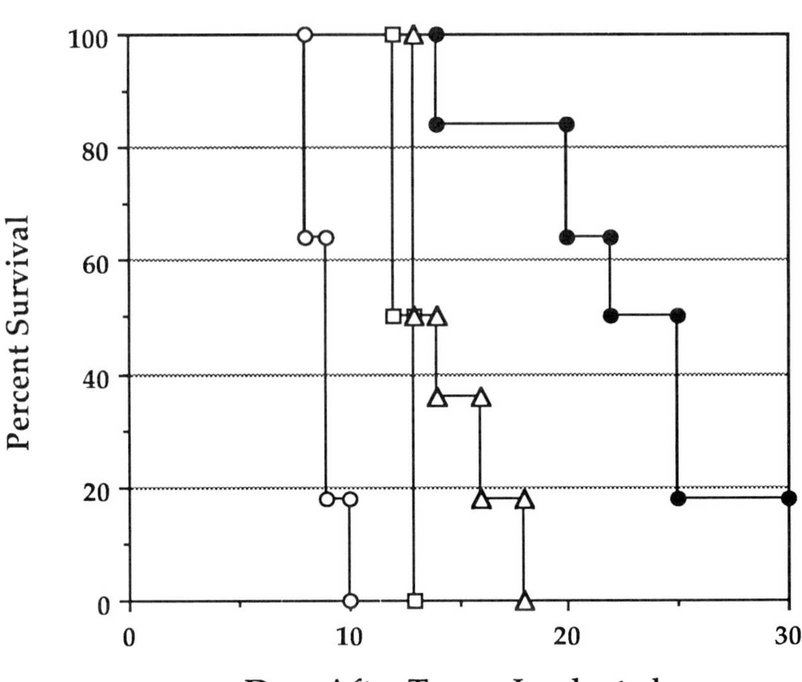

Days After Tumor Implanted

Figure 2. Effect of Brequinar sodium and adriamycin on the survival of mice with L1210 leukemia. One day after i.p implantation with L1210 leukemia, the mice was treated with vehicle (0); brequinar sodium, 6.25 mg/kg (□); adriamycin, 2 mg/kg (△); and brequinar sodium, 6.25 mg/kg + adriamycin, 2 mg/kg (●) daily for 9 consecutive days.

The combination of brequinar sodium and cisplatin was used to treat nude mice bearing s.c. MX-1 human breast tumor implants; tumor size was 50-100 mg at the start of treatment (Table 2). Suboptimal doses of brequinar sodium (3-12 mg/kg) alone caused 33-64% tumor growth inhibition; no tumor regression was observed. Cisplatin alone, at 1 and 2 mg/kg caused 0 and 87% grow inhibition, respectively, with two mice showing tumor regression. Curative activity was obtained (60% of the mice were observed to have complete tumor regression) when brequinar sodium (at all three doses) was combined with 2 mg/kg of cisplatin; however, this combination was also toxic to the mice (37% lethality). Better results were obtained when brequinar sodium was combined with a lower dose of

Table 2

The Combination of Brequinar Sodium and Cisplatin Against MX-1 Human Tumor Xenografts

Nude mice bearing MX-1 human breast carcinoma xenografts were treated with brequinar and/or cisplatin as indicated. Mice and tumors were evaluated on day 19 following initiation of treatment.

Groups, Dose (mg/kg)[a,b]	Number of Mice Per Group	Number Dead	Number CR Complete Regressions	Number PR (% Tumor Shrinkage)	Growth Inhibition (Number of Mice Evaluated)[c,d]
Brequinar, (12)	9	0	0	0	64% (9)
Brequinar, (6)	9	0	0	0	52% (9)
Brequinar, (3)	9	0	0	0	33% (9)
Cisplatin, (2)	9	1	1	0	87% (7)
Cisplatin, (1)	9	0	1	0	0% (8)
Brequinar, (12) Cisplatin, (2)	9	4	4	1 (20%)	–
Brequinar, (6) Cisplatin, (2)	9	4	5	0	–
Brequinar, (3) Cisplatin, (2)	9	2	7	0	–
Brequinar, (12) Cisplatin, (1)	8	1	7	0	–
Brequinar, (6) Cisplatin, (1)	8	0	5	1 (38%)	95% (2)
Brequinar, (3) Cisplatin, (1)	8	0	7	0	88% (1)

[a]Route:IP
[b]Schedule: brequinar sodium Q1DX9; Cisplatin Q4DX3
[c]Final tumor mass per control mouse = 1800 mg
[d]Initial tumor mass per control mouse = 51 mg

cisplatin (1 mg/kg); 80% of tumors regressed completely and only 1 of 24 mice died. Moreover, the durability of the complete regressions was also quite good. Four months after the administration of drugs, of the sixteen mice with complete regressions in the groups receiving 2 mg/kg of cisplatin + brequinar sodium, fourteen remained tumor free. In contrast, the combination of adriamycin and brequinar sodium against the MX-1 breast tumor was no more effective than brequinar sodium alone. Complete disappearance of tumor was also observed in nude mice which were implanted with human colon tumor DLD-2 when brequinar sodium was combined with melphalan; no tumor regressions were observed when either drug was administered as a single agent at the maximal tolerated dose (6). The data with brequinar and adriamycin against L1210 leukemia, and brequinar with cisplatin against the MX-1 breast tumor xenografts indicate that selected combinations produced more than additive efficacy against these two experimental tumors.

In summary, brequinar sodium is a water soluble anticancer agent with a novel structure and excellent bioavailability. The compound has demonstrated broad spectrum activity against a variety of experimental tumors. Brequinar sodium has also shown good activity when used in combination with selected anticancer drugs.

MECHANISM OF ACTION

The distinct structure of brequinar sodium, which is unrelated to any known anticancer agents, has precluded any _a priori_ prediction of its mode of action. Therefore studies were conducted to elucidate its mechanism of action (7).

Exposure of cultured clone A human colon tumor cells to 25 to 75 μM of brequinar sodium for 48 to 72 hr resulted in a 3 to 4 log cell kill as determined by clonogenic survival assay. Clone A cells exposed to brequinar sodium became depleted in intracellular pools of uridine 5′-triphosphate (UTP) and cytidine 5′-triphosphate (CTP) (Figure 3). Both UTP and CTP were decreased to 50% of the levels in control cells at 3 h and were undetectable at 15 h after addition of 25 μM of brequinar sodium to the cultures. Similar effects were observed in L1210 leukemia cells. Addition of 100 μM uridine or cytidine restored intracellular pools of UTP and CTP to control levels (Figure 3) and rescued clone A cells from brequinar sodium cytotoxicity. Unlike uridine or cytidine, other purine and pyrimidine bases and their respective ribonucleosides and 2′-deoxyribonucleosides cannot reverse the cytotoxicity of brequinar sodium. Similar results were obtained with L1210 cells when uridine was added concurrently with brequinar; however, addi-

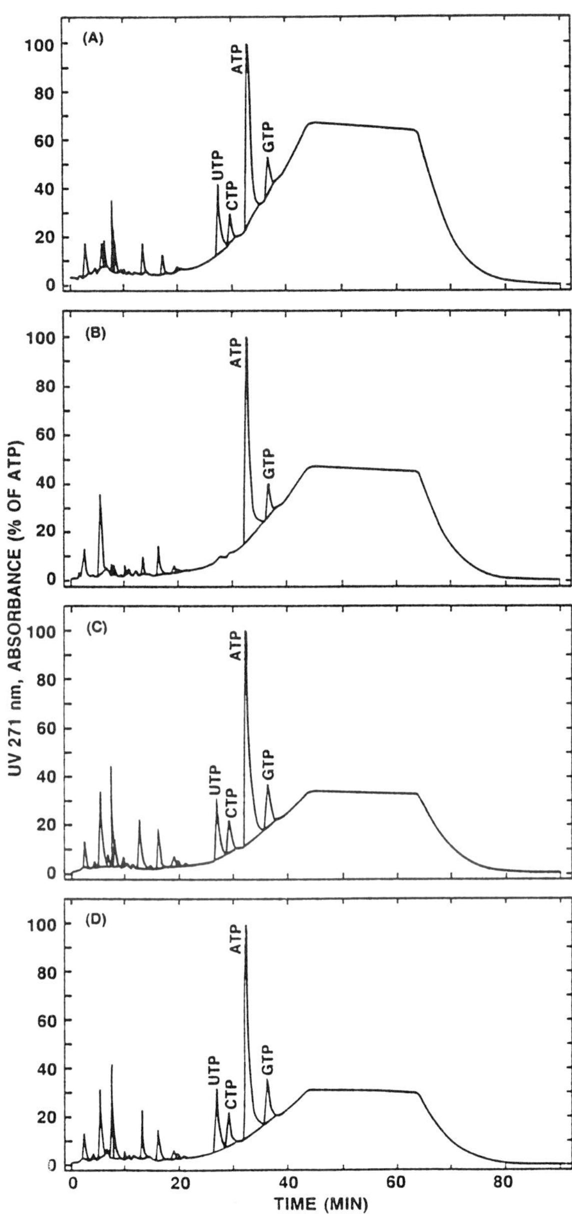

Figure 3. Pyrimidine nucleotide depletion by brequinar sodium and its reversal by uridine or cytidine in clone A cells. The cells were incubated with (A) RPMI-C medium, (B) brequinar sodium (25 μM), (C) brequinar sodium (25 μM) and cytidine (100 μM), and (D) brequinar sodium (25 μM) and uridine (100 μM) for 24 hr at 37°C. Acid-soluble nucleotides were analyzed by HPLC as described in Ref. 7.

tion of cytidine restored only intracellular CTP but not UTP (Figure 4). Thus cytidine was not able to rescue L1210 cells from brequinar cytotoxicity. This is consistent with the finding that L1210 cells lack cytidine deaminase and thus cannot form UMP from cytidine (8). Overall, these results indicated that brequinar sodium inhibits a step(s) in de novo pyrimidine nucleotide biosynthesis prior to the formation of UMP. Analysis of all six enzymes in the pathway subsequently demonstrated that only the mitochondrial enzyme, dihydroorotate dehydrogenase (DHO-DHase) is inhibited by brequinar sodium (Figure 1). The apparent K_i value of 23.5 $\pm$ 1.3 nM (SD) was estimated by Dixon's analysis, suggesting the brequinar sodium is a potent inhibitor of L1210 DHO-DHase (7).

Subsequently, Peters et al. (9) came to the same conclusion using a different approach. In addition to uridine and cytidine, these authors also found that orotate but not dihydroorotate or carbamyl aspartate can rescue L1210 leukemia and M5 melanoma cells from the cytotoxicity of brequinar sodium. This finding is in agreement with the fact that brequinar sodium inhibits DHO-DHase; orotate, the product of this enzyme-catalyzed reaction, should and does rescue cells and thus circumvents the cytotoxicity of brequinar sodium. Moreover, Peters et al. used a pyrazofurin test to demonstrate that brequinar sodium affects pyrimidine de novo biosynthesis. Pyrazofurin inhibits orotidylate decarboxylase, the last enzyme in the pyrimidine de novo biosynthesis leading to UMP. Addition of pyrazofurin to cultured cells leads to an accumulation of OMP and subsequently of orotate and orotidine. These authors found that the addition of brequinar sodium to the culture medium prevented the pyrazofurin-induced orotate and orotidine accumulation, a result similar to that reported for PALA, a potent inhibitor of aspartate carbamoyltransferase, the second enzyme involved in the pyrimidine de novo biosynthesis (10). Again, this result supports our finding that brequinar sodium inhibits pyrimidine de novo biosynthesis. Peters et al. found that brequinar sodium is an inhibitor of rat liver DHODHase; the mode of inhibition appeared to be linear mixed type with an apparent K_i of about 100 nM and an apparent K_i' of about 800 nM (9).

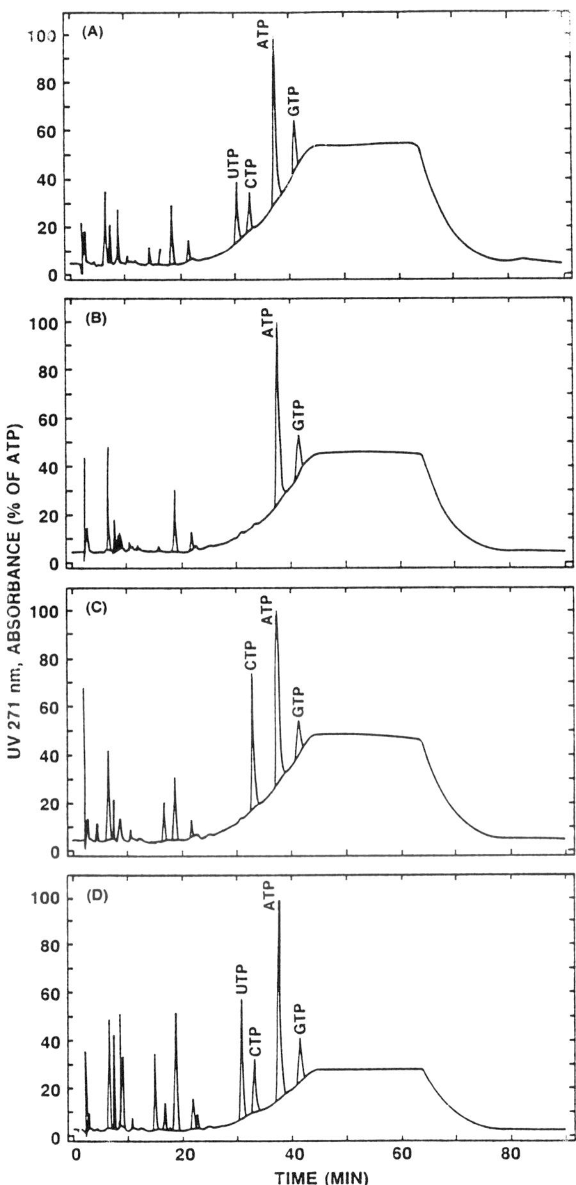

Figure 4. Pyrimidine nucleotide depletion by brequinar sodium and its reversal by uridine or cytidine in L1210 cells. The cells were incubated with (A) RPMI-C medium, (B) brequinar sodium (25 μM), (C) brequinar sodium (25 μM) and cytidine (100 μM), and (D) brequinar sodium (25 μM) and uridine (100 μM) for 24 hr at 37°C. Acid-soluble nucleotides were analyzed by HPLC as described in Ref. 7.

Anderson et al. developed a GC/MS (gas chromatography/mass spectrometry) method to quantitate dihydroorotate that accumulated in cultures of L1210 cells exposed to growth inhibitory concentrations of brequinar sodium (11). This method provides an important advantage as compared to an assay of partially purified DHO-DHase in broken cell preparations, in that the inhibition can be monitored in intact cells where normal regulatory controls on pathway activity remain in effect. A dose dependent accumulation of dihydroorotate in the culture media during exposure of L1210 cells to brequinar was observed. No accumulation of dihydroorotate in the culture media was observed in non-drug treated control cells. This study demonstrated a direct correlation between inhibition of de novo pyrimidine biosynthesis, changes in pyrimidine nucleotide concentrations, and cell proliferation following short (<24 h) drug exposure. Thus, the result of Anderson et. al (11) further confirmed that brequinar sodium inhibits the activity of DHO-DHase.

Schwartsmann et al. reported the effect of brequinar sodium on cell cycle (12). An exposure of L1210 cells to 25 μM of brequinar sodium for 12 hr caused an accumulation of cells in early S-phase. Brequinar sodium also caused WiDR human adenocarcinoma cells to accumulate in the S-phase of the cell cycle after 24 hr drug exposure. When WiDR cells were recultured in drug-free medium, cells continued to traverse through the cell cycle. The accumulation of cells in the S-phase of the cell cycle with brequinar is similar to that report with PALA and pyrazofurin (13). Thus the cell cycle effect of brequinar sodium is consistent with its mechanism as an agent that inhibits de novo pyrimidine biosynthesis.

ANTIPYRIMIDINE EFFECTS OF BREQUINAR SODIUM IN TUMOR-BEARING MICE

One prediction from the mechanism of brequinar would be that this agent, like PALA, should be effective in the biochemical modulation of tumor cells, which would enhance 5-fluorouracil (FUra) activity (14). This modulation, or "priming" action should occur when brequinar sodium is administered before, but not after, FUra.

Such an effect was indeed demonstrated by Pizzorno et al. (15). These workers, using a weekly schedule, showed that the administration of up to 140 mg/kg brequinar sodium only caused a marginal inhibition of colon 38 tumor growth. When FUra (100 mg/kg) was given 4 hr after brequinar sodium (80 mg/kg) on a weekly basis, there were regressions in these advanced tumors, whereas FUra alone had minimal effect.

The question of uridine (salvage pathway) rescue must also be considered when studying brequinar sodium. As described above, brequinar sodium inhibits the activity of mammalian DHO-DHases and leads to the depletion of intracellular pyrimidine nucleotides (UTP and CTP). Uridine can be incorporated into UTP and CTP by the salvage pathway and thus rescue the cells from the cytotoxicity of brequinar sodium. The _in_ _vitro_ activity of brequinar sodium can be demonstrated if the culture medium contains low concentration of uridine or cytidine. However, the _in_ _vivo_ activity of brequinar sodium could be dictated by (a) the dependency of each tumor type on the _de_ _novo_ pyrimidine pathway, (b) circulating plasma and intracellular uridine concentrations, and (c) any differential transport of uridine into normal and tumor tissues. These issues were addressed by Peters et al. (16) who reported that plasma and tumor tissue uridine levels in mice bearing implanted colon 38 carcinoma were depleted for several days. In contrast, uridine levels in the liver were not significantly affected following brequinar sodium administration. The colon 38 tumor was moderately sensitive to brequinar. Uridine nucleotide pools of colon 38 tumors were depleted by 50% after 1 and 2 days of brequinar sodium treatment. Colon 26 tumors were resistant to brequinar sodium, and tumor uridine levels were not appreciably affected by treatment with the agent. Moreover, no uridine nucleotide pool depletion was observed in colon 26 tumors implanted in mice treated with brequinar sodium (16). Thus there is a good correlation in this study among tumor response to brequinar sodium, uridine level in the tumor, and the biochemical effect on nucleotide pools, for two distinct murine colon carcinomas.

INTERACTION BETWEEN BREQUINAR SODIUM AND DHO-DHase

The finding that brequinar sodium inhibits the activity of DHO-DHase is interesting since its structure does not resemble either the substrate (dihydroorotate) or the cofactor (ubiquinone Q_6) involved in the enzyme reaction (Figure 1). Further studies were conducted to understand the interaction between brequinar sodium and its target enzyme.

DHO-DHase catalyzes the oxidation of dihydroorotate to orotate; this reaction is the single redox step in the pyrimidine _de novo_ biosynthetic pathway. Mammalian DHO-DHase is a mitochondrial enzyme and is located on the outer surface of inner membrane of the mitochondria (17). Several DHO-DHases from different species are known. The major difference in these enzyme forms appears to be the cofactor requirement. The commercially available DHO-DHase isolated from Z. _oroticum_ is a soluble enzyme that uses NAD^+ as cofactor. Prokaryotic DHO-DHase is a membrane-bound enzyme which uses ubiquinone Q_{10} as the natural cofactor (18). Eukaryotic DHO-DHases occur in both soluble and membrane-associated forms. Cytosolic enzymes have been isolated from the parasitic protozoan C. _fascicvlata_ and T. _brucei_ (19,20). Like the mammalian enzyme, the yeast DHO-DHase isolated from N. _Crassa_ is also a mitochondrial enzyme (21). Although brequinar sodium was shown to be a potent inhibitor of DHO-DHases isolated from L1210 or rat liver, it did not inhibit the enzymes isolated from S. _cerevisiae_, E. _coli_, and Z. _oroticum_ (22). Our finding that brequinar sodium does not inhibit the S. _cerevisiae_, and E. _coli_ DHO-DHase even though they also use dihydroorotate and ubiquinone as substrate and cofactor, respectively, suggests that brequinar sodium may not compete directly with either the substrate or the cofactor binding site on DHO-DHase.

In addition, brequinar sodium was found to inhibit the L1210 DHO-DHase noncompetitively with respect to either dihydroorotate (K_i = 6.5 nM) or ubiquinone (K_i = 6.2 nM) (23). These results further support our earlier findings, with various forms of the enzyme, that brequinar sodium may not compete directly with the substrate or cofactor binding sites on the enzyme.

The reaction catalyzed by DHO-DHase was reported to follow the pingpong mechanism based on the initial velocity pattern; dihydroorotate binding precedes ubiquinone binding (24). Recently, using highly purified DHO-DHase from bovine liver mitochondria, Hines and Johnston reported that the bovine enzyme may follow a nonclassical, two-site ping-pong mechanism (25). Orotate was shown to be a competitive inhibitor with respect to dihydroorotate. In a nonclassical ping-pong mechansim, the two substrates may not resemble each other chemically and therefore they may not bind to a single binding site, but probably bind to two adjacent sites that transfer the reactants. This mechanism is typical of an enzyme that contains two nonoverlapping and kinetically isolated substrate and cofactor binding sites (25). Our data suggest that L1210 DHO-DHase also follows a non-classical, two-site ping-pong mechanism.

The model that best fits our data is one in which DHO-DHase follows a non-classical two-site ping-pong mechanism; the substrate (dihydroorotate) and the cofactor (ubiquinone) binding sites are nonoverlapping and kinetically distinct. These two sites are probably linked by an intramolecular electron-transfer system involving FMN and perhaps iron or zinc. Brequinar sodium may bind to this electron transfer system and alter the conformation of the substrate and cofactor binding sites, and thus produce a noncompetitive inhibition pattern with respect to dihydroorotate and ubiquinone (26). Peters et al. have also reported that brequinar sodium is a linear mixed type inhibitor (noncompetitive with respect to dihydroorotate) of rat liver DHO-DHase (9).

STRUCTURE-ACTIVITY RELATIONSHIP

Chen et al. reported the apparent K_i of 69 analogs of 4-quinoline carboxylic acids as inhibitors of L1210 DHO-DHase (27 and Table 3). The study identified three critical regions on the brequinar sodium structure where specific substitutions are required for the inhibition of the activity of DHO-DHase. Other portions of the molecule were found to be sensitive to chemical modification for activity as well. The three principal regions are (i)

Table 3

Structure of selected 4-quinoline carboxylic acid analogs and their inhibition of DHO-DHase activity, *in vitro* growth inhibitory activity, and *in vivo* antitumor activity.

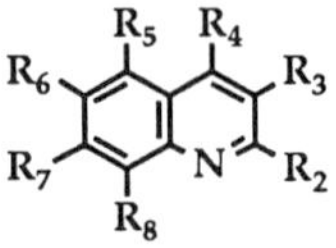

$$R_6 \quad R_5 \quad R_4 \quad R_3 \quad R_7 \quad N \quad R_2 \quad R_8$$

Compound No	R2	R3	R4	R5-R8	*App* K_i (nM)[a]	ID$_{50}$[b] (μg/ml)	%T/C[c]
S8577 Brequinar Sodium	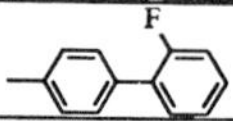 (2'-fluoro-biphenyl-4-yl)	-CH3	-COONa	6-F	25	0.132	179
X4544 NSC 339768	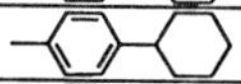 (biphenyl-4-yl)	-CH3	-COOH	6-F	27.5	0.077	181
S7243	(phenyl)	-CH3	-COOH	6-F	40,300	17.2	102
X3960	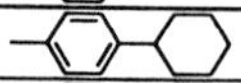 (biphenyl-4-yl)	-H	-COOH	6-F	122.0	0.047	141
S7911	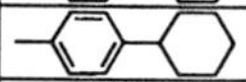 (biphenyl-4-yl)	-C2H5	-COOH	6-F	111	0.108	147
S8286	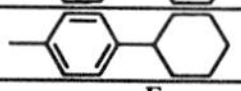 (biphenyl-4-yl)	-C3H7	-COOH	6-F	2,870	7.1	110
X9060	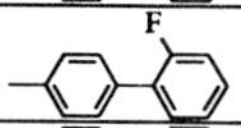 (2'-fluoro-biphenyl-4-yl)	-OH	-COOH	6-F	74.1	0.037	165
XA338	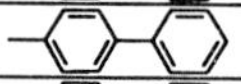 (biphenyl-4-yl)	-NH2	-COOH	6-F	18.0	0.11	157
S7741	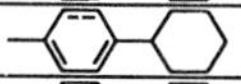 (biphenyl-4-yl)	-CH3	-COOC2H5	6-F	74,800	8.9	103
S7589	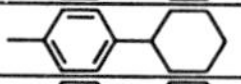 (biphenyl-4-yl)	-CH3	-CON(C2H5)2	6-F	13,300	6.8	94
S7680	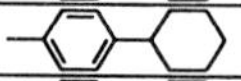 (biphenyl-4-yl)	-CH3	-CHO	6-F	3,900	1.03	104
S7678	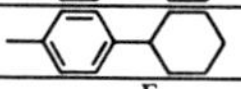 (biphenyl-4-yl)	-CH3	-CH2OH	6-F	3,130	1.99	118
X7335	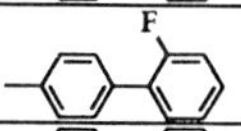 (2'-fluoro-biphenyl-4-yl)	-CH3	-SO3H	6-Cl	27,286	3.9	115
S8660	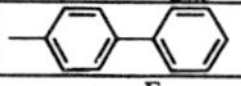 (biphenyl-4-yl)	-CH3	-COONa	5-Cl	65.8	0.57	180
S9665	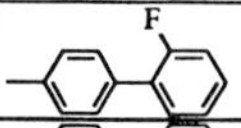 (2'-fluoro-biphenyl-4-yl)	-CH3	-COONa	6-Cl	36.6	0.186	173
S8412	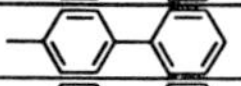 (biphenyl-4-yl)	-CH3	-COONa	7-Cl	4,750	8.6	104
S8409	(biphenyl-4-yl)	-CH3	-COONa	8-Cl	2,580	2.6	114
S8983	(biphenyl-4-yl)	-CH3	-COONa	5-Cl, 7 Cl	4,280	21.7	128

[a]Apparent Dixon Ki (nM) as inhibitor of L1210 Dihydroorotate Dehydrogenase (adapted from Ref. 27).
[b]Growth inhibitory activity against murine L1210 cells in culture as measured by MTT method.
[c]L1210 leukemia line is maintained by serial passage in DBA/2 mice; for drug evaluation tests, male or female DBA/2 or CD2F1 mice weighing 18-22 g were used. Test compounds were administered starting 1 day after i.p. tumor implantation. Drug efficacy is expressed as a percent of the mean survival time of the treated group vs that of the control group (T/C%). T/C% $\geq$ 125 is considered moderate activity, and a value of $\geq$ 150 is considered good activity.

the C(4) carboxylic acid, (ii) the C(2) position where bulky hydrophobic substituents are necessary, and (iii) the benzo portion of
the quinoline ring, with appropriate substitutions.

The carboxylic acid was found to be the only acceptable substituent at the C(4) position; the acid and its salts were equally
active. Other substituents (e.g. ester, amide, carboxaldehyde, hydroxymethyl, or sulfonic acid) at the C(4) position drastically reduced or totally abolished the inhibitory activity. These data
suggest that an important ionic interaction exists between the carboxylate group of the brequinar sodium analogs and a positively
charged group on DHO-DHase.

When the quinoline-4-carboxylic acid was substituted with a
smaller group at the C(2) position (e.g. a phenyl group), the analog was essentially inactive. However, when the quinoline-4-car-
boxylic acid was substituted with a bulky group at the C(2) position (e.g. biphenyl, substituted biphenyl, t-butyl phenyl, cyclo-
hexyl phenyl), the inhibitory activity increased 400-850 fold.
These data suggest that there is a strong hydrophobic interaction
between the enzyme and brequinar sodium at the C(2) position.

When the quinoline ring was replaced by a pyridine ring, that
compound did not inhibit the DHO-DHase activity (apparent K_i >
85,000 nM). This result indicates that the benzo portion of the
quinoline is necessary for the biological activity. We have found
that a chlorine substitution at the C(5) or C(6) position retained
the inhibitory activity. However, the compounds with a chlorine
substitution at the C(7) or C(8) position had greatly reduced inhibitory activity. It is of interest to note that the compound
with a chloro group substituted at both the C(5) and the C(7) position was also not active. These data suggest that the substituents
at the C(7) and C(8) position hinder the binding of the compound
to the enzyme.

The methyl group at the C(3) position was the best substituent. The inhibitory activity decreased as follow: methyl > ethyl
= hydrogen >> propyl. The effect of C(3) substitution on the inhibitory activity suggests that the C(3) substituent may interfere
sterically with the hydrophobic interaction of the C(2) group with

the enzyme or with the ionic interaction of C(4) carboxylic group
with the enzyme. We have also found that the methyl group can be
substituted with an hydroxy or amino group without affecting the
inhibitory activity. However, the inhibitory activity decreased
if the methyl group is substituted with the slightly bulkier methoxy group.

CORRELATION BETWEEN ENZYME INHIBITORY ACTIVITY, _IN_ _VITRO_ GROWTH INHIBITORY ACTIVITY, AND IN VIVO ANTITUMOR ACTIVITY

In addition to evaluating the analogs of 4-quinolinecarboxy-
lic acids as inhibitors of L1210 DHO-DHase, their _in_ _vitro_ growth
inhibitory activity and _in_ _vivo_ antitumor activity against murine
leukemia L1210 cells were also determined. Table 3 shows the
structure of selected analogs and the apparent K_i values, ID_{50}
values (concentration of drug that inhibits the growth of cultured
L1210 cells to 50% of the control), and %T/C values (mean survival
of mice bearing L1210 cells in the treated _vs_ control mice). The
data shown in Table 3 demonstrate a good correlation among the extent of enzyme inhibition, the _in_ _vitro_ growth inhibition of cultured L1210 cells, and the _in_ _vivo_ antitumor activity against murine L1210 leukemia. This good correlation between the cell-free
enzyme inhibitory activity and _in_ _vitro_ and _in_ _vivo_ antitumor activity is quite consistent with the mechanism of action of brequinar
sodium reported in this review. In addition, all of the weak inhibitors in this series of compounds are devoid of any _in_ _vivo_ antitumor activity. However, not all of the compounds that are good
inhibitors of DHO-DHase have _in_ _vivo_ activity. These results are
not unexpected, since various analogs might be expected to demonstrate different pharmacokinetics and metabolic fates.

SUMMARY

The salient features of the novel antitumor drug candidate
brequinar sodium have been described in this report. This substituted quinoline carboxylic acid salt has demonstrated excellent
activity against a panel of xenografted human carcinomas growing
in nude mice. Its efficacy in animal tumor models was schedule-

dependent; the agent showed high bioavailability and was equally active orally and parenterally.

Brequinar's unique structure as an anticancer agent precluded an _a priori_ identification or prediction of its mechanism. Subsequent to the demonstration of the compound's activity _vs_. solid tumor xenografts, its mechanism of action was determined to be the inhibition of the _de novo_ pyrimidine biosynthetic enzyme, dihydroorotate dehydrogenase. This mechanism explains why brequinar sodium acts in many ways like an antimetabolite, even though structurally the agent does not resemble an antimetabolite.

A more detailed investigation of the interaction between brequinar and its target enzyme has been completed. The enzyme DHO-DHase most likely follows a non-classical, two-site ping-pong mechanism. We propose that brequinar binds to the enzyme at a site distinct from either the substrate or the cofactor binding sites. A careful analysis of the kinetic data supports these conclusions.

SAR studies have demonstrated that the brequinar molecule has several sites where substitution patterns are crucial for enzyme inhibition. In particular, there is an absolute requirement for the carboxylic acid (or its salt) at the C(4) position of the quinoline ring. There are also strict requirements for a bulky substituent at the C(2) position, and for the benzo portion of the ring system. Substitutions that violate these strict requirements result in drastically reduced, or abolished, enzyme inhibitory activity.

Brequinar is currently undergoing phase 2 clinical trials as an anticancer agent. Our Discovery Groups have also determined recently that brequinar has excellent activity in animal models of arthritis, psoriasis and organ transplantation (28,29). Thus, this novel agent may have promise in disease indications other than cancer, such as organ transplant rejection.

ACKNOWLEDGEMENTS
The authors are grateful to Dr. R. C. Jackson for critically reading this manuscript. We also thank Drs. M. Forbes and N.A. Ackerman for their kind support during various stages of the dev-

elopment of brequinar sodium. We would also like to acknowledge many members of the Cancer Chemotherapy Group who have contributed significantly to the development of brequinar sodium. Drs. D.P. Hesson, R.J. Ardecky, G.V. Rao for their synthesis of many of the analogs, Ms. B.A. Dusak, and D.L. Behrens for their evaluation of the compounds _in vivo_, and to Ms. L.M. Papp for her outstanding technical assistance in biochemical evaluation of this series of compounds.

REFERENCES

1. Hesson DP: 2-Phenyl-4-quinolinecarboxylic acid and pharmaceutical compositions thereof. US Patent 4:680,299, 1987.
2. Dexter DL, Hesson DP, Ardecky RJ et al: Activity of a novel 4-quinolinecarboxylic acid, NSC 368390 [6-fluoro-2-(2'-fluoro-1,1'-biphenyl-4-yl)-3-methyl-4-quinolinecarboxylic acid sodium salt], against experimental tumors. Cancer Res. 45:5563-5568, 1985.
3. Goldin A, Venditti JM, MacDonald JS et al: Current results of the screening program at the Division of Cancer Treatment, National Cancer Institute. Europ. J. Cancer 17:129-142, 1981.
4. Braakhuis BJM, von Dongen GAMS, Peters GJ et al: Antitumor activity of brequinar sodium (DuP 785) against human head and neck squamous cell carcinoma xenografts. Cancer Lett. 49: 133-137, 1990.
5. Loveless SE, Neubauer RH: Antimetastatic activity of DuP 785. A novel anti-cancer agent. Proc. Am. Assoc. Cancer Res. 27:276, 1986.
6. Dexter DL, Dusak BA, Forbes M: Combination studies with brequinar sodium (DuP 785) and selected anticancer drugs against experimental tumors. Proc. Am. Assoc. Cancer Res. 29:333, 1986.
7. Chen SF, Ruben RL, Dexter DL: Mechanism of action of the novel anticancer agent 6-fluoro-2-(2'-fluoro-1,1'-biphenyl-4-yl)-3-methyl-4-quinolinecarboxylic acid sodium salt (NSC 368390): Inhibition of de novo pyrimidine nucleotide biosynthesis. Cancer Res. 46:5014-5019, 1986.
8. Boytek P, Beisler JA, Abbasi MM, Wolpert-DeFilippes MK: Comparative studies of the cytostatic action and metabolism of 5-azacytidine and 5,6-dihydro-5-azacytidine. Cancer Res. 37:1956-1961, 1977.
9. Peters GJ, Sharma SL, Laurensse E, Pinedo HM: Inhibition of pyrimidine de novo synthesis by DuP 785 (NSC 368390). Invest. New Drugs 5:235-244, 1987.
10. Moyer JD, Handschumacher RE: Selective Inhibition of pyrimidine synthesis and depletion of nucleotide pools by N-(phosphonacetyl)-L-aspartate. Cancer Res. 39:3089-3094, 1979.

279

11. Anderson LW, Strong JM, Cysyk RL: Cellular Pharmacology of DuP 785, a new anticancer agent. Cancer Comm. 1:381-387, 1989.
12. Schwartsmann G, Peters GJ, Laurensse E et al: DuP 785 (NSC 368390): Schedule-dependency of growth-inhibitory and anti-pyrimidine effects. Biochem. Pharmacol. 37:3257-3266, 1988.
13. Hunting D, Henderson JF: Relationship between ribo- and de-oxyribonucleotide concentrations and biological parameters in cultured Chinese hamster ovary cells. Biochem. Pharmacol. 31:1109-1115, 1982.
14. Grem JL, King SA, O'Dwyer PJ, Leyland-Jones B: Biochemistry and clinical activity of N-(phosphonacetyl)-L-aspartate: A Review. Cancer Res. 48:4441-4454, 1988.
15. Pizzorno G, Abate RA, Lentz SK, Handschumacher RE: Bre-quinar-5-Fluorouracil: A potent synergistic combination for anticancer therapy. Proc. Am. Assoc. Cancer Res. 31:426, 1990.
16. Peters GJ, Nadal JC, Laurensse EJ et al: Retention of in vivo antipyrimidine effects of brequinar sodium (DuP 785; NSC 368390) in murine liver, bone marrow and colon cancer. Biochem. Pharmacol. 39:135-144, 1990.
17. Chen JJ, Jones ME: The cellular location of dihydroorotate dehydrogenase: Relation to de novo biosynthesis of pyrimi-dine. Arch. Biochem. Biophys. 176:82-90,1976.
18. Karibian D: Dihydroorotate dehydrogenase (Escherichia coli). In: Methods in Enzymology, Purine and Pyrimidine Nucleotide Metabolism, PA Hoffee, ME Jones (eds.), Academic Press, Inc., New York, Vol. 51, pp. 58-63, 1978.
19. Pascal RA Jr, Trang NL, Cerami A, Walsh C: Purification and properties of dihydroorotate oxidase from Crithidia fasci-culata and Trypanosoma brucei. Biochem. 22:171-178, 1983.
20. Pascal RA Jr, Walsh CT: Mechanistic studies with deuterated dihydroorotates on the dihydroorotate oxidase from Crithidia fasciculata. Biochem. 23:2745-2752, 1984.
21. Miller RW: Dihydroorotate dehydrogenase (Neurospora). In: Methods in Enzymology, Purine and Pyrimidine Nucleotide Metabolism, PA Hoffee, ME Jones (eds.), Academic Press, Inc., New York, Vol. 51, pp. 63-69, 1978.
22. Chen SF, Papp LM, Dexter DL: Selective inhibition of dihydro-orotate dehydrogenase (DHO-DHase) by brequinar sodium. Proc. Am. Assoc. Cancer Res. 31:445, 1990.
23. Chen SF, Perrella FW, Behrens DL, Papp LM: Inhibition of L1210 mitochondrial dihydroorotate dehydrogenase by DuP 785 [6-fluoro-2-(2'-fluoro-1,1'-biphenyl-4-yl)-3-methyl-4-quino-linecarboxylic acid sodium salt]. Proc. Am. Assoc. Cancer Res. 28:320, 1987.
24. Jones ME: Pyrimidine nucleotide biosynthesis in animals: Genes, enzymes, and regulation of UMP biosynthesis. Ann. Rev. Biochem. 49:253-279, 1980.
25. Hines V, Johnston M: Analysis of the kinetic mechanism of the bovine liver mitochondrial dihydroorotate dehydrogenase. Biochem. 28:1222-1226, 1989.

26. Chen SF, Perrella FW, Behrens DL, Papp LM: Inhibition of dihydroorotate dehydrogenase by brequinar sodium (unpublished results).
27. Chen SF, Papp LM, Ardecky RJ et al: Structure-activity relationship of quinoline carboxylic acids: A new class of inhibitors of dihydroorotate dehydrogenase. Biochem. Pharmacol. 40:709-714, 1990.
28. Ackerman NR, Harris RR, Neubauer RH, Loveless SE: 4-Quinoline carboxylic acid derivatives useful for treating skin and muco-epithelial diseases. US Patent 4:861,783, 1989.
29. Ackerman NR, Jaffee BD, Neubauer RH, Loveless SE: 4-Quinoline carboxylic acid derivatives useful as immunosuppressive agents. US Patent 4:968,701, 1990.

17

DIPHTHERIA TOXIN-RELATED PEPTIDE HORMONE FUSION PROTEINS: NEW
TOXINS WITH THERAPEUTIC POTENTIAL

John R. Murphy, Diane P. Williams, Tetsuyuki Kiyokawa, Paige L.
Anderson and Terry B. Strom

INTRODUCTION

The genetic replacement of either the native diphtheria toxin
or _Pseudomonas_ exotoxin A receptor binding domain with eukaryotic
cell receptor-specific polypeptide hormones or growth factor sequences has resulted in the development of a new class of biological
response modifier - the fusion toxin (1-6). The first of these
fusion toxins, DAB_{486}-IL-2, is currently in human Phase I clinical trials and the early results clearly domonstrate that this
molecule is safe, well-tolerated, and biologically active in the
elimination of high affinity IL-2 receptor positive leukemia and
lymphoma cells without adverse side-effect (LeMaistre, personal
communication). DAB_{486}-IL-2 is a bipartite fusion protein composed of diphtheria toxin fragment A and fragment B sequences to
Ala^{486} linked to Pro^2 through Thr^{133} of human interleukin-2
(IL-2) (2). This chimeric protein is the product of a genetic
fusion between a truncated gene encoding fragment A and the membrane associating domains of fragment B of diphtheria toxin and a
synthetic gene encoding human IL-2 (7). DAB_{486}-IL-2 has been
shown to selectively bind to high affinity IL-2 receptors, be internalized by receptor-mediated endocytosis, and facilitate the
delivery of diphtheria toxin fragment A to the cytosol of target
cells (8,9). Recent studies have defined the minimal size of
fragment B that is required to deliver fragment A across the endocytic vesicle membrane in target cells, and defined the site of
proteolytic processing involved in the release of fragment A from
the intact fusion toxin molecule (10,11).

In an attempt to broaden the scope of the fusion toxin technology, we have recently focused our attention on the development of tripartite proteins in which diphtheria toxin fragment A sequences are being substituted with a variety of active polypeptides. While the application of protein engineering to the development of new biologicals is in its infancy, it is now clear that one can design and genetically construct a wide variety of fusion toxins that are extraordinarily selective and potent in the elimination of receptor-bearing target cells. Indeed, the early results from human Phase I/II clinical trials of DAB_{486}-IL-2 suggest that the fusion toxin technology will play an important role in the development of new biological agents for the treatment of specific human malignancies.

<u>Diphtheria Toxin</u>

Biochemical and genetic analyses of diphtheria toxin has clearly shown that the toxin molecule is composed of at least three functional domains: (i) the enzymatically active fragment A, (ii) the membrane associating domains and (iii) receptor binding domain of fragment B. Moreover, each domain of diphtheria toxin has been shown to play an essential role in the intoxication of intact sensitive eukaryotic cells (12). In mature form, diphtheria toxin is a single polypeptide chain of 585 amino acids in length, and contains four cysteine residues which form two disulfide bridges: Cys^{186}-Cys^{201} and Cys^{461}-Cys^{471} (13-15). The fourteen amino acid loop subtended by the first disulfide bridge contains three arginine residues (Arg^{190}, Arg^{192}, and Arg^{193}) and is extremely sensitive to proteolytic attack by serine proteases. Upon trypsin "nicking" and reduction of the first disulfide bridge, diphtheria toxin can be separated under denaturing conditions into two polypeptide fragments (16,17). Fragment A, the N-terminal 21.1 kDa polypeptide, carries the catalytic centers for the nicotinamide adenine dinucleotide (NAD+) dependent adenosine diphosphoribosylation (ADPR) of eukaryotic elongation factor 2 (EF-2) (18). The B fragment of diphtheria toxin, the 37.1 kDa polypeptide, carries at least two functional domains: the hydro-

283

phobic membrane associating domains which are responsible for the translocation of fragment A through the cell membrane and into the cytosol (19), and the native diphtheria toxin receptor binding domain (18). The toxin receptor binding domain has been recently located at the extreme C-terminal end of the toxin molecule (20,21).

Interactions between diphtheria toxin and toxin sensitive eukaryotic cells involve (i) the binding of intact toxin to the cell surface receptor (22), (ii) internalization of bound toxin by receptor-mediated endocytosis into acidification competent vesicles (23), and upon "nicking" of the toxin in this acidic environment [pH 5.3 - 5.1] (22,24), (iii) insertion of the hydrophobic domain(s) into the vesicle membrane (25,26), thereby facilitating the (iv) delivery of fragment A to the cytosol. Once delivered to the cytosol, fragment A catalyzed ADP-ribosylation of EF-2 abolishes cellular protein synthesis and as a result leads to the death of the cell. Yamaizumi et al. (27) have demonstrated that a _single_ molecule of fragment A delivered to the cytosol of a cell is sufficient to be lethal for that cell.

Since structure/function analysis of diphtheria toxin has shown that the toxin's receptor binding domain is positioned at the C-terminal end of the molecule, and that the first step in the intoxication process involves the binding of diphtheria toxin to its receptor, we reasoned several years ago that the replacement of the receptor binding domain with either a polypeptide hormone or cell specific growth factor should result in the formation of _new_ toxins. Moreover, the cellular target of these new toxins should be determined by the polypeptide hormone or growth factor used in its construction (1,2). Unlike the immunotoxins [i.e., fragments of microbial or plant toxins cross-linked to monoclonal antibodies], we chose to assemble these chimeric toxins at the level of the gene rather than by chemically coupling the toxophore with the ligand. The assembly of these fusion toxins at the level of the gene allows for (i) the precise linkage of the two components through a peptide bond, (ii) the modification of that structure through recombinant DNA techniques, and (iii) the production of the fusion toxins in recombinant _Escherichia coli_.

Thus, the approach that we have taken toward the development of targeted cytotoxins is fundamentally different from that of the immunotoxins. Rather than chemically cross-linking the toxophore and ligand components through a disulfide bond, we have employed protein and genetic engineering methods to create gene fusions whose chimeric products are joined by a peptide bond at a defined site. The precision of the genetic fusion strategy enables the assembly of isomeric fusion proteins, while chemical cross-linking yields racemic mixtures. Moreover, following interaction with cell surface receptors, the genetically engineered fusion toxins would by expected to be internalized by receptor mediated endocytosis which would deliver the toxin to the acidic environment of the endosome and facilitate the delivery of the ADP-ribosyltransferase to the cytosol. It should be noted that monoclonal antibodies can insure the delivery of immunotoxins to the cell surface; however, they do not provide assured delivery of the toxophore to either the endosome or the cytosol. Therefore, rather than to employ monoclonal antibodies as the cellular targeting component, we have used polypeptide hormones and growth factors whose receptors are known to undergo receptor-mediated endocytosis. Since peptide hormones and growth factors are known to be internalized into vesicles that become acidified, we reasoned that the internalization of a given toxin-related fusion protein should follow the same route of entry into the cell as diphtheria toxin itself.

IL-2-Toxin (DAB_{486}-IL-2)

Williams et al. (2) described the genetic construction and properties of a fusion toxin that was assembled from a truncated form of diphtheria toxin and human interleukin-2 (IL-2), DAB_{486}-IL-2. In this construct, the 3′-end of the _tox_ structural gene encoding the C-terminal receptor binding domain of diphtheria toxin was removed and replaced by a synthetic gene encoding amino acids 2 through 133 of mature human IL-2. Since the native diphtheria toxin receptor binding domain was replaced with IL-2 sequences, the resulting fusion toxin is directed towards cells bearing the IL-2 receptor. Importantly, cells which lacked the IL-2 re-

ceptor were found to be resistant to the inhibitory action of
DAB_{486}-IL-2. Bacha et al. (8) have confirmed and extended these
initial observations and have shown that the cytotoxic action of
this fusion toxin is mediated through the IL-2 receptor and can be
blocked by excess free recombinant IL-2, as well as by antibodies
that bind to the p55 subunit (Tac antigen) of the IL-2 receptor.
Moreover, since lysozomatrophic agents (e.g., chloroquine) also
block the cytotoxic action of DAB_{486}-IL-2, it is apparent that
the fusion toxin must pass through an acidic compartment in order
to deliver its ADP-ribosyltransferase to the cytosol of target
cells. Bacha et al. (8) also demonstrated that inhibition of protein syntheses in target cells was, in fact, due to the specific
ADP-ribosylation of elongation factor 2 in the target cell cytosol. Thus the cytotoxic action of DAB_{486}-IL-2 is (i) directed
through the IL-2 receptor, (ii) requires passage through an acidic
compartment in a manner analogous to native diphtheria toxin, and
(iii) catalyzes the ADP-ribosylation of elongation factor 2 in a
manner indistinguishable from that of native diphtheria toxin
fragment A.

More recently, Walz et al. (28) demonstrated that the sequential events following the binding of DAB_{486}-IL-2 to the IL-2 receptor on PHA activated T-cells reflects both the IL-2 and the ADP-
ribosyltransferase components of the fusion toxin. In a manner
identical to native IL-2, DAB_{486}-IL-2 was found to stimulate the
expression of c-_myc_, interferon gamma, IL-2 receptor, and IL-2
mRNA's for the first seven hours of exposure. However, after 7
hours exposure the action of the fusion toxin is analogous to that
of cycloheximide. By this time, the effects of inhibition of protein synthesis by the ADP-ribosylation of elongation factor 2 predominate and the steady state levels of c-_myc_ and IL-2 receptor
mRNA are decreased. Importantly, Walz et al. (28) have demonstrated that the ADP-ribosyltransferase defective mutant $DA(197)B_{486}$-
IL-2 does not inhibit protein synthesis and is capable of signal
transduction in PHA activated T-cells. This study has demonstrated that the functional activity of each of DAB_{486}-IL-2 component
parts are retained: (i) interaction of the fusion toxin with the

IL-2 receptor results in signal transduction, and (ii) the delivery of the ADP-ribosyltransferase to the cytosol results in an inhibition of protein synthesis and elicits a series of effects which are similar to those imposed by cycloheximide.

It is well known that the high affinity form of the IL-2 receptor is composed of at least two subunits: a low affinity 55 kDa glycoprotein (p55, Tac antigen) and an intermediate affinity 75 kDa glycoprotein (p75, Tic antigen) (29-34). Moreover, it is known that both the high affinity (p55 + p75) and intermediate affinity receptor, but not the low affinity receptor, undergo accelerated internalization after binding native IL-2 (33-36). Based on these observations, Waters el al. (9) have examined the receptor binding requirements of DAB_{486}-IL-2 for the efficient intoxication of target cells. As can be seen in Figure 1, dose response analysis of high, intermediate, and low affinity IL-2 re-

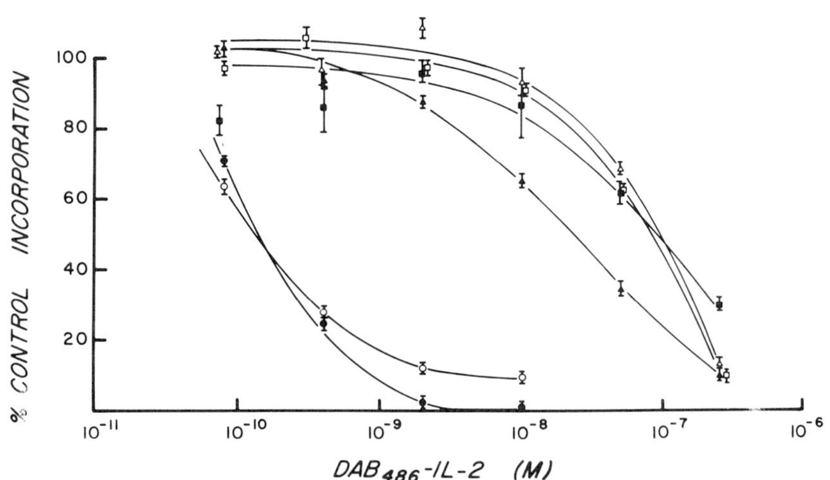

Figure 1. Comparison of sensitivity of high, intermediate, and low affinity IL-2 receptor bearing cell lines to DAB_{486}-IL-2. High affinity receptor bearing cell lines, HUT 102/6TG (●), C91/PL (O); intermediate affinity receptor bearing cell lines, YT2C2 (▲), SKW6.4 ([]), MLA-144 ( ); low affinity receptor bearing cell line, MT-1 (■) [adapted from Waters et al., 1990].

ceptor bearing cells demonstrates that only cell lines which bear the high affinity form of the IL-2 receptor are sensitive to the cytotoxic action of DAB_{486}-IL-2 ($IC_{50} \leq 1 \times 10^{-10}$ M). In marked contrast, cell lines which bear either isolated p55 chains or p75 chains are resistant to the action of the fusion toxin and require exposure to ca. 1,000-fold higher concentrations ($IC_{50} \geq 1 \times 10^{-7}$ M) of DAB_{486}-IL-2.

Since peripheral blood mononuclear cells (PBMC) with natural killer (NK) activity have been reported to bear only the p75 sub-unit of the IL-2 receptor on the cell surface and these cells are responsive to IL-2 and appear to be precursors of lymphokine acti-vated killer (LAK) cell activity, Waters el al. (9) examined the effect of DAB_{486}-IL-2 on NK cell activity. In these experiments, PBMC from healthy donors were cultured in the presence or absence of IL-2 and DAB_{486}-IL-2 and the subsequent NK cell activity was measured using K-562 target cells in a 4 hour [^{51}Cr]-release assay. Anti-CD3-induced T-cell cytotoxicity was measured in the same assay using an anti-CD3 mAb-producing target cell line. As shown in Table 1, concentrations of DAB_{486}-IL-2 greater than

Table 1

Effect of DAB_{486}-IL-2 on Human NK Cell Activity
(Adapted from Waters et al., 1990)

conditions	NK cell activity (% specific lysis) E / T ratio		
	40	20	10
medium	26	16	9
rIL-2	43	31	27
DAB_{486}-IL2 (10^{-7}M)	12	9	7
DAB_{486}-IL-2 (10^{-7}M) + rIL-2	20	14	10
DAB_{486}-IL2 (10^{-8}M)	27	18	14
DAB_{486}-IL-2 (10^{-8}M) + rIL-2	42	31	19

1×10^{-7} M are required to inhibit NK cell activity. Thus, human peripheral blood monocytes with NK activity are as resistant to the action of DAB_{486}-IL-2 as continuous cell lines which bear the p75 subunit of the IL-2 receptor.

Weissman et al. (35) have shown that the p55 subunit of the IL-2 receptor does not mediate efficient internalization of bound $[^{125}I]$-labeled IL-2. By comparison, native IL-2 bound to the p75 subunit of the receptor is known to be internalized as rapidly as the high affinity receptor [t1/2 = 15 min] (37). Since p75-only bearing cell lines were resistant to the action of DAB_{486}-IL-2, we reasoned that this resistance was due to altered binding of the fusion toxin to this subunit of the receptor. Waters et al. (9) have also determined the receptor binding properties of DAB_{486}-IL-2 by competitive displacement experiments using $[^{125}I]$-labeled IL-2. As shown in Table 2, approximately 200-fold higher concentrations of DAB_{486}-IL-2 are required to displace radio-

Table 2

Relative Ability of rIL-2 and DAB_{486}-IL-2
to Displace $[^{125}I]$-rIL-2 from the High,
Intermediate, and Low Affinity IL-2 Receptor
(Adapted from Waters et al., 1990)

| | | 50% displacement | |
cell line	IL-2 receptor	DAB_{486}-IL-2	rIL-2
HUT 102/6TG	p55, p75	8.1×10^{-9}M	3.8×10^{-11}M
YT2C2	p75	5.3×10^{-7}M	4.4×10^{-9}M
MT-1	p55	4.0×10^{-7}M	2.2×10^{-8}M

labeled IL-2 from the high affinity (p55 + p75) receptor. It is of interest to note that only 18-fold higher concentrations of DAB_{486}-IL-2 than native IL-2 are required to displace radio-labeled ligand from the p55 subunit; whereas, 120-fold higher concentrations are required for the p75 subunit.

The receptor binding experiments described above strongly suggest that the relative resistance of p75-only bearing cells to the cytotoxic action of DAB_{486}-IL-2 is due to altered binding to the p75 subunit of the receptor. Although both the p75 and the high affinity heterodimer share the common property of rapidly internalizing bound ligand, p75 binding is characterized by slow kinetics of association/dissociation. In contrast, the high affinity receptor displays the fast "on" rate of p55 and the slow "off" rate of p75 (38,39). Thus, an alteration in DAB_{486}-IL-2 binding to the p75 subunit may more dramatically influence the kinetics of this fusion toxin's binding to the intermediate vis-a-vis high affinity receptor. Clearly, the results of the competitive displacement studies described by Waters et al. (9) are consistent with this interpretation. As determined by the concentration of fusion toxin required to inhibit radiolabeled IL-2 binding, it is evident that DAB_{486}-IL-2 displays altered binding to <u>both</u> subunits of the IL-2 receptor; however, binding to the p75 subunit appears to be more significantly affected than binding to the p55 subunit.

Since Collins et al. (40) have reported that the N-terminal sequences of native IL-2, particularly Asp^{20}, are essential for binding to the p75 subunit of the IL-2 receptor, it is likely that the altered binding of DAB_{486}-IL-2 to this subunit results from stearic constraints imposed on the fusion toxin : p75 interaction. In the case of DAB_{486}-IL-2, human IL-2 sequences are fused to the C-terminal end of a truncated form of the toxin. Therefore, the fusion junction between diphtheria toxin-related and IL-2 sequences are likely to place Asp^{20} [Asp^{505} in DAB_{486}-IL-2] in an internal or less favorable position to bind to the p75 subunit. Consistent with this interpretation are the results of Lorberboum-Galski et al. (41) who have described the cytotoxic action of an analogous fusion toxin composed of a truncated form of <u>Pseudomonas</u> exotoxin-A and IL-2, IL-2-PE40. In this instance, cells which express the high affinity form of the IL-2 receptor have been found to be only 8 - 20 times more sensitive to the cytotoxic action of IL-2-PE40 than cell lines which express either isolated p75 or p55 chains of the receptor. Moreover, only 6-fold differences in binding to the p75 subunit were reported for IL-2-PE40 relative to native IL-2. In the case of IL-2-PE40, the fusion junction between the two proteins occurs at the C-terminal end of IL-2 and the N-terminus of PE40. Since the N-terminus of this fusion toxin consists of IL-2 sequences, Asp^{20} is likely to be more available for binding to the p75 subunit of the receptor than Asp^{505} in DAB_{486}-IL-2. The observed cytotoxicity of this fusion toxin for p75-only bearing cells supports this hypothesis.

Williams et al. (10) have demonstrated that the inframe deletion of 97 amino acids from Thr^{387} to His^{485} of DAB_{486}-IL-2 increases both the potency (IC_{50} = 2 - 5 x 10^{-11} M) and the apparent dissociation constant (K_d) of the resulting DAB_{389}-IL-2 for high affinity IL-2 receptor bearing T-cells (Figure 2 & 3). In marked contrast, the deletion of an additional 94 amino acids

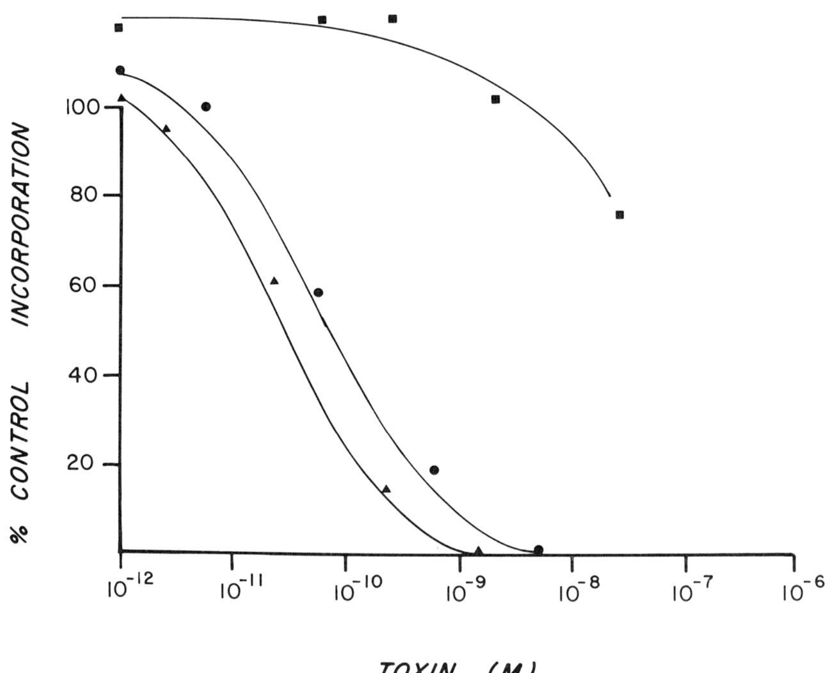

Figure 2. Dose response analysis of DAB_{486}-IL2 (●); DAB_{389}-IL-2 (▲); and DAB_{295}-IL-2 (■) on HUT 102/6TG cells. Results are presented as percent control incorporation of $[^{14}C]$-leucine into trichloroacetic acid precipitable material.

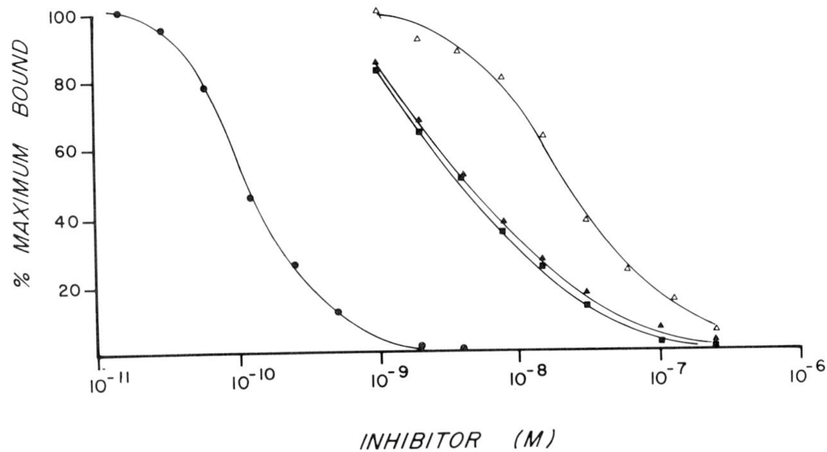

Figure 3.   Competitive displacement of [^{125}I]-rIL-2 from the high affinity IL-2 receptor by unlabeled rIL-2 (●), DAB$_{486}$-IL-2 (△); DAB$_{389}$-IL-2 (■); and DAB$_{295}$-IL-2 (△).

(Asp^{291} to Gly^{483}) results in a greater than 1,000-fold loss of cytotoxic potency in the fusion toxin DAB$_{295}$-IL-2. It should be noted that the structural regions between Asp^{291} and Gly^{483} include the hydrophobic putative membrane spanning helical regions of fragment B that have been postulated to facilitate the delivery of fragment A across the endocytic vesicle membrane (19). The results of experiments described by Williams et al. (10) strongly suggest that the putative membrane spanning helices of fragment B are essential in the intoxication process.

In addition, Williams et al. (10) have shown that the amphipathic membrane surface binding region of fragment B contained between Asn^{204} and Ile^{290} is also essential to the cytotoxicity of the DAB-IL-2 fusion toxins. It is important to note that the genetic deletion of this region of fragment B in both DAB(205-289)$_{486}$-IL-2 and DAB(205-289)$_{389}$-IL-2 also decreases biologic activity of the fusion toxin by ca. 1,000-fold. Most interestingly, these in-frame internal deletion mutations also effect the apparent K_d of the fusion toxin for the high affinity IL-2 receptor. Since the region that has been deleted carries an amphipathic domain(s) (42), it is reasonable to postulate that this region of fragment B associates with the T-cell membrane surface forming a non-specific secondary binding event and appears to stabilize the interaction of the fusion toxin with the target cell surface.

We have analyzed the primary amino acid sequence of DAB_{486}-IL-2 and DAB_{389}-IL-2 fusion toxins for predicted secondary structure using the PC GENE software (Intelligenetics, Mountain View, CA). In particular, the FLEXPRO program of Karplus and Schulz (43) was used to predict the flexibility of the DAB-IL-2 fusion toxins at each point of their sequence. This program calculates the theoretical flexibility of the peptide chain at each amino acid and is measured from the average value of the atomic temperature factor (B value) of the alpha carbon atom, as affected by the adjacent amino acids. The "neighbor-correlated" average normalized B values for each amino acid was found from a set of proteins whose three dimensional structural was known. The predicted flexibility at an amino acid is the weighted sum of the normalized B values (taking account of neighbors) of the seven amino acids closest to that point in the sequences.

It is of particular interest to note that this analysis of the DAB-IL-2 toxins has revealed a common predicted "most" flexible region - amino acids 1 through 10 of human IL-2 (Table 3).

Table 3

Position and Amino Acid Sequence of the Predicted Most
Flexible segments of DAB_{486}-IL-2 and DAB_{389}-IL-2

Fusion toxin	from	to	B-[norm]	Sequence
DAB_{486}-IL-2	487	493	1.135	Pro-Thr-Ser-Ser-Ser-Thr-Lys
DAB_{389}-IL-2	390	396	1.135	Pro-Thr-Ser-Ser-Ser-Thr-Lys

Since this region was also found to be unordered in the 5.5 A
crystal structure of IL-2 (44), we postulated that the apparent
flexibility of this region of the fusion toxin might allow for
some degree of mobility of the IL-2 component with respect to the
diphtheria toxin-related sequences. Were this the case, duplication of the flexible region might result in a fusion toxin with increased receptor binding affinity and potency. In order to test
this hypothesis, we have genetically constructed mutants of DAB_{486}-
IL-2 and DAB_{389}-IL-2 in which amino acids 1 through 10 of IL-2
were duplicated at the fusion junction (45). These constructions
were made by cloning a 33-mer oligonucleotide linker encoding
amino acids 1 through 10 of IL-2 into the unique SphI site which
defines the fusion junction between diphtheria toxin-related and
IL-2 sequences. It should be noted that codon usage in the linker
was changed with respect to that already present in the DAB_{486}-
IL-2 structural gene in order to insure genetic stability of the
insert.

Figure 4 shows the dose response curve of the duplication
mutant DAB_{389}-(1-10)IL-2 on high affinity IL-2 receptor bearing
HUT 102 6/TG cells. As can be seen, the IC_{50} for DAB_{389}-(1-10)
IL-2 (6 x 10^{-12} M) is 40 to 60-fold higher than that of DAB_{486}-
IL-2 and approximately 10-fold higher than DAB_{389}-IL-2. These
studies clearly demonstrate that the application of protein engineering methodologies towards the development of second generation DAB-IL-2 fusion toxins will result in variants with increased
biologic potency.

Tripartite Fusion Toxins: Shiga-A-DT"B"-IL-2

We (Anderson, Itoh, Nishibuchi, Takeda, and Murphy, in preparation) have selected the A chain of Shiga-like toxin to replace
diphtheria toxin fragment A in the construction of the first tripartite toxin for the following reasons: (i) both Shiga-like A
and diphtheria fragment A are similar in molecular mass, (ii) the
introduction of a single molecule of Shiga-like A chain to the cytosol of a target cell will result in an irreversible inhibition
of protein syntheses, and, as a result, the measurement of bio-

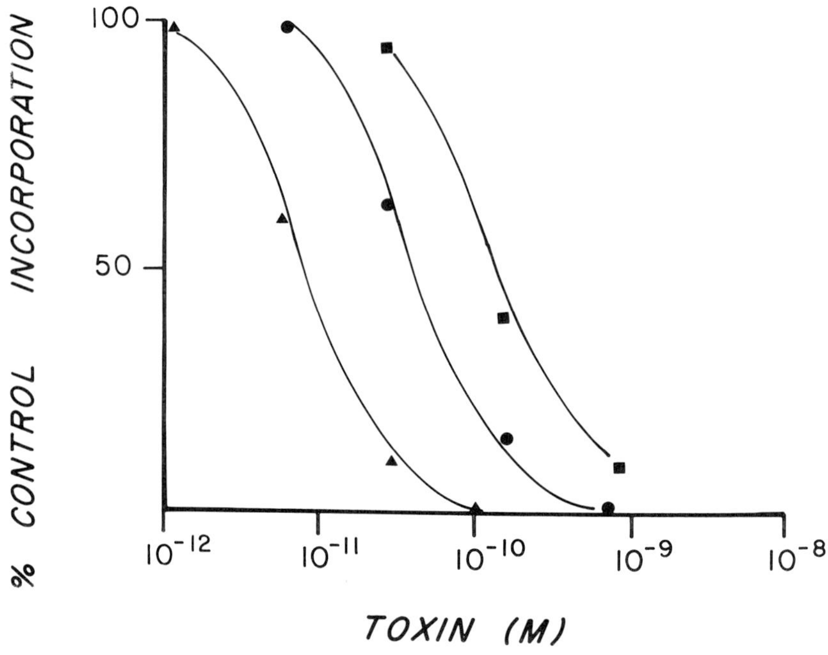

Figure 4. Dose response analysis of DAB_{486}-IL-2 (■); DAB_{389}-IL-2 (●); and DAB_{389}-(1-10)$_2$IL-2 (△) on HUT 102/6TG cells.

logic activity of the tripartite fusion would be both convenient and sensitive, and (iii) the modification of the gene for Shiga-like A chain required to construct the tripartite fusion toxin gene is straightforward and could be readily accomplished.

The gene for Shiga-like toxin has recently been cloned and sequenced (46,47). Shiga-like toxin is composed of an A subunit (32,225 Da) that is noncovalently bound to a pentameric B subunit (7,961 Da). The A subunit of Shiga-like toxin contains a single disulfide bridge that subtends a protease sensitive loop. Upon trypsin nicking an A1 and A2 fragment are released. The A1 fragment of Shiga-like toxin has been shown to be an enzyme which specifically cleaves the N-glycosidic bond at adenine 4325 in the 28S ribosomal RNA. Thus, Shiga-like toxin inhibits protein synthe-

sis in a manner that is identical to that of the plant toxin ricin
(48). It should be noted that the isolated chains of Shiga-like
toxin, like those of diphtheria toxin, are <u>not</u> toxic for intact
eukaryotic cells.

Biochemical/genetic analysis of DAB_{486}-IL-2 mutants has
recently shown that fragment A <u>must</u> be released from the fusion
toxin in order to intoxicate target lymphocytes. Williams et al.
(11) have found that the substitution of Arg^{194} with Gly results
in an approximate 5,000-fold loss of cytotoxic potency of the fusion toxin. Interestingly, pre-nicking the mutant fusion toxin
with trypsin restores full biologic activity. These results suggests that DAB_{486}-IL-2 binds to the IL-2 receptor, and is then
<u>processed</u> by a cellular protease at Arg^{194} in order to release
fragment A which is then delivered to the cytosol. These results
strongly suggest that an intact disulfide bridge between Cys^{187}
and Cys^{202} in DAB_{486}-IL-2 is essential for full biologic activity.

As a result of these observations, we have developed a vector
for the genetic construction of the tripartite fusion toxin which
retains the Cys^{187} : Cys^{202} disulfide bond. We have taken advantage of a unique <u>Nsi</u>I restriction endonuclease site that is positioned at Cys^{202} and the <u>Nco</u>I site that contains the ATG of the
translational initiation signal at the beginning of fragment A.
Following digestion of plasmid pABI6508 with <u>Nsi</u>I and <u>Nco</u>I, we
have cloned an <u>Nsi</u>I-<u>Apa</u>I-<u>Nco</u>I linker that restores the genetic information encoding the Cys^{187} : Cys^{202} disulfide loop. The modified plasmid has been designated pPA101. Importantly, this linker
also introduces a unique <u>Apa</u>I site immediately upstream of Cys^{187}.
As a result, <u>any</u> gene that can be modified at its 5′end by the introduction of an <u>Nco</u>I site, and at its 3′end by the introduction
of an <u>Apa</u>I site can be inserted into pPA101 giving rise to a tripartite fusion gene.

We have modified the structural gene for Shiga-like toxin A
chain by the introduction of a 5′ <u>Nco</u>I-<u>Taq</u>I linker, and a 3′ <u>Xmn</u>I-
<u>Apa</u>I linker. The modified gene for Shiga-like A chain was then
introduced into the <u>Nco</u>I and <u>Apa</u>I sites of pPA101 to form plasmid

pPASA101 (Anderson and Murphy, unpublished). Following growth and expression of the tripartite toxin gene, the Shiga-like A-DT"B"-IL-2 fusion toxin was purified by immunoaffinity chromatography on an anti-IL-2 matrix. As shown in Figure 5, the tripartite toxin can be readily purified to apparent homogeneity by immunoaffinity

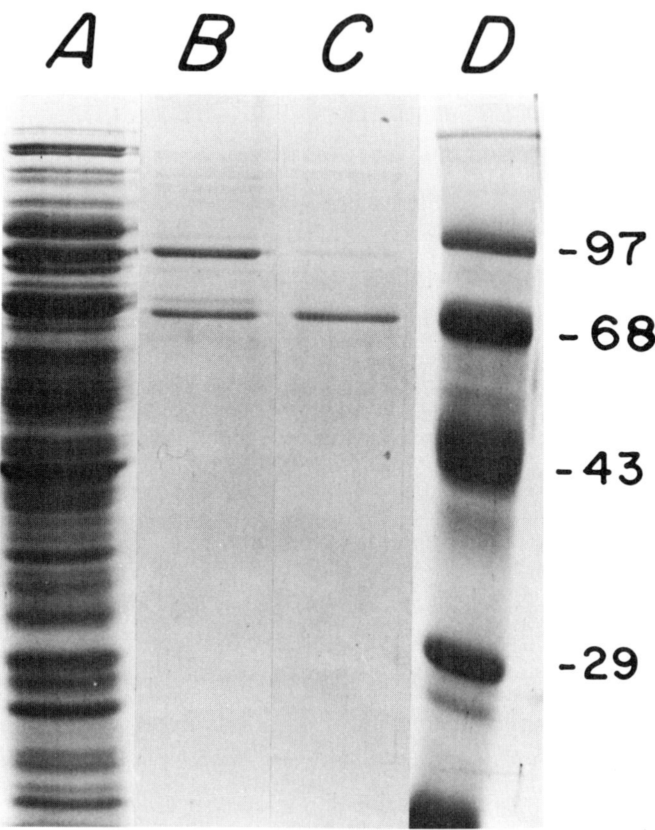

Figure 5. Sodium docelysulfate polyacrylamide gel electrophoresis of partially purified tripartite Shiga-like A-DT"B"-IL-2 fusion toxin. Lane A, crude extracts from recombinant _E. coli_; Lane B, peak fraction from anti-IL-2 affinity chromatography; Lane C, peak fraction from HPLC sizing column; Lane D, molecular weight standards. Apparent molecular weights are given as M_r x 10^{-3}.

chromatography followed by HPLC chromatography. Futhermore, the tripartite fusion toxin has been shown to carry determinants that are reactive on immunoblots probed with anti-Shiga-like A, anti-IL-2, and anti-diphtheria toxin sera. Thus, the three domains of the tripartite toxin fold in such a way as to present their own unique and characteristic immunodominant epitopes. Most exciting, however, is the observation that the tripartite toxin is biologically active against high affinity IL-2 receptor bearing T-lymphocytes (Figure 6). It should be noted that the biological activity of the tripartite toxin can be specifically blocked with either

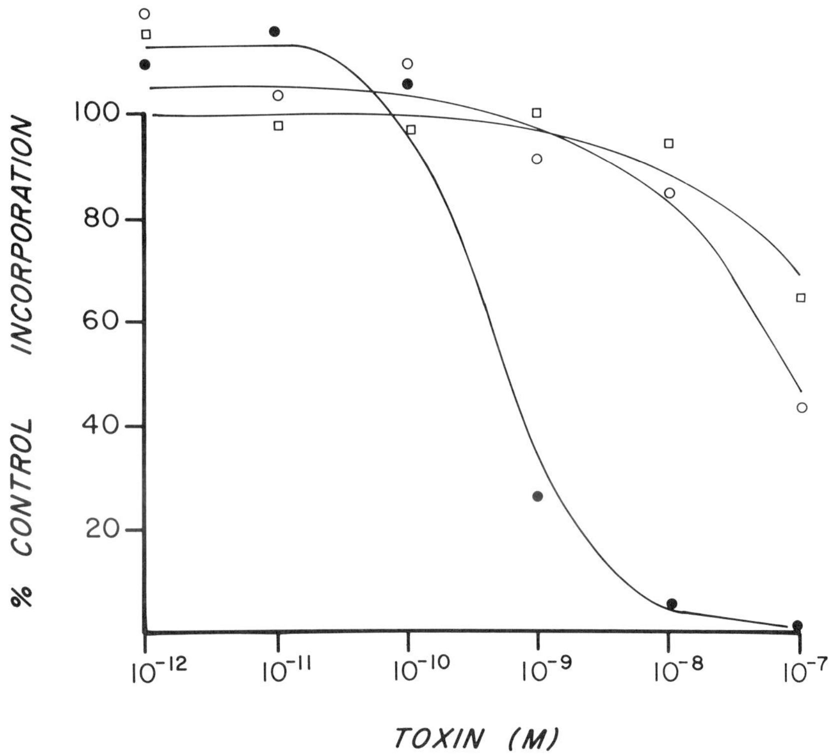

Figure 6. Comparison of sensitivity of high, intermediate, and low affinity IL-2 receptor bearing cell lines to the tripartite Shiga-like A-DT"B"-IL2 fusion toxin. High affinity IL-2 receptor bearing HUT 102/6TG cells (●), intermediate affinity IL-2 receptor bearing YT2C2 cells (O), and low affinity IL-2 receptor bearing MT-1 cells (▢).

excess IL-2 or monoclonal antibody to the p55 subunit of the IL-2 receptor. These results demonstrate that the action of this fusion toxin is mediated through the IL-2 receptor.

ACKNOWLEDGEMENTS

Preparation of this review was supported in part by Public Health Service grants RO1 CA-41746 and UO1 CA-48626 (J.R.M.) from the National Cancer Institute, and RO1 AI-22882 (T.B.S.) from the National Institute of Allergy and Infectious Diseases.

REFERENCES

1. Murphy JR, Bishai W, Borowski M et al: Genetic construction, expression and melanoma-selective cytotoxicity of a diphtheria toxin-related α-melanocyte stimulating hormone fusion protein. Proc. Natl Acad. Sci. 83:8258-8262, 1986.
2. Williams DP, Parker K, Bacha P et al: Diphtheria toxin receptor binding domain substitution with interleukin-2: Genetic construction and properties of a diphtheria toxin-related interleukin-2 fusion protein. Protein Engineering 1:493-498, 1987.
3. Chaudhary VK, FitzGerald DJ, Adhya S, Pastan I: Activity of a recombinant fusion protein between transforming growth factor type alpha and _Pseudomonas_ toxin. Proc. Natl. Acad. Sci. 84:4538-4542, 1987.
4. Loberboum-Galski H, FitzGerald DJ, Chaudhary V et al: Cytotoxic activity of an interleukin-2 Pseudomonas exotoxin chimeric protein produced in _Escherichia coli_. Proc. Natl. Acad. Sci. 85:1922-1926, 1988.
5. Chaudhary VK, Mizukami T, Fuerst TR et al: Selective killing of HIV-infected cells by recombinant human CD4-_Pseudomonas_ exotoxin hybrid protein. Nature (London) 335:369-372, 1988.
6. Siegall CB, Chaudhary VK, FitzGerald DJ, Pastan I: Cytotoxic activity of an interleukin-6-_Pseudomanas_ exotoxin fusion protein on human myeloma cells. Proc. Natl. Acad. Sci. 85:9738-9742, 1988.
7. Williams DP, Regier D, Akiyoshi D et al: Design, synthesis and expression of a human interleukin-2 gene incorporating the codon usage bias found in highly expressed _Escherichia coli_ genes. Nucleic Acids Res. 16:10453-10467, 1988.
8. Bacha P, Williams DP, Waters C et al: Interleukin-2 receptor targeted cytotoxicity: Selective action of a diphtheria toxin-related interleukin-2 fusion protein. J. Exp. Med. 167:612-622, 1988.
9. Waters CA, Schimke P, Snider CE et al: Interleukin-2 receptor targeted cytotoxicity: Receptor binding requirements for entry of IL-2-toxin into cells. Eur. J. Immunol. 20:785-791, 1990.
10. Williams DP, Snider CE, Strom TB, Murphy JR: Structure function analysis of IL-2-toxin (DAB_{486}-IL-2): Fragment B sequences required for the delivery of fragment A to the cytosol of target cells. J. Biol. Chem. 265:11885-11890, 1990.

11. Williams DP, Wen Z, Watson RS et al: Cellular processing of the fusion toxin DAB_{486}-IL-2 and efficient delivery of diphtheria toxin fragment A to the cytosol of target cells requires Arg194. J. Biol. Chem. 265:20673-20677, 1990.
12. Pappenheimer AM Jr.: Diphtheria toxin. Ann. Rev. Biochem. 46:69-94, 1977.
13. Kazcorek M, Delpeyroux F, Chenciner N et al: Nucleotide sequence and expression in _Escherichia coli_ of the _tox_228 diphtheria toxin gene. Science 221:855-858, 1983.
14. Greenfield L, Bjorn M, Horn G et al: Nucleotide sequence of the structural gene for diphtheria toxin carried by corynebacteriophage β. Proc. Natl. Acad. Sci. 80:6853-6857, 1983.
15. Ratti G, Rappuoli R, Giannini G: The complete nucleotide sequence of the gene coding for diphtheria toxin in the corynephage omega (_tox_+) genome. Nucleic Acids Res. 11:6589-6595, 1983.
16. Gill DM, Pappenheimer AM Jr.: Structure activity relationships in diphtheria toxin. J. Biol. Chem. 246:1492-1495, 1971.
17. Collier RJ, Kandel J: Structure and activity of diphtheria toxin. I. Thiol-dependent dissociation of a fraction of toxin into enzymatically active and inactive fragments. J. Biol Chem. 246:1496-1503, 1971.
18. Uchida T, Gill DM, Pappenheimer AM Jr: Mutation in the structural gene for diphtheria toxin carried by temperate phage β. Nature (New Biol.) 233:8-11, 1971.
19. Boquet P, Silverman MS, Pappenheimer AM Jr, Vernon WB: Binding of Triton X-100 to diphtheria toxin, cross-reacting material 45, and their fragments. Proc. Natl. Acad. Sci. 73: 4449-4453, 1976.
20. Greenfield L, Johnson V, Youle RJ: Mutations in diphtheria toxin separate binding from entry and amplify immunotoxin selectivity. Science 238:536-539, 1987.
21. Rolf JM, Gaudin HM, Eidels L: Localization of the diphtheria toxin receptor-binding domain to the carboxy-terminal $M^r \approx$ 6000 region of the toxin. J. Biol. Chem. 265:7331-7337, 1990.
22. Middlebrook JL, Dorland RB, Leppla S: Association of diphtheria toxin with Vero cells: Demonstration of a receptor. J. Biol. Chem. 253:7325-7330, 1978.
23. Moya M, Dautry-Versat A, Goud B et al: Inhibition of coated-pit formation in Hep2 cells blocks the cytotoxicity of diphtheria toxin but not that of ricin toxin. J. Cell Biol. 101:548-559, 1985.
24. Sandvig K, Tonnessen TI, Sand O, Olsnes S: Requirement of a transmembrane pH gradient for the entry of diphtheria toxin into cells at low pH. J. Biol. Chem. 261:11639-11645, 1986.
25. Donovan JJ, Simon MI, Draper RK, Montal M: Diphtheria toxin forms transmembrane channels in planar lipid bilayers. Proc. Natl. Acad. Sci. 78:172-176, 1981.
26. Kagan BL, Finkelstein A, Colombini M: Diphtheria toxin fragment forms large pores in phospholipid bilayer membranes. Proc. Natl. Acad. Sci. 78:4950-4954, 1981.

27. Yamaizumi M., Mekada E, Uchida T, Okada Y: One molecule of diphtheria toxin fragment A introduced into a cell can kill the cell. Cell 15:245-250, 1978.
28. Walz G, Zanker B, Brand K et al: Sequential effects of inter-leukin-2/diphtheria toxin fusion protein on T-cell activa-tion. Proc. Natl. Acad. Sci. 86:9485-9488, 1989.
29. Sharon M, Klausner RD, Cellen BR et al: Novel interleukin-2 receptor subunit detected by cross-linking under high-affi-nity conditions. Science 234:859-863, 1986.
30. Tsudo MR, Kozak W, Goldman CK, Waldmann TA: Demonstration of a non-Tac peptide that binds interleukin-2: A potential par-ticipant in a multichain interleukin-2 receptor complex. Proc. Natl. Acad. Sci. 83:9694-9698, 1986.
31. Teshigawara K, Wang HM, Kato K, Smith KA: Interleukin-2 high affinity receptor expression depends on two distinct binding proteins. J. Exp. Med. 165:223-238, 1987.
32. Dukovich M, Wano Y, Bich-Thuy LT et al: A second human interleukin-2 binding protein that may be a component of high-affinity interleukin-2 receptors. Nature (London) 237:518-522, 1987.
33. Robb RJ, Rusk CM, Yodoi J, Greene WC: Interleukin 2 binding molecule distinct from the Tac protein: Analysis of its role in the formation of high affinity receptors. Proc. Natl. Acad. Sci. 84:2001-2006, 1987.
34. Tanaka T, Saiki O, Doi S et al: Novel receptor-mediated in-ternalization of interleukin-2 in B cells. J. Immunol. 140:866-870, 1988.
35. Weissman AM, Harford JB, Svetlik PB et al: Only high affin-ity receptor for interleukin-2 mediates internalization of ligand. Proc. Natl. Acad. Sci. 83:1463-1466, 1986.
36. Fujii M, Sugamura K, Sano K et al: High affinity receptor-mediated internalization and degradation of interleukin-2 in human T-cells. J. Exp. Med. 163:550-562, 1986.
37. Robb RJ, Greene WC: Internalization of interleukin-2 is mediated by the β chain of the high affinity interleukin-2 receptor. J. Exp. Med. 165:1201-1206, 1987.
38. Wang HM, Smith KA: The interleukin-2 receptor: Functional consequences of its biomolecular structure. J. Exp. Med. 166:1055-1069, 1987.
39. Lowenthal JL, Greene WC: Contrasting interleukin-2 binding properties of the α (p55) and β (p70) protein subunits of the human high-affinity interleukin-2 receptor. J. Exp. Med. 166:1156-1161, 1987.
40. Collins L, Tsien WH, Seals C et al: Identification of speci-fic residues of human interleukin-2 that affect binding to the 70-kDa subunit (p70) of the interleukin-2 receptor. Proc. Natl Acad. Sci. 85:7709-7713, 1988.
41. Lorberboum-Galski H, Kozak RW, Waldmann TA et al: Interleukin-2 (IL-2) PE40 is cytotoxic to cells displaying either the p55 or p70 subunit of the IL-2 receptor. J. Immunol. 263:18650-18656, 1988.
42. Lambotte P, Falmagne P, Capiau C et al: Primary structure of diphtheria toxin fragment B: Structural similarities with lipid-binding proteins. J. Cell Biol. 87:837-840, 1980.

43. Karplus P, Shultz GE: Prediction of chain flexibility in proteins - A tool for the selection of peptide antigens. Natarwissenschaften 72:212-213, 1986.
44. Brandhuber BJ, Boone T, Kenney WC, McKay DB: Three dimensional structure of interleukin-2. Science 238:1707-1709, 1987.
45. Kiyokawa T, Williams DP, Snider CE et al: Protein engineering of diphtheria toxin-related interleukin-2 fusion toxins to increase biologic potency for high affinity interleukin-2 receptor bearing target cells. Protein Engineering. 1990, in press.
46. Calderwood SB, Auclair F, Donohue-Rolfe A et al: Nucleotide sequence of the Shiga-like toxin genes of _Escherichia_ _coli_. Proc. Natl. Acad. Sci. 84:4364-4368, 1987.
47. Strockbine NA, Jackson MP, Sung LM et al: Cloning and sequencing of the genes for Shiga toxin from _Shigella_ _dysenteriae_ type 1. J. Bacteriol. 170:1116-1122, 1988.
48. Endo Y, Tsurugi K. RNA-glycosidase activity of ricin A-chain: Mechanism of action of the toxin lectin ricin on eucaryotic ribosomes. J. Biol. Chem. 262:8128-8130, 1987.

18

ANTI-GROWTH FACTOR RECEPTOR ANTIBODIES AS THERAPY FOR CANCER

Raymond Taetle

INTRODUCTION

The idea of attacking cancer cells at the cell surface was revived in the past decade by the availability of monospecific heteroantisera. Phase I trials using monoclonal antibodies to most tumor cell antigens have shown little anti-tumor activity (Reviewed in 1,2). The reasons for these failures are complex, but include heterogeneity of tumor antigen expression; antibody-induced antigen modulation from the cell surface; formation of human anti-mouse antibodies; and the uncertain efficacy of the host cell anti-tumor response (1,2). Immunoconjugates employing monoclonal antibodies as carriers for toxins, drugs, or radio-isotopes and chimeric human-mouse monoclonal antibodies remain under investigation (1,2).

We have taken a slightly different approach to this problem by using cell surface growth and nutrient receptors as targets for monospecific antisera. For the past 5 years, these reagents have been developed under the auspices of a National Cooperative Drug Discovery Group with Dr. John Mendelsohn as the Project Leader and Hideo Masui at Memorial/Sloan Kettering Cancer Institute, Dr. Ian Trowbridge at the Salk Institute and myself, with the assistance of National Cancer Institute staff.

A variety of evidence suggests that many tumor cells require growth factors for proliferation, and that growth factor receptor display alters tumor cell behavior (3-5). Our goal has been to develop anti-cancer agents which inhibit tumor cell growth by both marshalling immune responses, and by directly depriving cells of epidermal growth factor (EGF) receptor stimulation or transferrin receptor function. In contrast to serotherapy targeting other cell surface antigens, in this setting, antibodies inducing antigen modulation may reduce available tumor cell growth factor receptors, and may be as effective as reagents which block or inhibit growth factor receptor action. These reagents have also been useful for studying tumor cell growth factor responses and antigen expression (6-12).

ANTIBODIES TO THE EPIDERMAL GROWTH FACTOR RECEPTOR
Background

The EGF receptor is the prototype ligand-stimulated, protein tyrosine kinase receptor and is highly homologous to the erb-b1 oncogene (13). In vitro studies indicate that the EGF receptor is over-expressed in many different tumor types, and suggest these receptors contribute to the transformed cell phenotype. In vitro, a variety of non-hematologic tumor cell lines express EGF receptors, including lung, bladder, breast, colon and vulvar squamous cell carcinomas (14-22). Many of these same tumors contain RNA for and express the polypeptide growth factor transforming growth factor-α (TGF-α), which binds to and stimulates EGF receptors, and induces a transformed cell phenotype in vitro (23). Recent studies showed that a membrane bound form of tumor cell TGF-α also mediates EGF receptor stimulation (24,25), and indicate that TGF-α can cause transformation without being secreted into the extracellular environment. This potential auto-secretory loop between TGF-α producing tumor cells and endogenous, overexpressed EGF receptors provides a strong rationale for attacking the EGF receptor with monoclonal antibodies (MAbs).

Expression of normal EGF receptors at high density in normal murine fibroblasts by transfecting these cells with a human EGF receptor gene construct causes EGF-dependent cell transformation (13,26), indicating that the native receptor can induce abnormal cellular behavior. When sublines of a squamous cell carcinoma xenograft were implanted in immune-deficient mice, tumor growth rate was positively related to surface EGF receptor number (27).

Recent data suggest that growth rates of human gastric carcinoma xenografts also correlate with levels of tumor cell EGF receptor expression (28). Thus, in experimental _in vitro_ and _in vivo_ systems, the native EGF receptor causes significant alterations in cancer cell growth.

When relative numbers of EGF receptors were compared in tumor and normal tissues from patients, overexpression of EGF receptors was detected in breast, non-small cell lung, gastric, esophageal, kidney, glial, and bladder tumors (14-22). For several tumors, the level of EGF receptor expression was related to clinical parameters of aggressive behavior. Thus, in carcinoma of the breast, EGF receptor expression was inversely related to clinical hormonal responses and tumor levels of cytoplasmic estrogen receptors (29-31) a variable which favors survival, but positively correlated with microscopic lymphatic invasion (31), an indicator of poor prognosis. In bladder carcinomas, EGF receptor levels were higher on invasive tumors (32), and in gastric cancers were associated with tumors presenting in advanced stage (33). Clinical studies in breast and esophageal cancers also suggest that EGF receptor display is associated with a poor prognosis (30,34). Recent studies showed that expression of the closely related neu (erb-b2) proto-oncogene is also a strong, independent predictor of poor prognosis in breast cancer patients with nodal metastases (35).

MONOCLONAL ANTIBODIES TO EGF RECEPTORS

Both IgG1 and IgG2a monoclonal antibodies to the polypeptide external domain of the EGF receptor were obtained (36). These antibodies bind to the EGF receptor with affinities similar to the natural ligand (Kd $\approx$ 3nM) (6,7), and block EGF binding to its receptor and EGF-induced receptor autophosphorylation (7). However, the antibodies induce EGF receptor internalization and the loss of EGF receptors from the cell surface (7). These reagents, therefore, have properties which we postulated would make anti-growth factor receptor MAbs effective anti-cancer agents, i.e. the ability to block ligand binding and modulate receptors from the cell surface.

In <u>vitro</u>, anti-EGF receptor MAbs inhibit growth of tumor cells with highly amplified (>5 x 10^5 receptors/cell) EGF receptor expression (37), but are also effective against normal fibroblasts and cell lines whose <u>in vitro</u> growth is strictly dependent on EGF (36,38) (Figure 1A). Recently, anti-EGF receptor MAbs were shown to inhibit estrogen-dependent growth of a breast carcinoma cell line (Figure 1B) (39). Similar inhibition was obtained with an anti-TGF- α peptide, suggesting that the MAb blocked estrogen-induced auto-stimulation mediated by TGF-α (39). Thus, <u>in vitro</u> studies indicate MAbs to the EGF receptor inhibit malignant cell growth, and in some cells, may act by blocking an autosecretory loop.

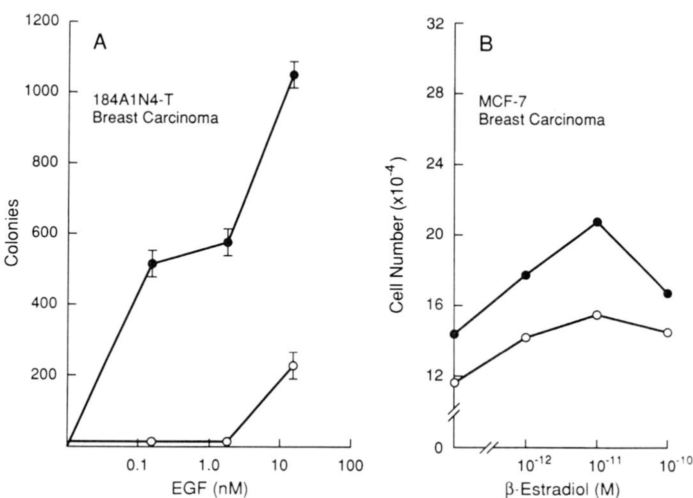

Figure 1. A) Effect of anti-EGF receptor MAb 225 (O) on colony growth of EGF dependent 184A1N4-T transformed breast cells. Control cells (●). Modified from Ennis BW et al. (38). With permission. B) Effects of anti-EGF receptor MAb 528 (O) on estrogen stimulated growth of MCF-7 breast carcinoma cells. Control cells (●). Nearly identical inhibitory effects were seen with an anti-TGF- α peptide. Modified from Eppstein DA et al. (39). With permission.

In <u>vivo</u> anti-EGF receptor MAbs administered to immune defic-
ient mice showed a serum half-life of approximately 3 days, allowing for sustained levels when MAb was administered every 2-3 days
(40). When cells from squamous cell or breast carcinoma and anti-
EGF receptor MAb were administered simultaneously to immune defic-
ient mice, xenograft growth was completely abrogated (Figure 2)
(40,41). When administered to animals with established tumors,
anti-EGF receptor MAbs caused reversible tumor growth arrest (40).

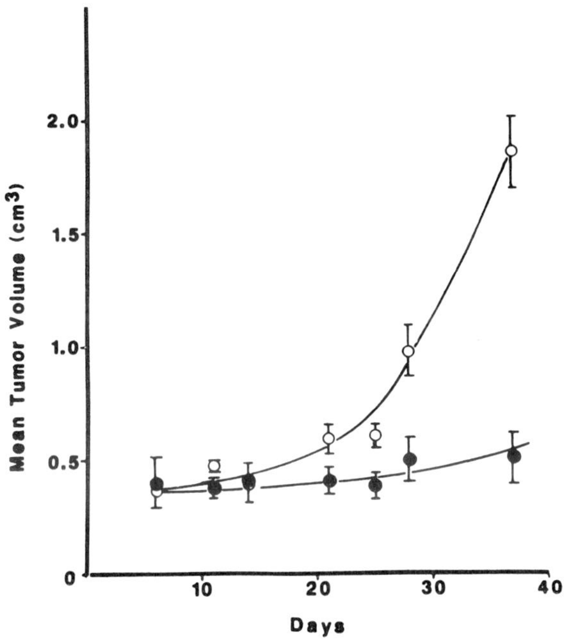

Figure 2. Effect of anti-EGF receptor IgG2a 528 MAb on growth of
MDA human breast carcinoma xenografts. Treatment was given with 2
mg of 528 intraperitoneally on the day of tumor inoculation, and
twice weekly thereafter. (●) MAb treated; (O) control. From Mendelsohn J. (41). With permission.

A comparison of host cell responses to IgG1 and IgG2 anti-EGF receptor MAbs showed the latter could mediate macrophage tumor cell
lysis, but suggested a direct inhibitory effect for the IgG1 MAb
(42). ^{111}In-labelled anti-EGF receptor MAbs were also used to
image squamous cell carcinoma xenografts in nude mice (41,43).

Tumor/blood ratios of approximately 4.5 and tissue/tumor ratios ranging from 6.7 to 41 were obtained (Table 1), indicating the radiolabelled MAb was concentrated in tumor tissues.

Table 1

Distribution Ratios of Labeled MAbs Between Tumors and Normal Tissues

Tissue	MAb225	KS1/4-S1
Blood	4.5±0.6	1.0±0.2
Liver	6.7±1.2	1.0±0.1
Spleen	13.0±2.5	1.3±0.2
Kidney	12.0±0.7	3.3±0.7
Lung	12.0±1.7	2.6±0.5
Muscle	41.0±7.2	12.0±8.4

Distribution ratios were calculated as ([cpm/mg in tumor]/[cpm/mg in normal tissue]) in specimens from six animals.

Reprinted from Mendelsohn J. (41). With permission.

These _in vitro_ and _in vivo_ pre-clinical studies provided a basis for a Phase I trial of radiolabelled IgG1 anti-EGF receptor MAb 225 (44).

An immunotoxin was also prepared by linking IgG2a anti-EGF receptor MAb 528 and recombinant ricin A chain (37,45). The resulting hybrid toxin was specifically toxic _in vitro_ to EGF receptor-bearing cells, and its toxicity increased with increasing EGF receptors/cell (37,45). However, kinetics of _in vitro_ cytotoxicity were protracted and, some cells required treatment for up to 48 hr to induce cell death (37). Although the immunotoxin was highly effective _in vitro_, a low therapeutic index was observed in tumor-bearing nude mice (45). Nevertheless, substantial _in vivo_ tumor regressions were observed, suggesting that the immunotoxin may be efficacious _in vivo_ if nonspecific toxicity can be controlled.

PHASE I TRIAL OF [111]IN-LABELLED ANTI-EGF RECEPTOR MONOCLONAL ANTIBODY

[111]In-labelled MAb 225 was prepared in collaboration with Hybritech, Inc., and a Phase I trial carried out at Memorial/ Sloan-Kettering Cancer Center (44). The goals of the trial were: 1) to define the pharmacokinetics and toxicity of anti-EGF receptor MAb, and 2) to determine whether radiolabelled MAb could localize and image tumors with EGF expression. Patients with Stage III or IV epidermoid carcinoma of the lung received infusions of 1-4 mg [111]-Indium labelled MAb with doses of unlabeled MAb ranging from 4-300 mg. At the highest dose of unlabeled MAb, both the primary tumor and metastases were visualized. Tumor accumulation of radioactivity reached 3.4% 72 hr after infusions of 120 mg. Liver uptake at the same dose was 27%, and liver imaging was prominent at all doses tested. As doses of MAb were escalated, the serum half-life increased from <5 min to more than 24 hr. No toxicity was observed, and the maximum tolerated dose of unlabeled MAb was not reached.

CONCLUSIONS AND FUTURE PROSPECTS

These studies have shown that MAbs to a normal cell surface growth factor receptor inhibit _in vitro_ and _in vivo_ growth of human solid tumors. Over-expression of EGF receptors and possible auto-secretion of TGF-α by some tumor cells continue to provide a strong rationale for this approach to cancer therapy. Other investigators also produced anti-EGF receptor MAbs and showed that these MAbs inhibit _in vitro_ tumor cell growth (46). A recent study examined anti-tumor effects of an anti-EGF receptor MAb combined with cisplatin in immune-deficient mice and showed synergistic antitumor effects (47). Some antibodies to the closely related neu (erb-b2) oncogene also inhibit _in vitro_ growth of solid tumor cells (46). Thus, in the future, combinations of antigrowth factor receptor MAbs, such as anti-EGF receptor and anti-neu MAbs, or combinations of MAbs and specific chemotherapeutic agents may increase the efficacy of anti-EGF receptor MAbs.

ANTI-TRANSFERRIN RECEPTOR MONOCLONAL ANTIBODIES

Background

In _vivo_ and _in vitro_ studies performed over a number of years indicate that Fe availability modulates tumor cell growth, and that proliferating normal and malignant cells express surface receptors for the Fe carrying protein, transferrin (Tf) (48,49). Interest in the role of Tf receptors in cell growth increased dramatically with demonstration by two groups (50,51) that a ubiquitous activation antigen identified by monoclonal antibodies was the cell surface Tf receptor. Using these reagents, surface Tf receptors were detected on virtually all cultured human cells (50,52), but on only a few normal tissues. These included proliferating cells, such as those of the intestinal crypts and epidermis, and a few others tissues, such as pituitary cells, islet cells of the pancreas, tissue macrophages, and liver (12). Bone marrow progenitor cells expressed varying numbers of Tf receptors (53,54), but Tf receptors were not detected on marrow stem cells (54).

When Tf receptor display was compared on tumor cells and their normal counterparts, Tf receptors were preferentially displayed by both solid and hemopoietic tumor cells (12). Certain blood cell tumors, such as thymic acute lymphoblastic leukemias (T-ALL) and non-immunoblastic large cell lymphomas constitutively express high levels of Tf receptors (50,52). The number of Tf receptor positive cells in such tumors exceeds their demonstrated or expected growth fractions. Recent evidence suggests that metastatic variants of melanoma cells may also preferentially express Tf receptors (55).

Several _in vitro_ strategies have been investigated for limiting Fe available to growing tumor cells, including culture with Fe chelators (56), Tf-Ga or Tf-In (57,58), and anti-Tf receptor monoclonal antibodies (10,11). The active form of the experimental chemotherapeutic agent Ga nitrate is a Tf-Ga complex whose antiproliferative effects are induced by Fe depletion (59). In clinical trials, Ga nitrate showed its greatest activity against large cell lymphomas, a tumor now known to express large numbers of Tf receptors (60, 61), suggesting Fe depletion may be an effective strategy against some tumors.

Most evidence suggests that cells require the Fe provided by Tf rather than the Tf or Tf receptor proteins for cell growth (11,48). Fe depleted cells undergo growth arrest followed by time-dependent cytotoxicity (62) (See Figure 4 following), and have decreased intracellular deoxynucleotide pools, reduced rates of DNA synthesis, and decreased activity of the enzyme ribonucleotide reductase (57,63). Although ribonucleotide reductase appears to be a major target of Fe depletion, Fe or Tf may also regulate activity of critical intracellular enzymes, such as RNA polymerase II and protein kinase C (64,65). These studies indicate that tumor cells, especially hemopoietic tumors, preferentially express Tf receptors, and that Fe depletion may be an effective strategy for limiting tumor cell growth.

Anti-Tf receptor MAbs have several potential advantages as a means of tumor cell Fe depletion. First, only cells expressing surface Tf receptors are potential targets for the Fe depletion. This avoids toxicity to critical, non-Tf receptor-bearing tissues, such as the retina, which incur damage from treatment with agents such as Fe chelators. Second, high levels of Tf receptor expression by some tumors (e.g. T-ALL) and their absence from marrow stem cells (54) may provide a therapeutic index for anti-Tf receptor MAbs. Finally, MAbs have the potential to marshall immune responses as well as affecting target cells by directly limiting Fe availability.

PRE-CLINICAL STUDIES OF ANTI-Tf RECEPTOR MONOCLONAL ANTIBODIES

From the outset, pre-clinical development of anti-Tf receptor MAbs was aided by availability of both murine MAbs reacting with the human receptor, and rat anti-mouse Tf receptor MAbs (10,66). While it is not yet possible to show that anti-human and antimouse MAbs react with similar functional domains of their respective Tf receptor targets, we have been able to conduct parallel in vitro studies of human and mouse cells, and in vivo investigations in

312

mice using MAbs whose _in vitro_ spectrum of action is virtually
identical to human reagents under development (67).

Early studies showed that anti-Tf receptor MAbs inhibited _in
vitro_ growth of many hemopoietic tumor cells (10,11,66) and normal
marrow progenitors (10,54,62), but did not affect growth of marrow
stem cells or solid tumor cells (54,68). The most effective antibodies were a rat anti-mouse IgM MAb and an unusual mouse IgA anti-
human Tf receptor (10,66), indicating that multivalency increased
the MAbs' effectiveness as _in vitro_ antiproliferative agents. Subsequent studies showed that IgG anti-Tf MAbs accelerated Tf receptor protein turnover and decreased surface and total cell Tf receptors (66,69), but had little effect on Tf internalization, Fe uptake, or cell growth (67,69,71). In contrast, multivalent IgM or
IgA anti-Tf receptor MAbs decreased surface Tf receptor binding,
caused surface Tf receptor cross-linking, inhibited Tf internalization and Fe uptake, and inhibited cell growth (66, 69,71). Because of these findings, the IgM anti-mouse Tf receptor and IgA
anti-human Tf receptor MAb (termed 42/6) have been subject to the
most extensive _in vivo_ and _in vitro_ pre-clinical studies. Recently, we developed IgG anti-Tf receptor MAbs which mediate antiproliferative effects, but their mechanism of action is less well
defined (71).

From the outset, it was apparent that some hemopoietic cells
and all solid tumors were resistant to _in vitro_ antiproliferative
effects of anti-Tf receptor MAbs (10,68). Since all cultured human cells express Tf receptors at high density (52,68), antigen
heterogeneity was an unlikely explanation for this finding. Originally, we suggested that surface Tf receptor display by some
cells might occur at lower density per unit of membrane area, making surface Tf receptor cross-linking less efficient (68). However, some cells can be grown _in vitro_ using elemental Fe sources
in lieu of Tf and are resistant to anti-Tf receptor MAb (11). A
specific, saturable, non-Tf mediated Fe uptake pathway has been
demonstrated in some of these cells (70), but it is unclear whether this pathway is involved in anti-Tf receptor MAb resistance.
Recently, we compared Fe uptake from Tf in 42/6-sensitive leu-

kemia cells and a 42/6 resistant solid tumor. Consistent with previous studies, 42/6 inhibited Fe uptake by the leukemia cells (Figure 3).

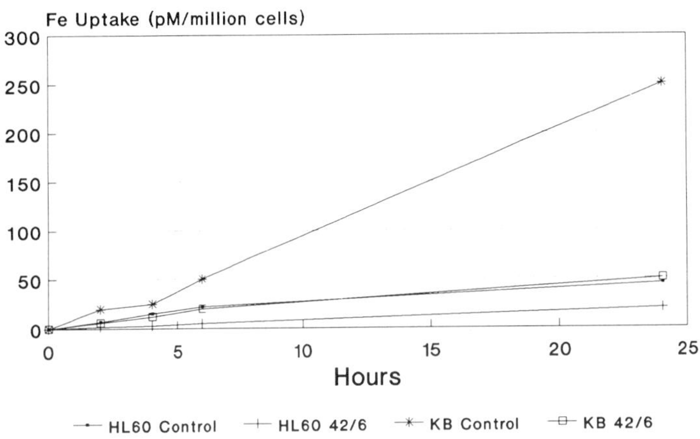

Figure 3. Effects of 10 ug/ml IgA anti-Tf receptor MAb 42/6 on Fe uptake from Tf in KB carcinoma (which are resistant to MAb 42/6) and HL60 myelocytic leukemia cells (which are sensitive to MAb 42/6). KB Control (*); KB with 42/6 ( ); HL60 Control (■); HL60 with 42/6 (+). Fe uptake was determined as described elsewhere (71).

42/6 also inhibited uptake by the solid tumor cells, but when Fe uptake was expressed on a per cell basis, the solid tumor cells showed much higher basal Fe uptake, and continued to take up as much Fe as untreated leukemia cells even after MAb treatment (Figure 3). Thus, resistance to anti-Tf receptor MAbs may result from extremely high basal rates of Fe uptake by some cells which cannot be reduced sufficiently by anti-Tf receptor MAbs to limit solid tumor cell growth. Whether some of this uptake occurs by non-Tf-dependent mechanisms remains unclear.

In _vitro_, IgA MAb 42/6 causes synergistic killing of 42/6-
sensitive target cells when combined with either an Fe chelator
(Figure 4) or Ga nitrate (62), but neither combination showed much
interaction against KB carcinoma cells (62).

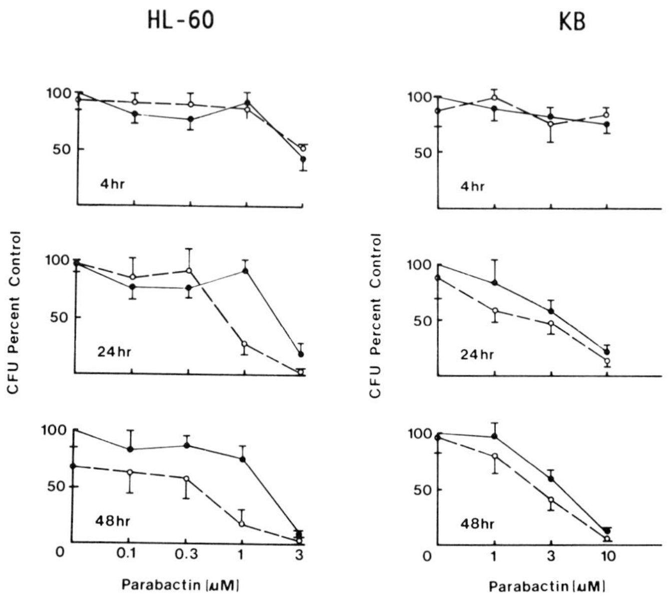

Figure 4.   Effects of anti-Tf receptor MAb 42/6 on HL60 leukemia
or KB carcinoma colony-forming cell survival in the presence (0)
or absence (●) of varying doses of the Fe chelator parabactin.
Colony-forming cell survival was determined as described (37).
Reprinted from Taetle R et al. (62).

In _vivo_, sustained levels (>10μg/ml) of IgM anti-murine Tf
receptor MAb could be maintained with twice weekly intraperitoneal
injections (67). Administration of anti-Tf receptor MAb on this
schedule was without toxicity, except for increased splenic and decreased marrow erythropoiesis (67). Similarly, administration anti-
Tf receptor MAb had no detectable effect on recovery of mice from
a single injection of cyclophosphamide (Trowbridge, unpublished
results). In contrast, twice weekly injections of anti-Tf receptor MAb increased the lifespan of mice bearing the SL2 transplantable leukemia/lymphoma (67) (Figure 5A).

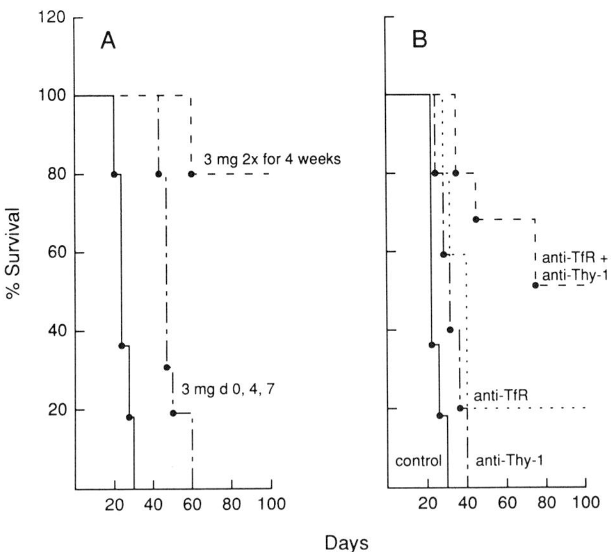

Figure 5.   A. Effects of IgM rat anti-mouse Tf receptor MAb on
survival of mice bearing the SL2 transplantable leukemia/lymphoma.
MAbs were administered at the doses and on the schedules shown. B.
Effects of therapy with anti-Tf receptor MAb or anti-Thy-1 MAb
alone or in combination on survival of mice bearing SL2 tumors.
Modified from Sauvage C et al. (67) With permission.

Synergistic effects in the SL2 model were noted when MAbs reacting
with the Tf receptor and Thy-1 (another surface antigen on SL2
cells) were administered simultaneously (Figure 5B) (67). Thus,
anti-Tf receptor MAbs showed _in vivo_ anti-tumor effects without
excess toxicity.

Although IgA anti-human Tf receptor MAb 42/6 is a potent _in
vitro_ anti-proliferative agent, administration of a large, multimeric MAb has potential drawbacks, such as poor tumor penetration.
For this reason, we developed a broader range of anti-Tf receptor
MAbs. Recombinant human Tf receptor protein was obtained from a
baculovirus expression system (72), and used to immunize mice.
From these immunizations, over 50 MAbs were obtained of which 30
reacted with the native Tf receptor (71). The vast majority of

these new MAbs were IgG1 subtype (71). One (MAb 65.3) showed
anti-proliferative effects when used alone against human leukemia
cells and synergistic growth inhibition when combined with other
IgG anti-transferrin receptor MAbs (Figure 6).

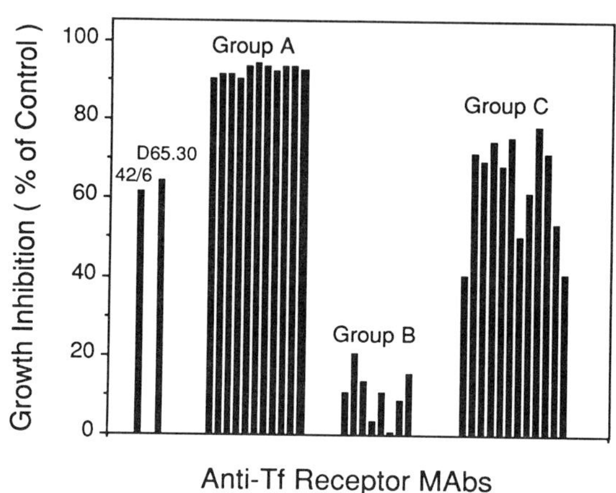

Figure 6. Effects of IgA anti-Tf receptor MAb 42/6 and IgG MAb
65.3 on <u>in</u> <u>vitro</u> growth of CEM human T leukemia cells. The effects of other IgG MAbs combined with 65.3 are also shown. Three
groups were defined: A) MAbs which had no effect or antagonized
antiproliferative effects of MAb 65.3; B) MAbs which showed synergistic growth inhibition when combined with MAb 65.3; and C)
MAbs which showed little or modest interaction with MAb 65.3.

Although most of these IgG anti-Tf receptor MAbs showed no
antiproliferative activity when used alone, when non-cross-block-
ing pairs of IgG anti-Tf receptor MAbs were used, <u>in</u> <u>vitro</u> antiproliferative and cytotoxic effects were observed (71). IgG anti-
Tf receptor MAbs also enhanced cell killing by 42/6 (71). The activity of these MAb combinations correlated with their ability to
inhibit Fe uptake from Tf (71). More important, active pairs of
IgG anti-Tf receptor MAbs inhibited in vivo growth of human leu-

kemia xenografts in nude mice (Figure 7) and caused regression of about 60% of established tumors.

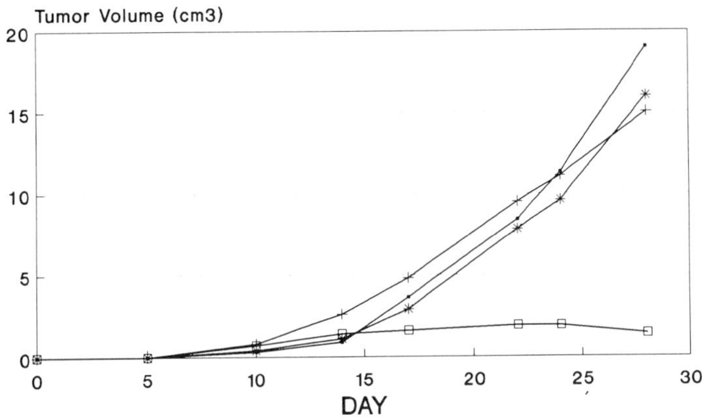

Figure 7. Effect of IgG anti-Tf receptor MAbs 65.3 or A27.15 alone or in combination on _in vivo_ growth of human CEM T cell leukemia xenografts. Results shown are mean tumor volumes of groups of five tumor-bearing mice. MAb administration was begun on day 10 and given every 3-4 d for a total of 6 doses. Control (■); 65.3 (*); A 27.15 (+); 65.3 combined with A27.15 (▢)

These data are very recent, and it is unclear whether _in vivo_ responses represent tumor cures. However, these studies indicate that combinations of IgG anti-Tf receptor MAbs are as active _in vitro_ and _in vivo_ as multimeric anti-Tf receptor MAbs, and tremendously expand the number of potentially active agents available. IgG anti-Tf receptor MAbs are also much more likely to mediate _in vivo_ anti-tumor immunologic responses.

PHASE I TRIAL OF MONOCLONAL ANTI-TRANSFERRIN RECEPTOR MAb 42/6

On the basis of _in vitro_ and _in vivo_ pre-clinical data, we propose a phase I trial of IgA anti-Tf receptor MAb 42/6. The goals of this trial will be: 1) To define pharmacokinetics of a murine IgA MAb in man; 2) To assess toxicities of an anti-Tf receptor MAb; 3) To determine whether 42/6 binds to or inhibits growth of bone marrow progenitors _in vivo_; 4) To assess effects of

318

anti-Tf receptor MAb on biochemical parameters of Fe balance (i.e.
serum Fe, transferrin saturation, and serum ferritin); and 5) To
correlate serum MAb levels with pretreatment levels of serum Tf
receptors. The last goal is of particular interest since several
groups recently showed (73,74) that immunoreactive Tf receptor protein circulates in blood. Whether these findings will impact delivery of anti-Tf receptor MAbs to cell targets remains unclear.

CONCLUSIONS AND FUTURE PROSPECTS

Anti-Tf receptor MAbs have potent anti-proliferative activity
against human hemopoietic tumor cells _in vitro_, and show _in vivo_
anti-tumor efficacy with minimal toxicity. As our recent studies
with combinations of IgG MAbs indicate, the optimal reagents for
this therapy have not yet been identified. This unusual approach
may provide an anti-tumor therapy which is non-cross-resistant
with anti-cancer drugs. Although some additive toxicity of drugs
and anti-Tf receptor MAbs is probable, identification of drugs
which show positive interactions with the MAbs is now a subject of
active study.

REFERENCES

1. Dillman RO: Monoclonal antibodies for treating cancer. Ann.
    Int. Med. 111:592-603, 1989.
2. Harris DT, Mastrangelo MI: Serotherapy of cancer. Semin
    Oncol. 16:180-198, 1989.
3. Heldin C-H, Westermark B: Growth factors: Mechanism of
    action and relation to oncogenes. Cell 37:9-20, 1984.
4. Goustin AS, Leof EB, Shipley GD, Moses HL: Growth factors
    and cancer. Cancer Res. 46:1015-1029, 1986.
5. Prehn RT: Tumor-specific antigens as altered growth factor
    receptors. Cancer Res. 49:2823-2826, 1989.
6. MacLeod CL, Masui H, Trowbridge IS, Mendelsohn J: Monoclonal
    antibodies directed towards growth-related receptors on human
    tumors. Monoclonal Antibody Therapy of Human Cancer, KA
    Foon, AC Morgan (eds), Martinus Nijhoff Publishing, pp.
    57-83, 1985.
7. Sunada H, Magun BE, Mendelsohn J, MacLeod CL: Monoclonal
    antibody against epidermal growth factor receptor is
    internalized without stimulating receptor phosphorylation.
    Proc. Natl. Acad. Sci. USA 83:3825-3829, 1986.
8. Yasui W, Sumiyoshi H, Hata J et al: Expression of epidermal
    growth factor receptor in human gastric and colonic carcin-
    omas. Cancer Res. 48:137-141, 1988.

9. Kawamoto T, Sato JD, Le A et al: Growth stimulation of A431 cells by epidermal growth factor: Identification of high-affinity receptors for epidermal growth factor by an anti-receptor monoclonal antibody. Proc. Natl. Acad. Sci. USA 80:1337-1341, 1983.

10. Taetle R, Honeysett JM, Trowbridge I: Effects of anti-transferrin receptor antibodies on growth of normal and malignant myeloid cells. Int. J. Cancer 32:343-349, 1983.

11. Taetle R, Rhyner K, Castagnola J et al: The role of trans-ferrin, Fe and transferrin receptors in myeloid leukemia cell growth: Studies with an anti-transferrin receptor monoclonal antibody. J. Clin. Invest. 75:1061-1067, 1985.

12. Gatter KC, Brown G, Trowbridge IS et al: Transferrin recep-tors in human tissues: Their distribution and possible clinical relevance. J. Clin. Pathol. 36:539-545, 1983.

13. Maihle NI, Kung H-I: c-erbB and the epidermal growth-factor receptor: A molecule with dual identity. Biochimica. Biophysica. Acta 948:287-304, 1988.

14. Real FX, Rettig WI, Chesa PG et al: Expression of epidermal growth factor receptor in human cultured cells and tissues: Relationship to cell lineage and stage of differentiation. Cancer Res. 46:4726-4731, 1986.

15. Lu S-H, Hsieh L-L, Luo F-C, Weinstein IB: Amplification of the EGF receptor and c-myc genes in human esophageal cancers. Int. J. Cancer 42:502-505, 1988.

16. Yao M, Shuin T, Misaki H, Kubota Y: Enhanced expression of c-myc and epidermal growth factor receptor (c-erbB-1) genes in primary human renal cancer. Cancer Res. 48:6753-6757, 1988.

17. Kamata N, Chida K, Rikimaru K et al: Growth-inhibitory effects of epidermal growth factor and overexpression of its receptors on human squamous cell carcinomas in culture. Cancer Res. 46:1648-1653, 1986.

18. Haeder M, Rotsch M, Bepler G et al: Epidermal growth factor receptor expression in human lung cancer cell lines. Cancer Res. 48:1132-1136, 1988.

19. Hollstein MC, Smits AM, Galiana C et al: Amplification of epidermal growth factor receptor gene but no evidence of ras mutations in primary human esophageal cancers. Cancer Res. 48:5119-5123, 1988.

20. Hendler FJ, Ozanne BW: Human squamous cell lung cancers express increased epidermal growth factor receptors. J. Clin. Invest. 74:647-651, 1984.

21. Ro I, North SM, Gallick GE et al: Amplified and overexpress-ed epidermal growth factor receptor gene in uncultured pri-mary human breast carcinoma. Cancer Res. 48:161-164, 1988.

22. Humphrey PA, Wong AJ, Vogelstein B et al: Amplification and expression of the epidermal growth factor receptor gene in human glioma xenografts. Cancer Res. 48:2231-2238, 1988.

23. Sporn MB, Roberts AB: Autocrine growth factors and cancer. Nature 313:745-747, 1985.

24. Wong ST, Winchell LF, McCune BK et al: The TGF-α precursor
    expressed on the cell surface binds to the EGF receptor on
    adjacent cells, leading to signal transduction. Cell
    56:495-506, 1989.
25. Brachmann R, Lindquist PB, Nagashima M et al: Transmembrane
    TGF-α precursors activate EGF/TGF-α receptors. Cell
    56:691-700, 1989.
26. Haley JD, Hsuan, JJ, Waterfield MD: Analysis of mammalian
    fibroblast transformation by normal and mutated human EGF
    receptors. Oncogene 4:273-283, 1989.
27. Santon JB, Cronin MT, MacLeod CL et al: Effects of epidermal
    growth factor receptor concentration on tumorigenicity of
    A431 cells in nude mice. Cancer Res. 46:4701-4705, 1986.
28. Yoshiyuki T, Shimizu Y, Onda M et al: Immunohistochemical
    demonstration of epidermal growth factor in human gastric
    cancer xenografts of nude mice. Cancer 65:953-957, 1990.
29. Nicholson S, Halcrow P, Farndon JR et al: Expression of
    epidermal growth factor receptors associated with lack of
    response to endocrine therapy in recurrent breast cancer.
    Lancet, January 28, 182, 1989.
30. Nicholson S, Sainsbury JRC, Needham GK et al: Quantitative
    assays of epidermal growth factor receptor in human breast
    cancer: Cut-off points of clinical relevance. Int. J.
    Cancer 42:36-41, 1988.
31. Toi M, Hamada Y, Nakamura T et al: Immunocytochemical and
    biochemical analysis of epidermal growth factor receptor
    expression in human breast cancer tissues: Relationship to
    estrogen receptor and lymphatic invasion. Int. J. Cancer
    43:220-225, 1989.
32. Smith K, Fennelly JA, Neal DE et al: Characterization and
    quantitation of the epidermal growth factor receptor in
    invasive and superficial bladder tumors. Cancer Res.
    49:5819-5815, 1989.
33. Sugiyama K, Yonemura Y, Miyazaki I: Immunohistochemical
    study of epidermal growth factor and epidermal growth factor
    receptor in gastric carcinoma. Cancer 63:1557-1561, 1989.
34. Ozawa S, Ueda M, Ando N et al: Prognostic significance of
    epidermal growth factor receptor in esophageal squamous cell
    carcinomas. Cancer 63:2169-2173, 1989.
35. Slamon DJ, Clark GM, Wong SG et al: Human breast cancer:
    Correlation of relapse and survival with amplification of the
    HER-2/neu oncogene. Science 235:177-182, 1987.
36. Sato JD, Kawamoto T, Le AD et al: Biological effects _in
    vitro_ of monoclonal antibodies to human epidermal growth
    factor receptors. Mol. Biol. Med. 1:511-529, 1983.
37. Taetle R, Honeysett JM, Houston LL: Effects of anti-epider-
    mal growth factor (EGF) receptor antibodies and an anti-EGF
    receptor recombinant-ricin A chain immunoconjugate on growth
    of human cells. J. Natl. Can. Inst. 80:1053-1059, 1988.
38. Ennis BW, Valverius EM, Bates SE et al: Antiepidermal growth
    factor receptor antibodies inhibit the autocrine-stimulated
    growth of MDA-468 human breast cancer cells. Mol. Endo-
    crinol. 3:1830-1838, 1989.

39. Eppstein DA, Marsh YV, Schryver BB, Bertics PJ: Inhibition of epidermal growth factor/transforming growth factor-α-stimulated cell growth by a synthetic peptide. J. Cell Physiol. 141:420-430, 1989.
40. Masui H, Kawamoto T, Sato JD et al: Growth inhibition of human tumor cells in athymic mice by anti-epidermal growth factor receptor monoclonal antibodies. Cancer Res. 44:1002-1007, 1984.
41. Mendelsohn J: Potential clinical applications of anti-EGF receptor monoclonal antibodies. Cancer Cells 7/ Molecular Diagnostics of Human Cancer 359-362, 1989.
42. Masui H, Moroyama T, Mendelsohn J: Mechanism of antitumor activity in mice for anti-epidermal growth factor receptor monoclonal antibodies with different isotypes. Cancer Res. 46:5592-5598, 1986.
43. Goldenberg A, Masui H, Divgi C et al: Imaging of human tumor xenografts with an indium-111-labeled anti-epidermal growth factor receptor monoclonal antibody. J. Natl. Can. Inst. 81:1616-1625, 1989.
44. Divgi CR, Welt S, Kris M et al: Phase I and imaging trial of indium-111 labeled anti-EGF receptor monoclonal antibody 225 in patients with squamous cell lung carcinoma. Submitted.
45. Masui H, Kamrath H, Apell G et all: Cytotoxicity against human tumor cells mediated by the conjugate of anti-epidermal growth factor receptor monoclonal antibody to recombinant ricin A chain. Cancer Res. 49:3482-3499, 1989.
46. Fendly BM, Winget M, Hudziak RM et al: Characterization of murine monoclonal antibodies reactive to either the human epidermal growth factor receptor or HER2/neu gene product. Cancer Res. 50:1550-1558, 1990.
47. Aboud-Pirak E, Hurwitz E, Pirak ME et al: Efficacy of antibodies to epidermal growth factor receptor against KB carcinoma _in_ _vitro_ and in nude mice. J. Natl. Can. Inst. 80:1605-1611, 1988.
48. Taetle R: The role of transferrin receptors in hemopoietic cell growth. Exp. Hematol. 18:360-365, 1990.
49. Weinberg ED: Iron withholding: A defense against infection and neoplasia. Physiol. Rev. 64:65-102, 1984.
50. Sutherland R, Delia D, Schneider C et al: Ubiquitous cell surface glycoprotein on tumor cells is proliferation-associated receptor for transferrin. Proc. Natl. Acad. Sci. USA 78:4515-4519, 1981.
51. Trowbridge IS, Omary MB: Human cell surface glycoprotein related to cell proliferation is the receptor for trans-ferrin. Proc. Natl. Acad. Sci. USA 78:3039-3043, 1981.
52. Omary MB, Trowbridge IS, Minowada J: Human cell-surface glycoprotein with unusual properties. Nature 286:888-891, 1987.
53. Sieff C, Bickwell D, Caine G et al: Changes in cell surface antigen expression during hemopoietic differentiation. Blood 60:703-713, 1982.

54. Lesley J, Domingo DL, Schulte R, Trowbridge IS: Effect of an antimurine transferrin receptor-ricin A conjugate on bone marrow stem and progenitor cells treated in vitro. Exp. Cell. Res. 150:400-407, 1984.
55. Nicolson GL, Inoue T, Van Pelt CS, Cavanaugh PG: Differential expression of a $M_r \approx 90,000$ cell surface transferrin receptor-related glycoprotein on murine B16 metastatic melanoma sublines selected for enhanced brain or ovary colonization. Cancer Res. 50:515-520, 1990.
56. Foa P, Maiolo AT, Lombari L et al: Inhibition of proliferation of human leukaemic cell populations by deferoxamine. Scand. J. Haematol. 36:107-111, 1986.
57. Chitambar CR, Matthaeus WG, Antholine WE et al: Inhibition of leukemic HL60 cell growth by transferrin-gallium: Effects on ribonucleotide reductase and demonstration of drug synergy with hydroxurea. Blood 72:1930-1936, 1988.
58. Moran PL, Seligman PA: Effects of transferrin-indium on cellular proliferation of a human leukemia cell line. Cancer Res. 49:4237-4241, 1989.
59. Chitambar CR, Seligman PA: Effects of different transferrin forms on transferrin receptor expression, iron uptake and cellular proliferation of human leukemic HL60 cells. J. Clin. Invest. 78:1538-1546, 1986.
60. Warrell RP, Coonley CJ, Straus DJ, Young CW: Treatment of patients with advanced malignant lymphoma using gallium nitrate administered as a seven day continuous infusion. Cancer 51:1982-1987, 1983.
61. Foster BJ, Clagett-Carr K, Hoth D, Leyland-Iones B: Gallium nitrate: The second metal with clinical activity. Cancer Treat. Rep. 70:1311-1319, 1986.
62. Taetle R, Honeysett JM, Bergeron R: Combination iron depletion therapy. J. Natl. Cancer Inst. 81:1229-1235, 1989.
63. Lederman HM, Cohen A, Lee JWW et al: Desferoxamine: A reversible 5-phase inhibitor of human lymphocyte proliferation. Blood 64:748-753, 1984.
64. Shoji A, Ozawa E: Necessity of transferrin for RNA synthesis in chick myotubes. J. Cell. Physiol. 127:349-356, 1986.
65. Phillips JL, Boldt DH, Harper J: Iron-transferrin-induced increase in protein kinase C activity in CCRF-CEM cells. J. Cell Physiol. 132:349-353, 1987.
66. Lesley JF, Schulte RJ: Inhibition of cell growth by monoclonal anti-transferrin receptor antibodies. Mol. Cell Biol. 5:1814-1821, 1985.
67. Sauvage CA, Mendelsohn JC, Lesley JF, Trowbridge IS: Effects of monoclonal antibodies that block transferrin receptor function on the in vivo growth of a syngeneic murine leukemia. Cancer Res. 47:747-753, 1987.
68. Taetle R, Honeysett JM: Effects of monoclonal anti-transferrin receptor antibodies on in vitro growth of human solid tumor cells. Cancer Res. 47:2040-2044, 1987.
69. Taetle R, Castagnola J, Mendelsohn J: Mechanisms of growth inhibition by anti-transferrin receptor monoclonal antibodies. Cancer Res. 46:1759-1763, 1986.

70. Sturrock A, Alexander J, Lamb J et al: Characterization of a
    transferrin-independent uptake system for iron in HeLa cells.
    J. Biol. Chem. 265:3139-3145, 1990.
71. White S, Taetle R, Seligman PA et al: Combinations of
    anti-transferrin receptor monoclonal antibodies inhibit human
    tumor cell growth in vitro and <u>in vivo</u>: Evidence for syner-
    gistic anti-proliferative effects. Cancer Res. In press.
72. Domingo DL, Trowbridge IS: Characterization of the human
    transferrin receptor produced in a baculovirus expression
    system. J. Biol. Chem. 263:13386-13392,1988.
73. Flowers CH, Skikne BS, Covell AM, Cook TD: The clinical
    measurement of serum transferrin receptor. J. Lab. Clin.
    Med. 114:368-378, 1989.
74. Kohgo Y, Niitsu Y, Kondo H et al: Serum transferrin receptor
    as a new index of erythropoiesis. Blood 70:1955-1958, 1987.

19

REGULATION OF POLYAMINE BIOSYNTHETIC ACTIVITY AND HOMEOSTASIS AS A
NOVEL ANTIPROLIFERATIVE STRATEGY

Carl W. Porter, Debora L. Kramer, Ralph J. Bernacki and Raymond J.
Bergeron

INTRODUCTION

Induction of polyamine biosynthetic activity and the subsequent increases in intracellular polyamine pools are well documented components of the proliferative response (reviewed in 1-3).
Indeed, several lines of evidence clearly indicate that sustained
polyamine biosynthesis is a critical component of cell growth and
not simply a consequence of it (2,4). In many ways, the association of polyamines with cell growth and, in particular, the properties of the enzyme proteins themselves bear intriguing resemblance
to proto-oncogenes and their encoded products. Two key biosynthetic enzymes, ornithine and S-adenosylmethionine decarboxylase (ODC
and AdoMetDC, respectively), are extremely short-lived with half-
lives of less than 1 hr, highly inducible and subject to sensitive
regulatory control. Increases in their activities are invariably
associated with the very early stages of cell growth and, somewhat
less consistently, with tumor promotion (5,6). Although the most
illustrative of the enzymes in this respect, ODC, has not been
shown to have transforming capabilities, cells which overexpress
the enzyme can be endowed with increased proliferative potential
(7) and/or tissue invasiveness (8). Moreover, induction of the
enzyme, like certain of the proto-oncogenes, is known to be critically important for initiating and sustaining cell proliferation.

Even prior to the discovery of proto-oncogenes and oncogenes
and our awareness of the above similarities, polyamines attracted
considerable attention as a potential chemotherapeutic target site
in antiproliferative strategies. Since cell growth is associated

with increases in polyamine anabolic activity, initial approaches
by most laboratories focussed on interference with the biosynthetic pathway and ultimately produced specific and potent inhibitors
of all four enzymes (reviewed in 3). Best known of these, is
α-difluoromethylornithine (DFMO), an irreversible inhibitor of
ODC (9) which has been studied clinically as an anticancer agent
(reviewed in 3) and used, with greater success, as an antiparasitic agent (reviewed in 10). As an alternative approach to the
use of enzyme inhibitors, we have attempted to identify polyamine
analogs which interfere with polyamine biosynthesis by exploiting
pathway regulatory mechanisms and thereby restrict the synthesis
of key enzymes. The strategy, (described in greater detail below), is dependent upon the extreme rapidity of enzyme turnover
and the high sensitivity of their synthesis to feedback control by
the polyamine pools (11). While the inhibitor, DFMO, is finding
utility in the therapy of parasitic diseases, such as African try-
panosomiasis, and also as a possible chemopreventive agent for
high-risk cancer populations (12), potentially meaningful applications for the regulatory analogs are only now being identified.

No matter the approach, initiatives targeting polyamines have
been hindered by major uncertainties regarding the nature of the
role(s) of these molecules in the proliferative process and tumor
cell biology. Although polyamines accumulate to relatively high
(mM) concentrations in proliferating cells, traditional methods of
inquiry have been confounded by the fact that, unlike other molecules of similar size, such as sugars and amino acids, polyamines
do not incorporate into macromolecules but rather bind tenuously
to them via electrostatic interactions. Accordingly, one of the
most consistently fruitful approaches to their study has been the
use of inhibitors and analogs of defined mode of action to alter
polyamine pools and evaluate the cellular consequences. Our polyamine program has been guided by two primary goals: (1) to identify and develop polyamine analogs and/or inhibitors of defined
mode of action as potential anticancer agents and (2) to utilize
those agents to study cellular responses which may be related to
polyamine function and/or mechanisms of polyamine homeostasis --

327

binding, biosynthesis, catabolism and transport. For the purposes
of this volume, emphasis will be given, to our progress towards
the first of these goals as it pertains to our studies with the
polyamine analogs. Specifically we will review the rationale for
our analog strategy, its proof of principle, relevant mechanisms,
anticipated and unanticipated cellular responses, and the <u>in vitro</u>
and <u>in vivo</u> antiproliferative activity in selected tumor model
systems.

METABOLIC CONSIDERATIONS
     All cells are equipped with the polyamine biosynthetic path-
way shown in Figure 1 and contain the three polyamine species
shown in Figure 2. Various terminally N-acetylated forms of the

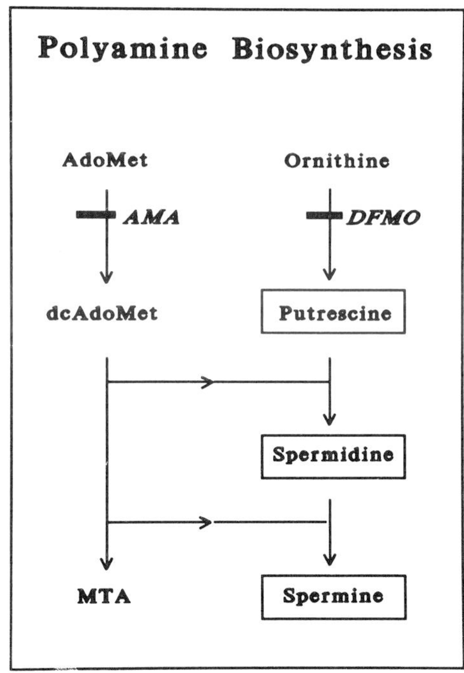

Figure 1. Polyamine biosynthetic pathway showing the site of
action of the irreversible inhibitors, α -difluoromethylornithine
(DFMO) and S-(5′-adenosyl)methylthioethylhydroxylamine (AMA), at
the two lead-in enzymes, ornithine decarboxylase (ODC) and
S-adenosylmethionine decarboxylase, respectively. Other enzymes
include spermidine and spermine synthase. Abbreviations are
dcAdoMet, decarboxylated S-adenosylmethionine and MTA, 5′-deoxy-
5′-(methylthio)adenosine.

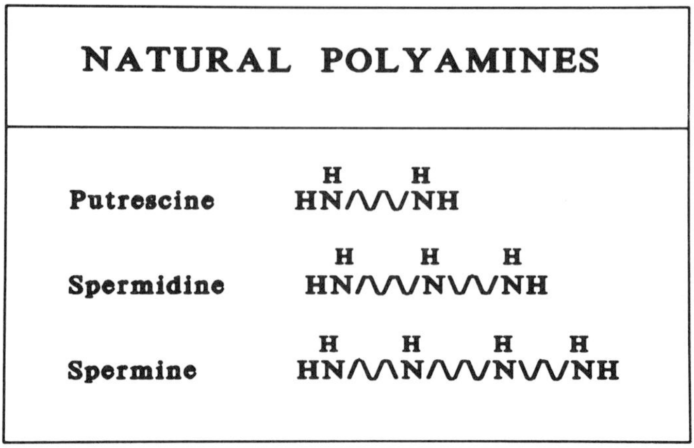

NATURAL POLYAMINES

Putrescine

H   H

HN/\/\/NH

Spermidine

H   H   H

HN/\/\/N\/\/NH

Spermine

H   H   H   H

HN/\/\N/\/\/N\/\/NH

Figure 2. Structural representation of the three polyamine species found in eukaryotic cells.

two higher polyamines, spermidine (SPD) and spermine (SPM) are found in trace quantities inside cells but predominate in the serum. With only minor exceptions involving the initiation factor, hypusine (13,14), polyamines do not incorporate into macromolecules but exist as electrostatically bound and unbound pools which are acid extractable and quantifiable by chromatography. Thus, intracellular pools represent functional entities rather than macromolecular precursors. Although cells are dependent on the availability of polyamines for growth from either de novo synthesis or, to a lesser extent, from exogenous sources, this dependence differs significantly from that for precursor pools of DNA, for example. Whereas antimetabolite-induced depletion of nucleotide pools has readily deducible consequences, comparable perturbations involving polyamine pools are not so obviously interpretable since their function is uncertain.

Until recently, at least part of this problem was due to our relative inability to selectively modulate the individual polyamine pools. While it has been possible to use the ODC inhibitor, DFMO (Figure 1), to deplete PUT and SPD pools, it has not been possible to concomitantly deplete SPM pools which typically increase during DFMO treatment. In 1989, however, Kramer et al (15) used DFMO in combination with AMA, an irreversible inhibitor of AdoMetDC (Figure 1), to define the relative importance of the individual polyamines to cell growth and plating efficiency. The strategy involved metabolically "freezing" the pathway with the two inhibitors, depleting the various polyamine pools and then selectively increasing individual pools with exogenous polyamines. These manipulations led to the following conclusions: (a) all three of the polyamines are capable of individually supporting cell growth to some degree, (b) only spermidine can fully support cell growth by itself, (c) maximum growth inhibition is achieved by maximum depletion of all three polyamine pools, (d) the latter is best accomplished by concomitant inhibition of <u>both</u> ODC and AdoMetDC, and (e) as determined by plating efficiency, inhibition of ODC has greater antiproliferative potential than inhibition of AdoMetDC (due to substantial compensatory increases of the precursor polyamine, PUT). Thus, it is not sufficient to simply block flux through the pathway by inhibiting a single enzyme. Rather, the cell must be depleted of polyamines to achieve maximum growth inhibition. With inhibitors of polyamine biosynthesis, pools are largely depleted by daughter cell dilution until a critically low level of one or more of the pools is achieved. Depending on the inhibitor and where it acts in the pathway, depletion of one pool can lead to increases in another which in turn, may counter the effects of reductions made elsewhere.

Although not usually relevant with enzyme inhibitors, other mechanisms can contribute to polyamine depletion during a pathway blockade. Polyamines can be catabolized intracellularly by an inducible polyamine-specific pathway involving the sequential steps of N-acetylation followed by oxidation. In addition, their excretion out of the cell may be enhanced by what appears to be a metabolically-linked transport mechanism (16,17). Thus, activation of one or both of these latter two mechanisms by polyamine analogs could also play a contributing role in depleting polyamine pools and, hence, in inhibiting cell growth.

REGULATORY STRATEGY

A major disadvantage in the use of enzyme inhibitors to deplete polyamine pools is that the two lead-in and rate-limiting enzymes, ODC and AdoMetDC, are sensitively regulated by intracellular polyamine pools (3,4). Thus, perturbations which lower SPD and/or SPM pools, in particular, invoke compensatory increases in one or both of these enzyme activities. Inhibition of AdoMetDC with AMA (Figure 1), for example, produces several-fold increases in ODC and its product, PUT (15) while inhibition of ODC by DFMO leads to increases in AdoMetDC and its product, decarboxylated AdoMet (Figure 1) (9,18). As a result, the pathway typically is primed to recover from the enzyme effect as soon as the inhibitor diffuses away. The high accumulation of the polyamine precursor, PUT, seems to account for the relatively weak effect of AMA on plating efficiency (15). Likewise, increases in AdoMetDC during DFMO treatment, allows the pathway to adjust to near-normal flux levels in the absence of total ODC inhibition.

It has also been recognized for many years that the reverse of this phenomenon can also take place (4,19). That is, these same enzymes can be down-regulated by _increases_ in polyamine pools. Thus, exposure of cells to exogenous SPD or SPM reduces ODC and AdoMetDC activities to very low levels in a relatively short time. Cells so treated, however, avoid becoming growth inhibited by utilizing the exogenous polyamines in place of those which they would otherwise synthesize. The objective of our regulatory strategy has been to synthesize and identify polyamine analogs which, in similarity to the natural polyamines, regulate ODC and/or AdoMetDC activities, but which are incapable of substituting for the natural polyamines in those unidentified functions required for cell growth (4). Thus, by suppressing polyamine biosynthesis, intracellular pools would be depleted and ultimately replaced with a potentially dysfunctional analog. The end result of this strategy differs substantially from that attained with enzyme inhibitors where various polyamine pools are simply depleted but not replaced with an analog. The strategy, therefore, offers the additional potential of having the cellular effects of polyamine depletion further enhanced by dysfunctional replacement of the analogs at vacated polyamine binding sites.

PROOF OF PRINCIPLE

Due to the availability of synthetic schemes for triamines (20) but not tetraamines at the outset of our studies, verification of the regulatory strategy initially focussed on systematically modified SPD analogs (21). From a large series of analogs in which modifications involved substituent size, location of the derivatized amine and bond species (i.e. alkyl versus acyl), it was determined that the relatively simple bis(ethyl) derivatives best fulfilled the proposed criteria for the regulatory strategy. Namely, they penetrated cells well, negatively regulated ODC as effectively as SPD itself and were ineffective in substituting for SPD in SPD-depleted (DFMO-treated) cells (21). In a subsequent study (22), it was determined that the spermine analog, N^1,N^{12}-bis-(ethyl)spermine (BESPM), was even more effective than BESPD since it suppressed ODC and AdoMetDC and reduced all three polyamine pools to the lowest levels achieved by any single agent. It had an IC_{50} in L1210 cells of 10 μM as compared to 100 μM for BESPD. Thus, although BESPD served as the original prototype for the regulatory strategy, the much more effective BESPM and its homologs were adapted as the agents of choice for further development as antiproliferatives. In addition, comparative studies between BESPD and BESPM and other analogs have provided valuable structure-function data relevant to polyamine biology (23). On the basis of antitumor activity in the L1210 murine system (24), the homolog N^1,N^{14}-bis(ethyl)homospermine (Figure 3) was advanced to Phase I clinical trial by Drs. Bergeron and Streiff at the University of Florida, Gainesville.

MECHANISMS INVOLVED

In order to verify that the analogs were indeed behaving in a manner identical to the natural polyamines in suppressing ODC and/ or AdoMetDC, mechanistic studies were undertaken comparing BESPD

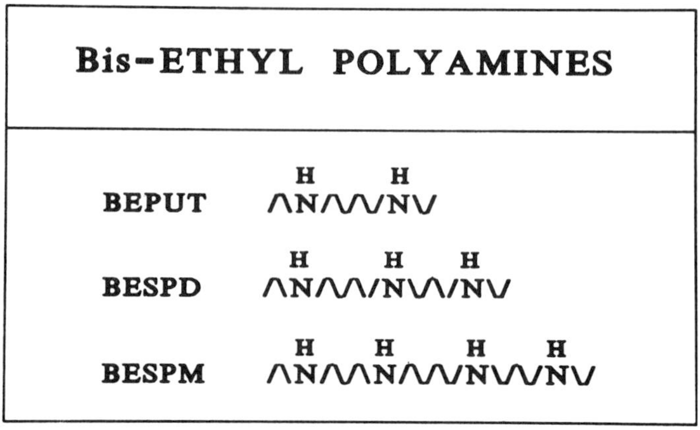

Bis-ETHYL POLYAMINES

BEPUT   H   H
          ∧N∧∨∨∨N∨

BESPD   H   H   H
          ∧N∧∨∧∨N∨∧∨N∨

BESPM   H   H   H   H
          ∧N∧∨∧N∧∨∨∨N∨∨∨N∨

Figure 3. Structural representation of three bis-ethyl homologs of SPM which differ according to the length of methylene bridges separating the four amines. Abbreviations are (BENSPM, N^1N^{11}-bis(ethyl)norspermine; BESPM, N^1,N^{12}-bis(ethyl)-spermine; and BEHSPM, N^1,N^{14}-bis(ethyl)homospermine.

with SPD (25) and BESPM with SPM (26). The studies revealed that, in both cases, the analogs were as effective as the natural polyamines and shared the same kinetics of enzyme suppression. ODC regulation was more sensitively controlled than AdoMetDC with the major enzyme decline occurring within two hours in response to BESPM at intracellular concentrations comparable to only a 7 to 13% rise in the combined SPD and SPM pools (26). In similarity to the natural polyamines, neither analog had any greater direct inhibitory effects on the enzymes than did the natural polyamines. In further support of this, it was observed that decline in enzyme activity was accompanied by a decrease in enzyme protein, indicating that decreased enzyme synthesis and/or increased enzyme degradation was probably responsible for the loss in activity. Northern blot analyses of analog-treated cells revealed no changes in enzyme-specific RNA levels suggesting post-transcriptional control if decreased synthesis were involved. Of particular relevance was the observation initially made by Pegg _et al_. (27) and later by Porter _et al_. (26) that the analogs in similarity to the polyamines could preferentially inhibit the _in vitro_ translation of ODC and AdoMetDC relative to total protein or albumin synthesis in a reticulocyte-lysate system and at concentrations (75-100 μM) much lower than those achieved in cells. Further, on a concentration basis, there was agreement between the abilities of BESPD and BESPM to inhibit AdoMetDC translation _in_ _vitro_ (26,27) and their relative effects on this enzyme in cells (22,25). Considerable effort has been expended by several groups in studying the molecular aspects of ODC regulation (reviewed in 28). There is a correlative indication that the rapid turnover of both ODC and AdoMetDC may relate to the presence of runs of basic amino acids termed PEST sequences which are known to be associated with rapidly turning-over proteins (29). To date, however, there is no direct linkage between these observations and polyamine-induced enzyme suppression.

Thus, to the extent they have been compared with polyamines, the analogs seem to behave identically with respect to the mechanism(s) by which they suppress ODC and/or AdoMetDC. This demonstrates at least one instance in which the analogs can fully substitute for the natural molecules in a biological function. Since the end result of exposure to analogs, however, is growth inhibition, they are apparently unable to substitute for other cellular functions and particularly those required for growth. A negative finding with respect to enzyme suppression is that upon removal of the analog, cells rapidly recover enzyme activity (25,26). Analogs with greater binding affinity might, therefore, prove more effective as antiproliferative agents. However, until the nature of the binding site is defined, the current search for such agents must be based on semi-random structural variation in analog synthesis.

GROWTH INHIBITION

Initially, all polyamine analogs were evaluated in L1210 cells where appropriate test systems had been developed to evaluate analog function and mode of action [i.e. uptake, enzyme suppression, polyamine depletion, polyamine substitution and growth inhibition (4,21)]. Of the various analogs studied in this system, bis(ethyl) analogs of SPD and SPM gave the greatest growth inhibition while still fulfilling criteria consistent with the regulatory strategy. In the case of homologs of bis(ethyl)spermine (Figure 3), IC_{50} values were typically in the low micromolar range depending upon culture conditions. Growth inhibition was invariably cytostatic in nature except under extended treatment conditions (i.e. >48 hr) where it tended to become irreversible.

Evaluation of certain of the analogs in the NCI human tumor screening panel (Figure 4) provided interesting and useful information. In confirmation of previous findings by Casero _et al._,

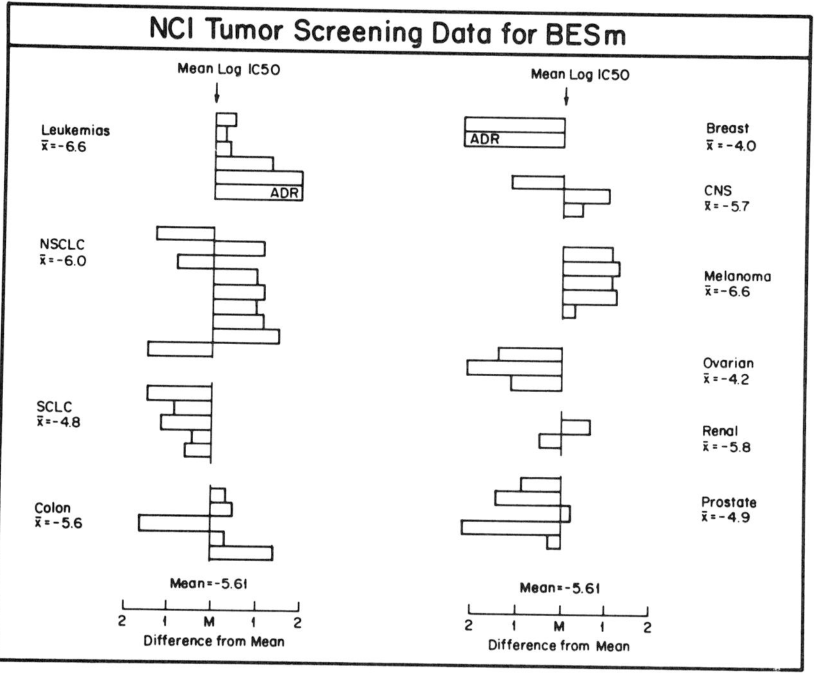

Figure 4. Data from NCI human tumor panel testing of BESPM. Each horizontal bar represents a single cell line. The center vertical line represents the mean IC_{50} value at 96 hr for all cell lines taken together. Bars projecting to the right of the vertical center line indicate lower IC_{50} values (and hence, greater sensitivity) and those to the left, higher IC_{50} values. Data provided by Drs. M.E. Boyd, R.J. Shumaker, A. Monks and colleagues (NCI Biological Testing Branch, Frederick, MD).

(30), 6 of 9 human non-small cell lung lines showed high sensitivity to BESPM while 4 of 4 small cell carcinomas were about 2 logs less sensitive by IC_{50} values. Unexpectedly, the screening data revealed that five of five human melanoma lines were one to two logs more sensitive than all other cell lines together. We have since confirmed this sensitivity in MALME-3 human melanoma cells and find further that in similarity to large cell lung carcinoma H-157 cells (30), a comparable but somewhat less impressive cytotoxic response. Thus, our subsequent studies involving preclinical development of these analogs have focussed on large cell lung and melanoma model systems.

HOMEOSTATIC EFFECTS

In the interest of determining the basis for the high sensitivity of large cell lung carcinoma and melanoma cell lines to SPM analogs, we compared MALME-3 cells with LOX, an amelanotic human melanoma line found to be inherently resistant to the analog (32) while Casero et al. (31) undertook studies comparing BESPM effects in large cell lung with small cell lung carcinoma lines. In both cases, it was observed that polyamine pools in the sensitive cell lines were more rapidly and extensively depleted by BESPM treatment than pools in the insensitive cell lines. The finding implicated involvement of spermidine/spermine N^1-acetyltransferase (SSAT, Figure 5), an enzyme known to be critically involved in the catabolism of polyamines (33-35) and proposed to play a role in polyamine excretion by cells (16,36). Further, it had been shown previously that exposure to analogs of SPD (37) and SPM (38,39) led to a profound (i.e. 10 to 15-fold) increase in SSAT activity.

SSAT is a cytosolic enzyme which catalyzes the transfer of an acetyl group from acetyl coenzyme A to a terminal aminopropyl nitrogen of SPM or SPD. These, in turn, are then acted upon by a FAD-dependent polyamine oxidase to produce SPD and PUT, respectively, along with 3-acetamidopropanal. Because acetylation effectively reduces the net charge of SPD or SPM by one, SSAT has been proposed to modulate intracellular binding and to influence their excretion out of the cell (16). Support for this derives from the

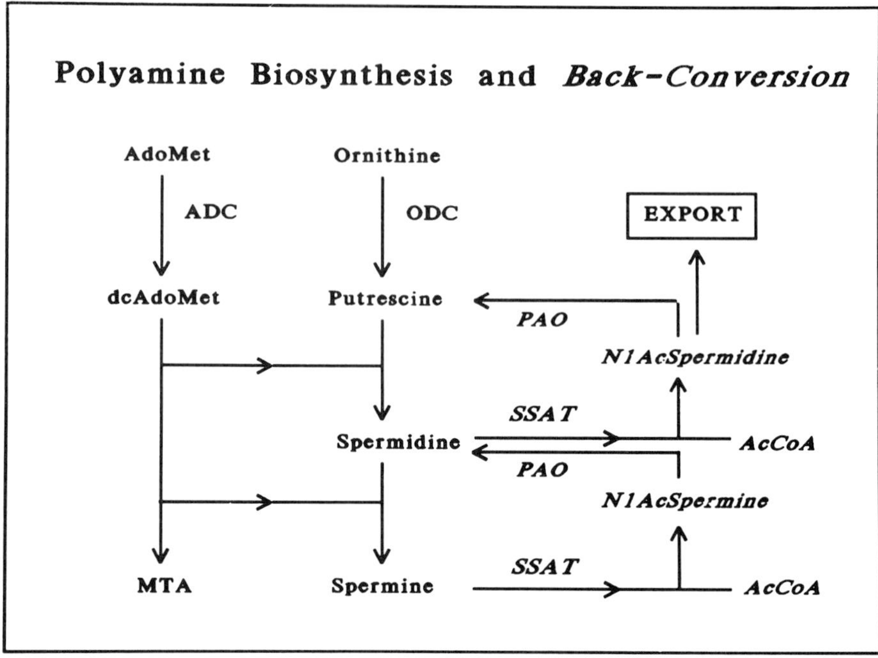

Figure 5. Polyamine biosynthetic pathway extended to show the role of spermidine/spermine-N^1-acetyltransferase (SSAT) in the back-conversion pathway and its possible participation in polyamine excretion. Abbreviations not defined in Figure 1 include PAO, polyamine oxidase.

observation that in whole animal systems, acetylated SPD and SPM constitute the predominant extracellular polyamines (16).

Measurement of SSAT activity in BESPM-treated sensitive melanoma and large cell lung carcinoma cell lines provided dramatic results. Whereas in other cell lines, the analog typically produced increases of enzyme activity up to 200 pmol/min/mg (38-40), SSAT rose to approximately 40,000 in H-157 large cell lung carcinoma cells (31) and to 10,000 in the MALME-3 melanoma cells (32). In correlation with effects on growth, SSAT rose minimally in the insensitive cell lines. In the absence of other comparably different polyamine effects between growth sensitive (H-157 and MALME-3) and insensitive (H-82 and LOX) cells, it is tempting to causally relate the 80- to 100-fold greater accumulation in SSAT activity in the former to their sensitivity to the analogs. This was further supported mechanistically by the observation that cells treated with BESPM or its homologs (Figure 3) excrete substantially greater quantities of polyamines into the culture medium (32,40) and, therefore, become more rapidly depleted of polyamines.

There is indication that SSAT induction may represent one of several compensatory mechanisms constituted in a broader homeostatic response. Bergeron <u>et al</u>. have observed that L1210 cells treated with bis(ethyl) spermine homologs maintain a total cationic charge balance between the intracellular homolog concentration and the decreasing natural polyamine pools. Whereas modest increases in SSAT might be expected to help maintain this balance by contributing to the efflux of polyamines during analog influx, massive increases such as seen in MALME-3 and H-157 cells could cause a major disruption in this equilibrium. Such perturbations would be expected to contribute significantly to homeostatic imbalances and ultimately to the nature of the cellular growth response.

The mechanistic basis for this unusual enzyme effect has yet to be defined. Libby <u>et al</u>. (42) have purified and characterized human SSAT and determined that the various bis(ethyl) homologs of SPM (Figure 3) are all inhibitors of SSAT and that the potency of their inhibition correlates qualitatively with their ability to induce SSAT activity. Thus enzyme stabilization may partially account for the increase, particularly since the uninduced enzyme has a half-life of only 20-30 min (3). Although reversibly inhibited by the analogs, the SSAT would be presumed to rise to a level where the unbound (functional) enzyme would be substantially above the basal activity levels. Since enzyme induction can be fully blocked with cycloheximide and partially blocked with actinomycin D (31,32,39), increased transcription and protein synthesis also seem to be involved. The intriguing question is why one cell type should differ so dramatically from another in this enzyme response.

ANTITUMOR ACTIVITY

Depending on the prevalence of the SSAT hyper-induction among other human melanomas, large cell lung carcinomas or even unrelated tumor types, the phenomenon could have relevant implications as a determinant of tumor sensitivity to bis(ethyl) polyamine analogs. Pending a detailed survey of various clinically-derived cell lines of recent origin, we have proceeded with _in vivo_ evaluation of analog efficiency against the MALME-3 tumor growing in athymic mice. Although these studies are still on-going, distinct trends have emerged. As determined by Bergeron _et al_. (24), the analogs are relatively ineffective when administered once per day. Optimal effectiveness was achieved on a schedule of 3 times/ day for 6 days. The basis for this is uncertain at present but may be related to the rapid clearance of the analogs from the circulation. When administered in the MALME-3 system under this schedule and at levels approximately 50% the lethal dose, a distinct tumor regression was apparent within 6 days, which in the case of BEHSPM at 5 mg/kg/injection, amounted to a 65% reduction in tumor volume (unpublished data). At equal dosages, BESPM and BENSPM were less effective but were tolerated at higher doses where they gave similar results to 5 mg/kg BEHSPM. Unfortunately, the effect was not sustained in any of the three treatments. Approximately 10 days after the last treatment, tumor growth resumed at a rate comparable to the untreated tumor. Multiple treatment strategies are now under evaluation.

In 1989, Drs. Bergeron and Richard Streiff initiated a Phase I clinical evaluation of the BESPM homolog, BEHSPM (Figure 3, known in that study as homoDES) at the University of Florida (Gainesville). In the seven patients evaluated, there has been minimal toxicity at doses administered to date. Although distinct symptomatic improvement was observed in most cases, antitumor activity has been difficult to quantitate due to heavy tumor burdens. The study is still underway.

339

RETROSPECTIVE

We have described a novel approach to a non-traditional chemotherapeutic target, the polyamines, and demonstrated some measure
of success in both mechanistic and antitumor objectives. To our
knowledge, the use of enzyme products or substrates to negatively
regulate a metabolic pathway as an antiproliferative strategy is
entirely unique. Our ability to apply this strategy effectively
to the polyamine biosynthesis is due, in part, to unusual properties inherent to the pathway which we only now appreciate. Pathway properties favoring the regulatory strategy include (a) the
existence of post-transcriptional product control mechanisms for
both of the key pathway enzymes, (b) the high sensitivity of these
mechanisms to product control, (c) the rapid turnover of ODC and
AdoMetDC, (d) the differential structural specificity of enzyme
regulation and growth dependent functions for the analogs, and (e)
the direct dependence of growth on sustained polyamine biosynthesis. Thus, by virtue of these unusual properties, we were able
to achieve our intended goals in controlling polyamine biosynthesis and inhibiting cell growth with the analogs.

An unanticipated effect of the polyamine analogs was their
ability in certain melanoma and large cell lung carcinoma cell
lines, to cause massive increases in SSAT activity. This and the
resulting effects on polyamine catabolism and excretion played a
contributing role in our main goal of maximizing polyamine depletion. Ultimately, given the magnitude of the enzyme induction and
its extreme heterogeneity among tumor cell types, the phenomenon
may provide a determinant for tumor selectivity for this class of
polyamine analogs. From the tumor regression observations seen in
the MALME-3 <u>in</u> <u>vivo</u> system, it would seem that a measure of selectivity has been achieved. While SSAT induction and its various
ramifications may account in part for this effect, other determinants that could also contribute include differential responses in
one or more of the following: analog uptake, polyamine dependence,
ODC/AdoMetDC regulatory mechanisms, polyamine function and/or
analog metabolism.

Recently, the apparent basis for the sensitivity of trypanosomes to DFMO and the relative clinical success of DFMO in treating African sleeping sickness has been discerned (43). Whereas in mammalian systems the half-life of ODC is in the order of 20 minutes, it has been found to be greater than 12 hr in trypanosomes. Thus, following treatment of DFMO, the host cells could regenerate their ODC very rapidly and recover from drug exposure while the trypanosomes could not. This and a predicted relationship for regulatory analogs are portrayed in Table 1. Interestingly, for BESPM to be effective, the opposite half-life relationship would have to prevail since it inhibits enzyme synthesis rather than the

Table 1

Relationship between Enzyme Half-life and Probable Efficacy
of Enzyme Inhibitors and Regulatory Analogs

		Enzyme Half-life		
Antagonist	Example	Target Tissue	Host Tissues	Predicted
Irreversible Inhibitor	DFMO	Short Long*	Long Short	Poor Good*
Regulatory Analog	BESPM	Short Long	Long Short	Good Poor

*i.e. _Trypanosoma brucei_ (43)

enzyme itself. Thus, a shutdown in enzyme synthesis by the analogs would impact most on cells with shorter enzyme half-lives and least on those with longer half-lives. Because the half-life of ODC is in the order of 20 minutes in mammalian cells, it is unlikely that any tumor might be found to have a much shorter half-life. None-the-less, the phenomenon in the trypanosomes provides an worthwhile example of how, even in the absence of absolute rationale at the outset, mechanism-directed drug discovery initiatives can emerge, with thorough exploration, as sound and useful strategies. It is our belief that polyamine analogs have that potential.

ACKNOWLEDGEMENTS

The authors gratefully acknowledge the secretarial assistance of Anne Culligan and Jessie Crowe. This work was supported by grants CA-51524, CA-22153, CA-37606, CA-13038, and CA-244538 from the National Cancer Institute, Department of Health and Human Services.

REFERENCES

1. Janne J, Poso H, Raina, A: Polyamines in rapid growth and cancer. Biochim. Biophys. Acta 473:241-293, 1978.
2. Porter CW, Sufrin JR: Interference with polyamine biosynthesis and/or function by analogs of polyamines or methionine as a potential anticancer chemotherapeutic strategy: A review. Anticancer Res. 6:525-542, 1986.
3. Pegg AE: Perspectives in Cancer Research. Polyamine metabolism and its importance in neoplastic growth and as a target for chemotherapy. Cancer Res. 48:759-774, 1988.
4. Porter CW, Bergeron RJ: Enzyme regulation as an approach to interference with polyamine biosynthesis -- an alternative to enzyme inhibition. In: Advances in Enzyme Regulation. G Weber (ed), Pergamon Press, New York and Oxford, Vol. 27, pp. 57-79, 1988.
5. Kingsnorth AN, King WWK, Diekema KA et al: Inhibition of ornithine decarboxylase with 2-difluoromethylornithine: Reduced incidence of dimethylhydrazine-induced colon tumors in mice. Cancer Res. 43:2545-2549, 1983.
6. O'Brien TG, Simsiman RC, Boutwell RK: Induction of the polyamine-biosynthetic enzymes in mouse epidermis by tumor-promoting agents. Cancer Res. 35:1662-1670, 1975.
7. Sistonen L, Keski-Oja J, Ulmanen I et al: Dose effects of transfected c-Ha-ras$^{val 12}$ oncogene in transformed cell clones. Exp. Cell Res. 168:518-530, 1987.
8. Alhonen-Hongisto L, Kallio A, Sinervirta R et al: Tumorigenicity, cell-surface glycoprotein changes and ornithine decarboxylase gene pattern in Ehrlich ascites-carcinoma cells. Biochem. J. 229:711-715, 1985.
9. Mamont PS, Duchesne M-C, Grove J, Bey P: Antiproliferative properties of DL-α-difluoromethylornithine in cultured cells. A consequence of irreversible inhibition of ornithine decarboxylase. Biochem. Biophys. Res. Commun. 81:58-66, 1978.

10. Schechter PJ, Barlow JLR, Sjoerdsma A: Clinical aspects of inhibition of ornithine decarboxylase with emphasis on therapeutic trials of eflornithine (DFMO) in cancer and protozoan diseases. In: Inhibition of Polyamine Metabolism. PP McCann, AE Pegg, A Sjoerdsma (eds), Academic Press, New York, pp. 345-364, 1987.
11. Porter CW, Bergeron RJ: Regulation of polyamine biosynthetic activity by spermidine and spermine analogs -- a novel antiproliferative strategy. Progress in Polyamine Research. V Zappia, AE Pegg (eds), Plenum Press, New York, pp. 677-690, 1988.
12. Verma AK: The enzyme-activated irreversible inhibitor of ornithine decarboxylase, DL-α-difluoromethylornithine: A chemopreventive agent. Preventative Medicine 18:646-652, 1989.
13. Park MH, Cooper HL, Folk JE: Identification of hypusine, an unusual amino acid, in a protein from human lymphocytes and of spermidine as its biosynthetic precursor. Proc. Natl. Acad. Sci. U.S.A. 78:2869-2873, 1981.
14. Park MH, Liberato DJ, Yergey AL, Folk JE: The biosynthesis of hypusine (N'-[4-amino-2-hydroxybutyl]lysine). Alignment of the butylamine segment and source of the secondary amino nitrogen. J. Biol. Chem. 257:12123-12127, 1984.
15. Kramer DL, Khomutov RM, Bukin YV et al: Cellular characterization of a new irreversible inhibitor of S-adenosylmethionine decarboxylase and its use in determining the relative abilities of individual polyamines to sustain growth and viability of L1210 cells. Biochem. J. 259:325-331, 1989.
16. Seiler N: Functions of polyamine acetylation. Can. J. Physiol. Pharmacol 65:2024-2035, 1987.
17. Seiler N, Dezeure F: Polyamine transport in mammalian cells. Int. J. Biochem. 22:211-218, 1990.
18. Alhonen-Hongisto L: Regulation of S-adenosylmethionine decarboxylase by polyamines in Ehrlich ascites-carcinoma cells grown in culture. Biochem. J. 190:747-754, 1980.
19. Clark JL, Fuller JL: Regulation of ornithine decarboxylase in 3T3 cells by putrescine and spermidine: Indirect evidence for translational control. Biochem. 14:4403-4409, 1975.
20. Bergeron RJ: Synthesis and solution structure of microbial siderophores. Acc. Chem. Res. 19:105-113, 1986.
21. Porter CW, Cavanaugh Jr, PF, Stolowich N et al: Biological properties of N^4- and N^1, N^8-spermidine derivatives in cultured L1210 leukemia cells. Cancer Res. 45:2050-2057, 1985.
22. Porter CW, McManis J, Casero RA, Bergeron RJ: Relative abilities of bis(ethyl) derivatives of putrescine, spermidine and spermine to regulate polyamine biosynthesis and inhibit cell growth. Cancer Res. 47:2821-2825, 1987.
23. Vertino PM, Bergeron RJ, Cavanaugh PF Jr, Porter CW: Structural determinants of spermidine-DNA interactions. Biopolymers 26:691-703, 1987.
24. Bergeron RJ, Neims AH, McManis JS et al: Synthetic polyamine analogues as antineoplastics. J. Med. Chem. 31:1183-1190, 1988.

25. Porter CW, Berger FG, Pegg AE et al: Regulation of ornithine
     decarboxylase activity by spermidine and the spermidine ana-
     log, N^1,N^8-bis(ethyl)-spermidine (BES). Biochem. J.
     242:433-440, 1987.
26. Porter CW, Pegg AE, Ganis B, et al: Combined regulation of
     ornithine an S-adenosylmethionine decarboxylases by spermine
     and the spermine analog, N^1,N^{12}-bis(ethyl)spermine.
     Biochemical Journal 268:207-212, 1990.
27. Pegg AE, Madhubala R, Kameji T, Bergeron RJ: Control of
     ornithine decarboxylase activity in -difluoromethylor-
     nithine-resistant L1210 cells by polyamines and synthetic
     analogues. J. Biol. Chem. 263:11008-11014, 1988.
28. Seiler N, Heby O: Regulation of cellular polyamines in mam-
     mals. Acta Biochim. Biophys. Hung. 23:1-36, 1986.
29. Rechsteiner M: Regulation of enzyme levels by proteolysis:
     The role of PEST regions. In: Advances in Enzyme Regula-
     tion. G Weber, (ed), Pergamon Press, Volume 27, pp. 135-151,
     1988.
30. Casero R, Go B, Theiss HW et al: Cytotoxic response of the
     relatively difluoromethylornithine-resistant human lung tumor
     cell line NCI H157 to the polyamine analogue N^1,N^8-bis(ethyl)-
     spermidine. Cancer Res. 47:3964-3967, 1987.
31. Casero RA Jr, Celano P, Ervin SJ et al: Differential induc-
     tion of spermidine/spermine N^1-acetyltransferase in human
     lung cancer cells by the bis(ethyl)polyamine analogues.
     Cancer Res. 49:3829-3833, 1989.
32. Porter CW, Ganis B, Libby PR, Bergeron RJ: Correlations be-
     tween polyamine analog-induced increases in spermidine/
     spermine N^1-acetyltransferase activity, polyamine pool dep-
     letion and growth inhibition in human melanoma cell lines.
     Cancer Res. (In Press).
33. Bolkenius FN, Seiler N: Functions of polyamine acetylation.
     Int. J. Biochem. 13:287-292, 1981.
34. Pegg AE, Matsui I, Seely JE et al: Formation of putrescine
     in rat liver. Med. Biol. 59:327-333, 1981.
35. Mamont PS, Seiler N, Siat M et al: Metabolism of acetyl de-
     rivatives of polyamines in cultured polyamine-deficient rat
     hepatoma cells. Med. Biol. 59:347-353, 1981.
36. Wallace HM: Polyamine catabolism in mammalian cells: Excre-
     tion and acetylation. Med. Sci. Res. 15:1437-1440, 1987.
37. Erwin BG, Pegg AE: Regulation of spermidine spermine N^1-
     acetyltransferase in L6 cells by polyamines and related com-
     pounds. Biochem. J. 238:581-587, 1986.
38. Libby PR, Bergeron RJ, Porter CW: Structure-function correla-
     tions of polyamine analog induced increases in spermidine/
     spermine acetyltransferase activity. Biochem. Pharmacol.
     38:1435-1442, 1989.
39. Libby PR, Henderson MA, Bergeron RJ, Porter CW: Major increa-
     ses in spermidine/spermine-N'-acetyltransferase activity by
     spermine analogs and their relationship to polyamine deple-
     tion and growth inhibition of L1210 cells. Cancer Res.
     49:6226-6231, 1989.

40. Pegg AE, Wechter R, Pakala R, Bergeron RJ: Effect of N^1, N^{12}-bis(ethyl)spermine and related compounds on growth and polyamine acetylation, content, and excretion in human colon tumor cells. J. Biol. Chem. 264:11744-11749, 1989.

41. Bergeron RJ, Hawthorne TR, Vinson JRT et al: Role of the methylene backbone in the antiproliferative activity of polyamine analogues on L1210 cells. Cancer Res. 49:2959-2964, 1989.

42. Libby PR, Ganis B, Bergeron RJ, Porter CW: Characterization of human spermidine/spermine N^1-acetyltransferase purified from cultured melanoma cells. Arch. Biochem. Biophys. (In Press).

43. Phillips MA, Coffino P, Wang CC: Cloning and sequencing of the ornithine decarboxylase gene from _trypanosoma_ _brucei_. J. Biol. Chem. 262:8721, 1987.

20

ESPERAMICIN A_1 (BMY28175) - A NOVEL POTENT ANTITUMOR AGENT OF
THE DIYNE-ENE CLASS

Terrence W. Doyle, Jerzy Golik, Henry Wong, Kin Sing Lam, David
Langley, Salvatore Forenza, Dolatrai Vyas and Susan Kelley

Preclinical antitumor research at Bristol-Myers Squibb
Company is concentrated on four major areas: programs for the
discovery and development of novel chemotypes, analog research,
novel drug delivery systems (e.g. monoclonal antibodies) and the
exploitation of newer biotechnological approaches to cancer
therapy. Historically, the discovery and development of novel
chemotypes especially natural products or compounds synthesized
based on natural product models has resulted in most of the
important antitumor agents in current clinical use. While it is
hoped that biotechnology will provide newer and less toxic
treatment modalities in the future it is our belief that conventional chemotherapy will continue to have an important role.

In the past ten years, our natural product based effort has
resulted in the discovery of several compounds currently in
clinical trials or in the late stages of preclinical development;
BMY28175, BMY28090 in the former category and BMY25067, BMY27557
and BMY40481, in the latter. In addition to these in house
discoveries we are also involved in the development of bryostatin
and taxol which are marine and plant derived natural products,
respectively. In order to maximize our chances for clinical
success we have made our selection criteria for project status
more stringent. Novel chemotypes are expected to show reasonably
broad spectrum activity in murine and human tumor models, activity
in distally implanted tumors and novel mechanisms of action.

This paper will review the current status of BMY28175
(esperamicin A_1, ESP A) which was isolated from cultures of

<u>Actinomadura verrucosospora</u> (1-3). The organism was isolated from a soil sample collected at Pto Esperanza, Missiones, Argentina, thus the trivial name. While the initial yield of esperamicin A$_1$ was less than 1 mcg/ml subsequent fermentation development resulted in a 50-fold improvement (4-6) making adequate quantities available for structure elucidation and further biological evaluation. Esperamicin A$_1$ showed an interesting profile of activity in experimental tumor models (7). It was active in a variety of ip-ip models (P388 and L1210 leukemias, B16 melanoma, M109 lung carcinoma, C26 colon carcinoma, M5076 sarcoma and Lewis Lung carcinoma). The activity of BMY28175 in a number of distal tumor models also met our criteria (active in iv P388 and L1210 leukemias, sc B16 melanoma, sc M109, and MX-1 mammary xenograft in subrenal capsule of nude mice).

Structure Elucidation

The structures of the naturally occurring esperamicins isolated to date are recorded in Figure 1. The isolation and elucidation of the gross structure of esperamicins A$_1$, A$_{1b}$ and A$_2$ was reported earlier (1-3). More recently esperamicins A$_{1c}$, P, A$_{2b}$ and A$_{2c}$ and have been isolated and their structures determined (8,9). The esperamicins consist of a bicyclic core to which are attached a trisaccharide and a sub-stituted 2-deoxy-L-fucose. The individual sugars of the tri-saccharide were previously undescribed and contained an unusual hydroxylamino sugar (HAS) linked to a thiomethyl sugar (TMS) via an O-glycosidic linkage at the 4 position. The HAS is further linked to an isopropylamino sugar (IAS) at the 2 position. The bicyclic core contained the very unusual ene-diyne, an allylic trisuffide and a bridgehead enone. Subsequent mechanistic work has established that the interaction of these three function-alities results in a bioreductively activated, highly efficient, DNA strand scission.

At the time of our earlier publications only the absolute configuration of the 2-deoxy-L-fucose had been determined (3). More recent work has confirmed this assignment and has resolved

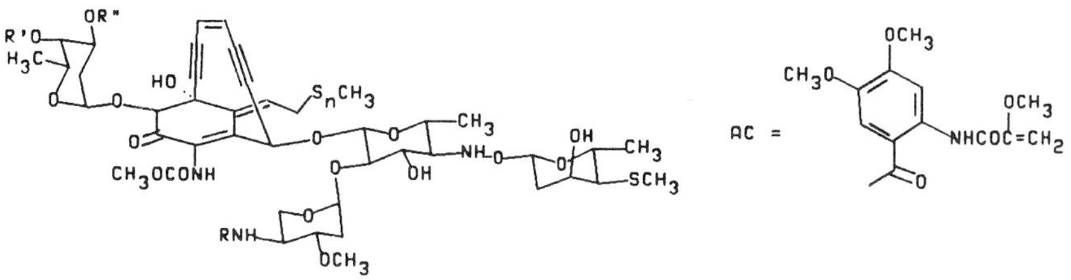

Esperamicin	n	R	R'	R"
A_1	3	$CH(CH_3)_2$	H	AC
A_{1b}	3	CH_2CH_3	H	AC
A_{1c}	3	CH_3	H	AC
P	4	$CH(CH_3)_2$	H	AC
A_2	3	$CH(CH_3)_2$	AC	H
A_{2b}	3	CH_2CH_3	AC	H
A_{2c}	3	CH_3	AC	H

Figure 1. Naturally occuring esperamicins.

the remaining questions concerning the absolute configurations of
each of the novel sugars and the bicyclic core. Thus stepwise
acid catalysed degradation of ESP A was carried out as shown in
Figure 2. Methanolysis yielded esperamicin C (ESP C) plus the
acylated deoxyfucose (DF-AC). Hydrolysis of DF-AC followed by
acylation of the sugar gave the bisbromobenzoate which was shown
to be of the L configuration by both single crystal x-ray and the
CD chirality method (3,10). Further methanolysis of ESP C gave
esperamicin D (ESP D) and the methyl glycoside of the thiomethyl-
sugar (TMS) the structure of which had been established earlier.
Conversion of TMS to its p-bromobenzoate followed by oxidation
gave the sulfone. The single crystal x-ray analysis of the
acylated sulfone established the D-ribo configuration (11). More
recently this has been confirmed by total synthesis (12). Methanolysis of ESP D gave esperamicin E (ESP E) plus the IAS. Reaction of the IAS with p-bromophenyl isocyanate gave the urea
which unfortunately failed to crystalize. Total syntheses of both

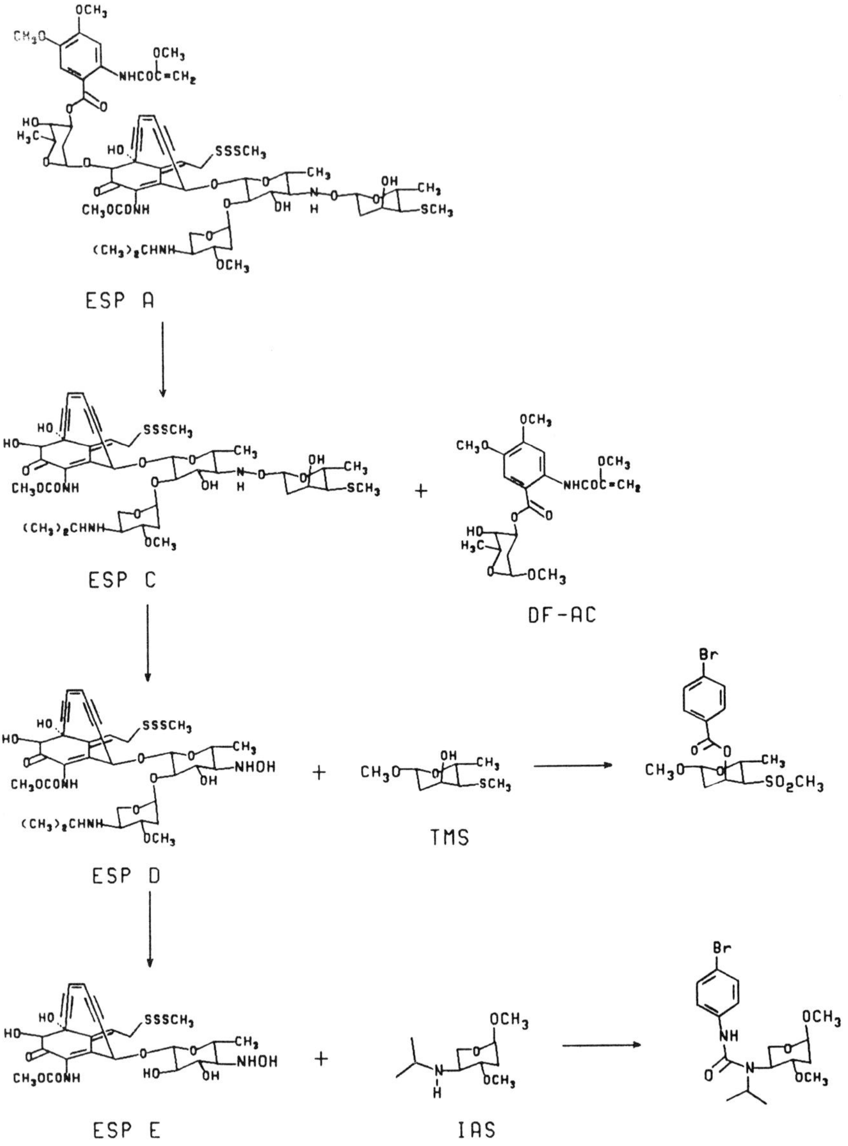

Figure 2. Stepwise acidic methanolysis of esperamicin A_1.

optical isomers of the urea were completed and the synthetic and natural compounds compared by circular dichroism. This established the L-threo configuration of the IAS (13). Attempts to further degrade ESP E to yield the core plus the HAS led to extensive degradation. Consequently, the alternate strategy depicted in Figure 3 was initiated. Treatment of ESP A with sodium borohydride in ethanol at pH 10 gave a novel trisaccharide in which the HAS had undergone a rearrangement to yield the N-alkoxyhexafuranose form shown. Methanolysis of the rearranged N-acetylated trisaccharide yielded the previously isolated methyl glycosides (TMS and N-Ac IAS) and a nitrone. The independent synthesis of the nitrone starting from D-fucose and L-fucose has established the D-gluco configuration of the HAS (14).

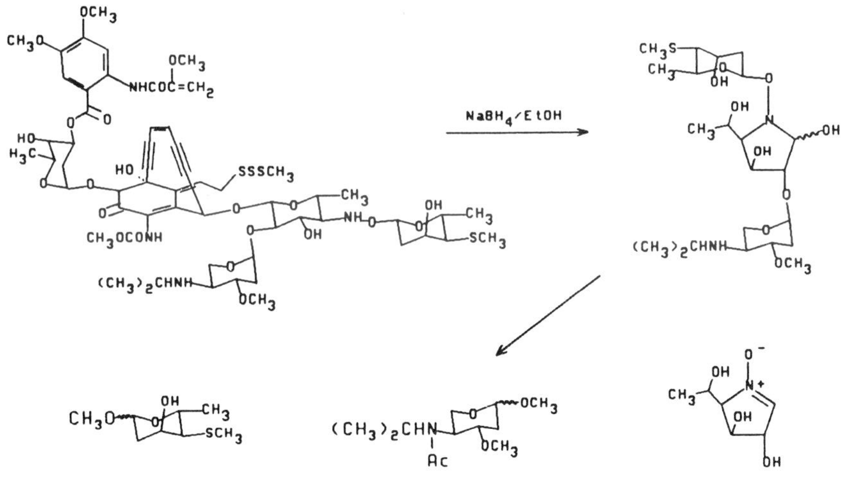

Figure 3. Reductive cleavage of trisaccharide.

The absolute configuration of the core of Esp A rests upon a comparison of esperamicin X (ESP X) with esperamicin Z (ESP Z). Treatment of ESP A with thiols results in cleavage of the trisulfide, Michael addition to the enone and subsequent aromatization of the ene-diyne to yield ESP Z (see Figure 6). In our earlier work we had isolated ESP X from the fermentation broths and had established its gross structure based on the x-ray analysis of its hydrolysis product (2). Recently, ESP X itself has been analysed by single crystal x-ray analysis. Since the absolute configuration of the deoxyfucose in ESP X is known this in turn unequivocally established the absolute configuration of the core. Comparison of the circular dichroism curves of ESP X and ESP Z confirmed that both have curves of similar sign thus establishing them to be of the same absolute configuration (Figure 4) (10) and completing the assignment of absolute configuration to ESP A itself.

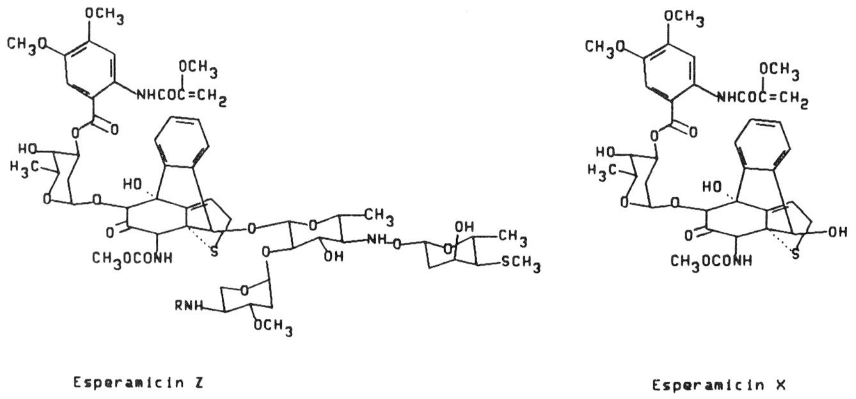

Figure 4. Structures of esperamicins X and Z.

Mechanism of Action

The mechanism of action of esperamicin and several related compounds (i.e. calicheamicin, neocarzinostatin) has been extensively studied (15-19). More recently the isolation of yet another member of this class, dynemicin, has been reported (20) (Figure 5). The proposed mechanism of action for the esperamicin-calicheamicin class is outlined in Figure 6. Within the intact

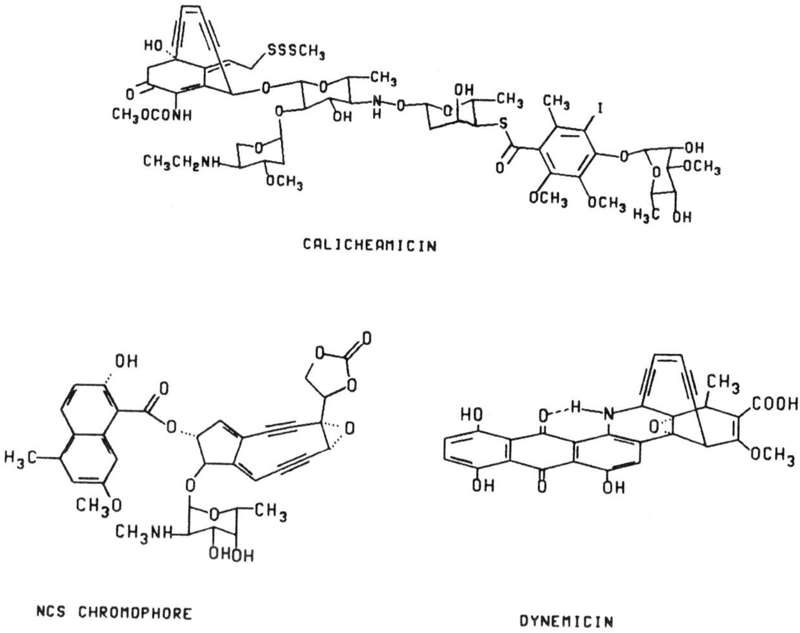

Figure 5. Structures of calicheamicin, NCS chromophore and dynemicin.

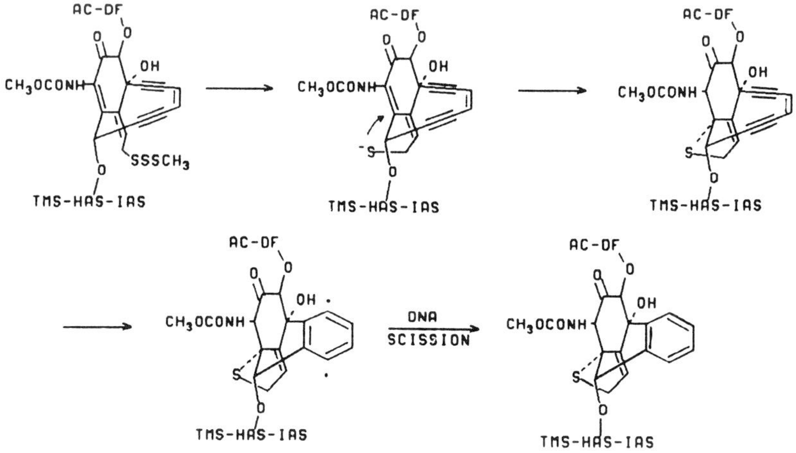

Figure 6. Esperamicin - mechanism of action.

ESP A the ends of the diyne-ene system are constrained from undergoing a cyclization to yield a benzene 1,4-diradical species. Reductive cleavage of the trisulfide yields a mercaptide anion which adds to the bridgehead enone yielding a tricyclic intermediate in which the ends of the diyne-ene come into closer proximity. Cyclization yields the diradical which can abstract hydrogen atoms from the deoxyribose backbone of DNA and results in DNA scission. In the case of neocarzinostatin (Figure 7) a diradical is also produced via nucleophilic addition of mercaptide to the cross conjugated diyne-diene system, generation of an yne-ene-cumulene system and cyclization to give the indenyl diradical (18). Similarly, dynemicin undergoes reductive opening

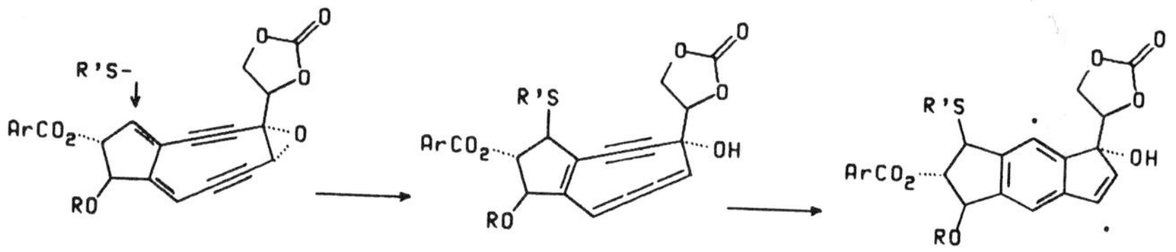

Figure 7. NCS chromophore - mechanism of action.

of the epoxide ring to yield a quino-methide structure which upon reduction or hydration gives an intermediate alcohol or diol capable of 1,4-diradical formation (Figure 8) (21,22). It would therefore appear that esperamicin is a member of a broad class of agents capable of cleaving DNA via direct carbon radical abstraction of deoxyribose hydrogen atoms. Further investigation of ESP A together with ESP C, ESP D, ESP E, ESP X, and ESP Z has established the following (15,16,23):
- Esperamicins can induce both single and double strand DNA breaks.
- Esperamicin A, induces primarily SSB while ESP C induces primarily DSB.

353

- Drug binding occurs in the minor groove of the DNA.
- Reductive activation is necessary to the activity.
- The presence of the diyne-ene function is a prerequisite to potent _in_ _vitro_ and _in_ _vivo_ activity.
- DNA cleavage most likely occurs via abstraction of the 5' hydrogen atom of the 2-deoxy ribose.
- The trisaccharide in esperamicin plays a crucial role in DNA binding. The 2-deoxy fucose substituent facilitates drug transport but may actually inhibit DSB formation.

Mechanistic and molecular modeling work on esperamicins is continuing with the goal of further refining our understanding of this unusual molecule.

Development Issues

Inasmuch as esperamicin A (BMY28175), fully met our criteria of novelty, broad spectrum of activity, and novel mechanism of action, a decision was made to proceed with clinical development.

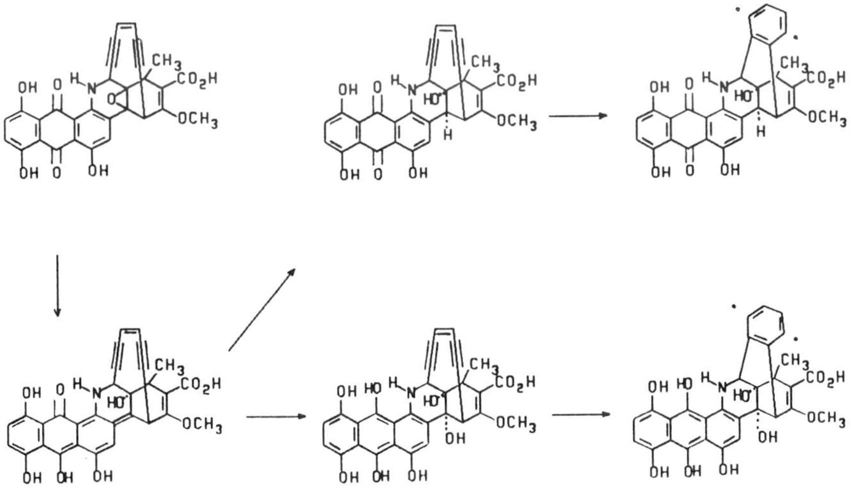

Figure 8. Dynemicin - mechanism of action.

Requirements for initiation of clinical trials with BMY28175 included: assuring an adequate supply of drug, preparation and stabilization of a clinical dosage form, completion of animal toxicology studies and design of appropriate Phase I clinical safety studies.

As indicated earlier, the initial fermentation yields of esperamicin A_1 were quite low. Several years of fermentation development have reliably increased those yields from approximately 0.2 ug/ml to 15-20 ug/ml. This was judged adequate for commercialization given the extreme potency of the compound (mouse LD_{10} = 9 ug/M^2). A collaborative effort of the NCI's Frederick Cancer Research Facility and Bristol-Myers Squibb has ensured adequate drug supply (24).

The development of a clinical formulation was complicated by the relatively small amount of drug/vial initially chosen i.e. 5 ug/vial of ESP A. Problems of both light sensitivity and absorption to glass surfaces were observed. The formulation eventually chosen consisted of 5 ug of BMY28175 and 20 mg lactose in 5 ml silanized amber vials. The reconstitution vehicle chosen was 40% ethanol in D5W.

Toxicologic evaluation of BMY28175 revealed myelosuppression affecting all cell types. The major nonhematologic toxicities were phlebitis, pyrogenicity, and delayed elevation of BUN and liver enzymes. In dogs clear cell foci were seen in the liver. Renal changes including nephrosis were also observed.

Phase I Clinical Trials

Based upon the results of preclinical toxicology studies, especially the delayed bone marrow, hepatic and renal toxicities, the design of the initial Phase I (safety) trials incorporated a six week observation period between doses in any individual patient. Two Phase I trials incorporating a single dose intermittent schedule and one Phase I trial with a five daily dosing schedule were initiated in mid 1988 and early 1989. Seventy patients with a variety of advanced malignancies have been treated so far.

Single-dose studies are underway in Bellinzona, Switerzland (25) and at the University of Maryland Cancer Center. The BMY28175 starting dose of 1.0 ug/M^2 was based on 1/10 the mouse LD_{10}. Dosage has been escalated to 8.9 ug/M^2 with toxicities including asymptomatic hypotension, fever, nausea, vomiting, phlebitis, myelosuppression, hepatic dysfunction and proteinuria (Table 1). Cumulative, delayed hepatotoxicity with fulminant

Table 1

BMY28175 - Phase I Single Intermittent Schedule

Dose ug/M^2	No Pts/Cycles	Fever	Chills	ꜜBP	Proteinuria
1	3/7	5	-	-	-
1.5	3/5	4	1	-	-
2.25	3/6	4	-	-	-
3	3/5	3	2	-	-
4	4/8	8	1	1	4
5.5	4/4	4	4	-	1
7	4/4	4	1	3	2

hepatic necrosis was encountered in one patient. A Phase I study using the five-daily dose schedule is in progress at the University of Texas in San Antonio (26). The starting dose of 0.15 ug/M^2/Dx5 has been escalated up to 1.35 ug/M^2/Dx5, administered on 4-week interval. Toxicities encountered so far include asymptomatic hypotension, fever, nausea, phlebitis, proteinuria and mild elevations of hepatic enzymes (Table 2). All studies are still ongoing in an attempt to delineate the extent and pattern of hepatic toxicity and to determine a suitable dose and schedule for Phase II efficacy studies.

Table 2

BMY28175 - Phase I Five-Daily Dosing

Dose $uG/M^2/DX5$	No Pts/Cycles	Fever	|BP	Proteinuria
0.15	4/10	2	-	-
0.30	3/5	-	-	2
0.60	3/3	-	-	2
0.75	4/10	-	2	4
1.0	4/7	1	1	-
1.35	1/1	-	-	-

ACKNOWLEDGEMENTS

We gratefully acknowledge the support of the National Cancer Institute both in the discovery phase of this research (NCI-CM-37556) and in its development with the Frederick Cancer Research Facility.

REFERENCES

1. Konishi M, Ohkuma H, Saitoh K et al: Esperamicins, a novel class of potent antitumor antibiotics.· I. Physico-chemical data and partial structure. J. Antibiot. 38:1605-1609, 1985.
2. Golik J, Clardy J, Dubay G et al: Esperamicins, a novel class of potent antitumor antibiotics. II. Structure of esperamicin X. J. Am. Chem. Soc. 109:3461-3462, 1987.
3. Golik J, Dubay G, Groenewold G et al: Esperamicins, a novel class of potent antitumor antibiotics. III. Structure of esperamicins A_1, A_2 and A_{1b}. J. Am. Chem. Soc. 109:3462-3464, 1987.
4. Forenza S, Claridge CA, Titus JA et al: Esperamicins, a novel class of potent antitumor antibiotics: Taxonomy and fermentation. Abstract O-23, 87th Annual Meeting of the American Society for Microbiology, Atlanta, GA, March 1-6, 1987.
5. Lam KS, Titus JA, Kimball DL: Isolation of esperamicin-hyperproducing strains of _Actinomadura verrucosopora_. Abstract O-40, 87th Annual Meeting of the American Society for Microbiology, Atlanta, GA, March 1-6, 1987.

6. Lam KS, Gustavson DR, Forenza S: Isolation of blocked mutants of esperamicin A_1 from <u>Actinomadura</u> <u>verrucosospora</u>. Abstract P-84, 46th Annual Meeting of Society of Industrial Microbiology, Seattle, WA, August 13-18, 1989.

7. Schurig JE, Rose WC, Kamei H et al: Experimental antitumor activity and toxicity of esperamicin, a new antitumor antibiotic. Invest. New Drugs 8:7-15, 1990.

8. Golik J, Beutler JA, Clark P et al: Esperamicin P, a novel antitumor antibiotic (BMY-41339), U.S. Patent applied (USSN323648), 1989.

9. Lam KS, Veitch JA, Gustavson DR et al: Unpublished observations.

10. Golik J, Doyle TW, Clardy J, VanDuyne G: Stereochemical studies on esperamicin A_1: An absolute configuration of the bicyclic aglycone. Submitted to Tetrah. Letters.

11. Golik J, Krishnan B, Doyle TW et al: Structural studies on esperamicin A_1: A single crystal x-ray structure of thiosugar moiety. Tetrah. Letters, in press.

12. Whitman MD, Halcomb RL, Danishefsky SJ et al: A route to glycols in the allal and gulal series: Synthesis of the thiosugar of esperamicin A_1. J. Org. Chem. 55:1979-1981, 1989.

13. Golik J, Wong H, Vyas DM, Doyle TW: Stereochemical studies on esperamicins: Determination of the absolute configuration of isopropylamino sugar moiety. Tetrah. Letters 30:2497-2500, 1989.

14. Golik J, Wong H, Vyas DM: Stereochemical studies on esperamicins: Determination of the absolute configuration of hydroxyamino sugar moiety. Submitted to Tetrah. Letters.

15. Long BH, Golik J, Forenza S et al: Esperamicins, a novel class of potent antitumor antibiotics. IV. Mechanism of action and cross-resistance properties. Proc. Nat. Acad. Sci. (USA) 86:2-6, 1989.

16. Sugiura Y, Uesawa Y, Takahashi Y et al: Nucleotide-specific cleavage and minor grove interaction of DNA with esperamicin antitumor antibiotics. Proc. Nat. Acad. Sci. (USA) 86:7672-7676, 1989.

17. a) Zein N, Sinha AM, MacGahren WJ, Ellestad GA: Calicheamicin γ_1: An antitumor antibiotic that cleaves double-strand DNA site specifically. Science 240:1198-1201, 1988.

    b) Zein N, Poncin M, Nilakantin R, Ellestad GA: Calicheamicin γ_1^I and DNA: Molecular recognition process responsible for site-specificity. Science 244:697-699, 1989.

18. Myers AG: Proposed structure of the neocarzinostatin chromophore - methyl thioglycolate adduct; a mechanism for the nucleophilic activation of neocarzinostatin. Tetrah. Letters 28:4493-4496, 1987.

19. Kappen LS, Goldberg IH: Identification of 2-deoxyribonolactone at the site of neocarzinostatin - induced cytosine release in the sequence d(AGC). Biochemistry 28:1027-1032, 1989, and references therein.

20. Konishi M, Ohkuma H, Matsumoto K et al: Dynemicin A_1 a novel antibiotic with the anthraquinone and 1,5-diyn-3-ene subunit. J. Antibiot. 42:1449-1452, 1989.
21. Sugiura Y, Shiraki T, Konishi M, Oki T: DNA intercalation and cleavage of an antitumor antibiotic dynemicin that contains anthracycline and enediyne cores. Proc. Nat. Acad. Sci. (USA) 87:3831-3835, 1990.
22. Langley DR, Doyle TW, Beveridge DL: The dynemicin-DNA intercalation complex, a model based on DNA affinity cleavage and molecular dynamics simulation. J. Am. Chem. Soc., submitted.
23. Dabrowiak J: Personal communication.
24. Beutler JA, Clark P, Roach J et al: Isolation and purification of Esperamicin A_1, ASP Congress on Natural Products, San Juan, Puerto Rico, 1989.
25. Sessa C, Drozd E, Gumbrell L et al: Phase I study of BMY-28175 (Esperamicin A_1 on a single intermittent schedule. Proc. ASCO, Washington DC, 1990.
26. Brown T, Havlin K, Weiss K et al: A Phase I clinical trial of BMY-28175, a novel antitumor antibiotic. Proc. ASCO, Washington DC, 1990.

21

MODIFIED 2-TUMOR (L1210, COLON 38) ASSAY TO SCREEN FOR SOLID TUMOR
SELECTIVE AGENTS

K.S. Smith, G.J. Badiner, E.G. Adams, D.K. Wilson, L.H. Li and
B.K. Bhuyan

INTRODUCTION

In 1983, the Cancer Research Department of The Upjohn Company
and Dr. Tom Corbett (then at Michigan Cancer Foundation) initiated
a collaborative effort to screen for agents selectively toxic to
solid tumors. The need for this assay arose from the fact that
the leukemic (L1210 and P388) cell lines used _in_ _vitro_ and _in_ _vivo_
as the primary screen for antitumor agents had produced substances
that were primarily active against leukemias and lymphomas. This
leukemia-oriented strategy had not generated agents significantly
active against the common solid tumors such as lung, colon, pancreas, stomach, etc. For example, of more than 100 agents which
were active against P388, only about 2% were active against Lewis
lung carcinoma or colon 38 or human xenograft CX-1 (1,2). Corbett
et al. (1,4) hypothesized that the vulnerability of P388 was different from that of the solid tumors. Therefore, they suggested
that the specific vulnerability of tumor of a particular organ
system would be detected only by models appropriate for that organ
system (3). They proposed the 2-tumor assay to screen for compounds selectively toxic against solid tumors (4). In this assay,
the lethality of the agent for L1210 cells was compared to lethality to cells from a drug-insensitive solid tumor (e.g. pancreatic
adenocarcinoma 02, colon 38, etc.). The L1210 cells will identify
agents toxic to rapidly growing cells, whereas the solid tumor
cells will select new agents that are possibly solid tumor specific. This assay had two other advantages: (i) Primary explants
of tumor (instead of a cell line) were used in the assay. Cells

from primary explants are much more likely to retain the characteristics of the original tumor than a cultured cell line. (ii) The
ability of the cells to survive and form colonies was used as the
end point. This is preferable to an indirect end point such as a
colorimetric protein determination or a trypan-blue viability
assay.

In the 2-tumor assay, cell suspensions, prepared by mechanical disruption of tumor, were planted in a 2-layer soft-agar medium. Cells from both tumor types were planted on the same plate.
Drug was applied via a paper disk. After several days of incubation, colony-forming units in the tumor cell population had grown
to form visible colonies. Drug effects were visualized microscopically as zones of inhibition around the paper disk. Since colonies from the 2 cell types (L1210 and colon 38) could be distinguished morphologically, the zones of inhibition could be determined on the same plate. We were concerned that planting both
cell types in the same plate may result in false values. For example, this could occur if the drug is metabolized only by L1210
to an active species. If the 2 cell types are planted together,
the drug will inhibit both cell types, whereas if they are planted
separately, only L1210 cells will be inhibited. Therefore, we decided to plant the 2 cell types on separate plates. We have since
been informed that for different cell types, Dr. Corbett's laboratory also uses separate plates.

Based on cell kinetic considerations, faster growing leukemic
cells would be expected to be more drug sensitive than slower growing solid tumor cells. Therefore, we were surprised at Corbett's
finding of several compounds (e.g. acivicin) which were more cytotoxic in this assay to solid tumor cells than leukemic cells. We
undertook to investigate this assay by: (a) optimizing cloning efficiency of the L1210 and solid tumor (colon 38) cells. It would
not have been possible to do this when the cells were planted together on one plate. (b) Quantitating cell survival by enumera-
ting surviving colonies rather than measuring zones on inhibition. Parts of this paper were previously presented as an abstract (5).

MATERIALS AND METHODS

Much of the procedures described here were adapted from those described originally by Corbett (ref. 4, and this volume). All media mentioned below were supplemented with serum as described by Corbett.

Tumor Cells

Corbett et al. (1984) used cells harvested from s.c. implanted L1210 in this assay. However, we obtained low cell yield and low plating efficiency for cells from s.c. tumor. Therefore, we decided to use L1210 ascitic cells in our assay.

L1210, a leukemic cell line, was maintained by injecting i.p. about 5×10^4 cells into 6 week old (≈ 15 g weight) DBA/2 male mice. Cells were harvested on the 7th day and transplanted to maintain stock. For the assay, cells were collected in a heparinized syringe on the 5th day. L1210 ascitic cells were centrifuged at 1,000 rpm for 3 min. The cells were washed twice with RPMI 1640 by centrifuging and resuspending the cell pellet in this medium. The cells were finally suspended in CMRL 1066 and were counted in the Coulter counter. An aliquot of cells was used in the assay.

Colon 38 (obtained from Dr. Tom Corbett, Wayne State University) was maintained in 6 week old C57BL/6 male mice weighing approximately 18 g. Tumor was transplanted by implanting a tumor fragment (2x3x3 mm) subcutaneously in the axillary region with a puncture in the inguinal region. Tumor was harvested either for the assay or for maintaining stock on day 14.

Mechanical Disaggregation of Colon 38

The tumor (500-3,000 mg) was sliced into 200-300 mg fragments which were suspended in 10 ml of RPMI 1640. The fragments were disaggregated mechanically in a Stomacher 80 (Tekmar Company, Cincinnati, OH) for 20 sec. The cell suspension was poured through a 45 mesh (355 µm) sieve; residual material was pushed through the sieve with a glass rod. The sieve was then rinsed with 10 ml RPMI 1640. The cell suspension was further disaggregated by pipeting

10 times through a glass pipette. The cells were then sieved through a 100 mesh (150 μm) sieve and the sieve washed twice with RPMI 1640. The cells were centrifuged at 150xg for 5 min and re-suspended in 15 ml RPMI 1640. Finally, the cell suspension was filtered through a sterile gauze. The cells were counted either in a hemocytometer or by a Coulter counter.

Enzymatic Disaggregation of Colon 38

In order to improve cell yield and cloning effciency, we tested several enzymes to disaggregate colon 38 tumor. A mixture of collagenase V and DNAase I (both from Sigma) gave the highest cell yield and was used in all experiments. The tumor was placed in a glass petri plate in a solution of the enzyme mixture and minced with crossed scalpels. One g of tumor was mixed with 2 ml of RPMI 1640 containing 20 mg collagenase type V and 50 μg of DNAase I. The minced mixture was transferred to a capped tube and rocked for 1 hr at 37°C. The supernatant cell suspension was removed after the large pieces of undigested tumor had settled. The large tumor pieces were washed with RPMI 1640 and the wash added to the supernatant cell suspension. The cell suspension was centrifuged and washed twice with RPMI 1640 to remove enzymes and then filtered through 150 μm Nitex filter. Cells were then counted in a Coulter counter.

Counting Cells

Cells were counted both by hemocytometer and the Coulter counter. For hemocytomer counting, 1 ml of cells in HBSS were stained with 0.1 ml of 0.4% trypan blue following which viable dye-excluding cells were counted. In general, cell suspension produced by enzymatic disaggregation contained <5% of cells that were not viable, i.e. stained blue. Therefore, in all further experiments the cells were counted with a Coulter counter.

Preparation of 2-Layer Agar Plate

The 2-layer agar plate was prepared by pipetting 3 ml of a soft-agar top layer over 3 ml of hard agar bottom layer in a 35 mm plate. To prepare the bottom layer, 40 ml of RPMI 1640 was mixed with 40 ml CMRL 1066 and 20 ml of 3% tryptic soy broth and 0.6 ml of 50 mg/ml DEAE-dextran. This mixture was warmed to $45^{\circ}C$ and then 20 ml of sterile Difco Bactoagar (3.5%) at $43^{\circ}C$ was added. The mixture was stirred and 3 ml aliquots were pipetted into 35 mm petri plates. The agar was allowed to harden and the plates stored in $37^{\circ}C$ incubator for 3-5 days prior to use.

To prepare the top layer, 2 ml of enriched RPMI 1640 and 2 ml of Fischers medium was mixed with 2 ml of colon 38 or L1210 cell suspension and 1.0 ml of 3% Difco agar and 3 ml were pipetted on top of the bottom layer in 35 mm plates. For top layer containing L1210 cells, 1 ml of 1% agar was used instead. It is necessary that the agar be maintained at $45^{\circ}C$ during use. The plates should be at room temperature prior to pouring the top layer.

Medium Preparation

Enriched CMRL 1066, enriched RPMI 1640, and enriched Fischers medium are referred to as CMRL 1066, RPMI 1640, and Fischers in the text. Enriched CMRL 1066 contained 500 ml CMRL 1066, 75 ml heat inactivated ($56^{\circ}C$, 40 min) horse serum, 20 ml of 100 mM $CaCl_2$, 4.3 ml of 10 mg/ml insulin, 5 ml 30 mM vitamin C, 1.7 ml of 200 mM L-glutamine. Penicillin, streptomycin, and Garamycin (0.5 ml of 40 mg/ml) were added to the medium. Enriched RPMI 1640 contained 500 ml RPMI 1640, 55 ml fetal calf serum, 5.1 ml of 200 mM L-glutamine, and 0.36 ml of 40 mg/ml Garamycin. Enriched Fischer's medium contained 500 ml Fischer's medium, 55 ml horse serum, 3.5 ml of 200 mM L-glutamine, and 0.36 ml of 40 mg/ml Gara-mycin.

Disk-Plate Assay

Filter-paper disks (6 mm, Whatman #1) were sterilized and placed on a wire grid. Drug solutions, up to 50 ul, were placed on the disk and allowed to dry. The disk was then placed on the top agar layer containing tumor cells and the plates incubated until colonies became visible. L1210 cells were incubated in a humidified incubator at 37° and gassed with 5% O_2, 6% CO_2 and

89% N_2. Colon 38 plates were incubated in a humidified incubator at 37° and gassed with an 8% CO_2 and 92% air mixture. The plates were examined by an inverted microscope usually at 65x magnification. A zone of inhibition was measured from the edge of the disk to the first colony and expressed in units where 1 unit = 150 μm. Maximum zone size was 120 units.

Cell-Survival Assay

In this assay the survival of cells was measured after either a 1 hr exposure to drug or a long term exposure (drug incubated with cells until colony formation) to drug.

For long-term exposure, the drug was mixed with the cells during the preparation of the top agar layer. The top layer was then pipetted over the hard agar bottom layer as described previously. The plates were incubated until colonies were visible. Colonies were counted with an inverted microscope at 65x magnification. Sufficient numbers of cells were planted to give between 10 to 200 colonies per plate. The cloning efficiency of the untreated (control) was normalized to 100% and the cloning efficiency of the drug-treated cells was expressed as a percentage of the control survival.

For 1 hr drug exposure, 2 ml of $2x10^6$ cells/ml were mixed with 4 ml of medium and drug in a 15 ml tube. The mixture was then rocked at 37^oC for 1 hr following which the cells were centrifuged at 1200 rpm x 5 min and washed twice with medium. The cells were then suspended in 7 ml medium (1:1 mixture of RPMI 1640 and Fischers). An aliquot was counted. Six ml of the cell suspension was mixed with 1.0 ml of melted agar (3% agar for colon 38, 1% agar for L1210) and 3 ml pipetted over the bottom layer. Colonies were counted and the percent survival calculated as described above.

L1210 and colon 38 cells were incubated in a humidified incubator at 37° and gassed with either 5% O_2-6% CO_2-89% N_2 (L1210) or 8% CO_2-92% air (colon 38).

Survival of Cells in Colon 38 Tumor Slices

For these studies, colon 38 tumor slices were exposed to drug following which the tumor was enzymatically disaggregated and cells planted to determine survival. Colon 38 tumor was minced with scalpels into approximately 2 mm cubes, which were washed with RPMI 1640 to remove any disaggregated cells. The tumor cubes were distributed to 15 ml centrifuge tubes, suspended in 6 ml medium and drug, tubes gassed with 8% CO_2 and incubated at $37^{\circ}C$ for 1 hr. The contents were mixed gently 4 times during the hour. Following incubation, the tubes were centrifuged and the tumor cubes washed twice with RPMI 1640. The tumor cubes were then digested with 0.5 ml of collagenase-DNAase mixture for 1 hr at $37^{\circ}C$. Following incubation, 10 ml of RPMI 1640 was added and the cell suspension filtered through 150 um Nitex filter. The cells were centrifuged and washed twice to remove enzymes. The cells were then suspended in 6 ml of medium plus 1 ml of 3% agar and 3 ml aliquots dispersed on top of the bottom agar layer.

Courtney-Mills Modification (6) of Colon 38 Survival Assay

After drug exposure cells were washed and resuspended in 5 ml of 1:1 mixture of CMRL 1066 and Fischers medium, then 1 ml of heat inactivated rat erythrocytes was added, followed by 1 ml of 3% agar. Three ml aliquots were planted on top of the hard agar bottom layer. To prepare rat erythrocytes, heparinized rat blood was centrifuged and the buffy coat was removed. The pellet of erythrocytes was washed and resuspended to original volume with CMRL 1066. They were then heated at $44^{\circ}C$ for 1 hr and diluted 8-fold with CMRL 1066 and stored in the refrigerator.

Flow Cytometry

Cell samples were prepared for DNA flow cytometry as previously described (7). Stained samples were analyzed for DNA content using a FACStarPLUS flow cytometer (Becton Dickinson Immunocytometry Systems (BDIS), San Jose, CA). Data from the FACStarPLUS were acquired in list mode on a Micro VAXII computer, and analyzed to exclude debris and cell doublets, using Consort40 software (BDIS).

DNA histograms were transferred to a PC computer and analyzed for cell cycle phase distribution using MODFIT (Verity Software House, Inc., Topsham, Maine).

Drug Preparation

U-73975 (The Upjohn Company) was stored frozen at 1 mg/ml in dimethylacetamide (8). Adriamycin (obtained from National Cancer Institute, U.S.A.) was stored frozen at 1 mg/ml in 0.01 M glucuronic acid. Acivicin was dissolved in saline at 1 mg/ml and stored frozen (9). Piercidin C_1 was dissolved in DMSO and stored frozen (10). The drugs were diluted in medium prior to adding to the cells. Acivicin and piercidin C_1 were obtained from Dr. Dave Martin of The Upjohn Company.

RESULTS

Growth Characteristics of L1210 and Colon 38 Tumors

Since our initial premise was that L1210 was a faster growing tumor than colon 38, we decided to determine their growth characteristics. The histology of colon 38 showed that the tumor is densely cellular consisting of mostly tumor cells. Tumor cells were pleomorphic and anaplastic and seemed to have a high mitotic rate. Very little stroma and very little inflammatory reaction was observed.

Colon 38 tumor implanted s.c. doubled about every 8 days, compared to 0.5-1 day doubling time for L1210 ascites. The DNA histograms of colon 38 and L1210 ascites is shown in Figure 1. Single cell suspension of colon 38 tumor was prepared by enzymatic digestion. Analysis of these histograms showed that the % of L1210 in G_0/G_1, S, G_2-M and polyploidy was 36.9, 47.3, 16.2, 3.2, and 0.0 respectively. The % of colon 38 cells in G_0/G_1, S, G_2-M and polyploidy was 45.9, 20.9, 9.0, and 24.2, respectively. The 2-fold difference in proportion of S phase cells in the two tumor types (L1210, 47.3% vs. Colon 38, 20.9%) may not explain the 8-16 fold difference in growth rate _in vivo_. This difference in growth rate may be due to higher rate of cell loss from colon 38 tumors. Colon 38 also contained a larger (up to 24%) proportion of cells

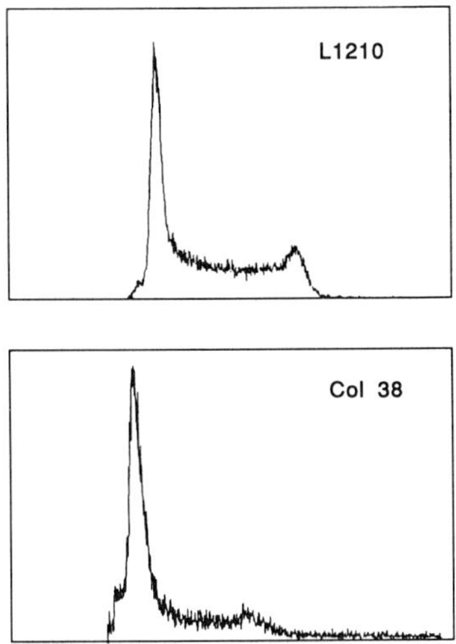

Figure 1. DNA histograms of L1210 and colon 38.

which were polyploid.

Comparative Cytotoxicity of Drugs for Colon 38 and L1210 in the Disk-Plate Assay

Prior to embarking on the more quantitative cell-survival assay (in which viable colonies are counted) we wanted to confirm Corbett's observation that certain compounds (e.g. acivicin and piercidin) were more cytotoxic to colon 38 than L1210 in a disk-plate assay. These results are presented in Table 1 and examples of dose response curves shown in Figure 2. We confirmed Corbett's observation that several compounds are indeed more cytotoxic to colon 38 than L1210 cells. For example, acivicin and its analogs were about 9 to 12 times more cytotoxic to colon 38 than L1210. Piercidin C_1 was unique in its specific cytotoxicity for colon 38 as compared to L1210. It was 4,000-times more cytotoxic to colon 38 than L1210. U-73975 was about 6 times more cytotoxic to L1210 whereas Adriamycin and flavone acetic acid were 4 times more cytotoxic.

Table 1

Cytotoxicity of Drugs for Colon 38 and L1210 in the Disk-Plate Assay

	Drug (μg/disk) for 50 unit zone	
	L1210	Colon 38
More active against colon 38		
Acivicin	0.7	0.08
Piercidin C_1	50	0.0125
More active against L1210		
U-73975	0.006	0.04
Adriamycin	0.1	0.4
Flavone acetic acid	50	100

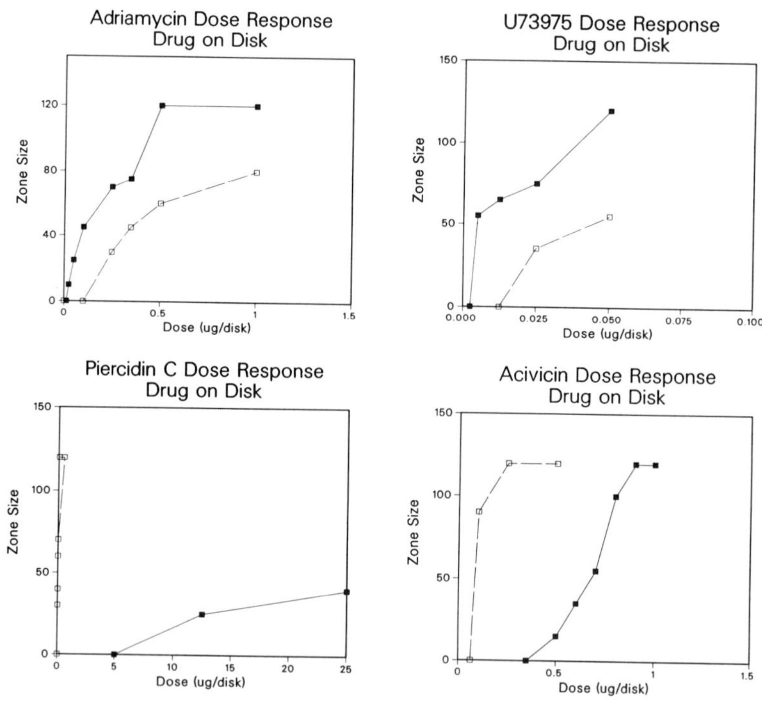

Figure 2. Zones of inhibition of different agents in the disk-plate assay using L1210 and colon 38. Zone size given in um. L1210, ■, colon 38, [ ].

Improving Plating Efficiency of L1210 and Colon 38

Table 2 shows the different modifications that increased the plating efficiency of L1210 cells about 50-fold. The original protocol (4) used 0.43% agar in the soft-agar layer and incubated the cells in an atmosphere of 8% CO_2-air mixture. In our laboratory, this resulted in a plating efficiency of less than 1% for L1210 ascites cells. By decreasing the agar percentage to 0.14% and by using an atmosphere of 6% CO_2, 5% O_2, 89% N_2, the plating efficiency was increased to about 20%. Further increase in plating efficiency was obtained by harvesting a younger (5 day old) tumor.

Table 3 shows the modifications that increased the plating efficiency of colon 38 cells about 12-fold. The major increases in plating efficiency occurred when (i) the tumor was dissociated by enzymatic treatment, (ii) a younger (14 day vs 21 day) tumor was used and the (iii) medium was supplemented with rat erythrocytes (Courtney-Mills modification). In contrast to L1210 cells, lowering the % O_2 to 5% or the % agar to 0.1% did not improve plating efficiency. Different agar preparations (BioRad, Seakem, etc.) were tried but did not result in improved plating efficiency. Therefore, in all subsequent studies, Difco agar was used.

Figure 3 shows the linear relationship between the number of colon 38 cells planted and the number of colonies counted. A similar linear correlation was obtained for L1210 cells. A linear relationship is necessary in order to obtain meaningful results in the cell-survival assay.

Comparative Cytotoxicity of Drugs for Colon 38 and L1210 Cells in a Clonogenic Cell Survival Assay

It is not possible to obtain quantitative values of drug cytotoxicity (i.e. LD_{50} and LD_{90}) values from a disk plate assay. Therefore, a survival assay in which surviving colonies are counted was done. In this assay, the drug was incorporated in the medium resulting in continuous exposure of cells to drug. Colonies formed after 7-12 days incubation were counted. Dose-response curves for several drugs are shown in Figure 4 and LD_{90} values are listed in Table 4. The results clearly show that acivicin

370

Table 2

Improvement of Plating Efficiency of L1210 Ascitic Cells[*]

Age of Tumor[***] (Days)	% Agar in Top Layer	% O_2[**]	% Plating Efficiency
7	0.43[*]	20	<1
7	0.21	20	2
7	0.14	20	5
7	0.14	5	20
5	0.14	5	30-45

[*]Parameters being compared are inside the rectangle.
[**]The 20% O_2 condition actually consisted of a mixture of 8% CO_2, 92% air. The 5% O_2 condition actually consisted of a mixture of 6% CO_2 and 5% O_2 and 89% N_2.
[***]Age of tumor refers to the day of tumor harvest after being implanted i.p. on day zero.

Table 3

Improvement of Plating Efficiency (P.E.) of Colon 38 Cells[*]

Age of Tumor (Days)	% of Agar in Top Layer	% O_2+	Tumor Dissociation	Fold Increase in P.E.
21	0.43	20	Mechanical[*]	1 (0.003%)
21	0.43[*]	20	Enzymes	3.3
21	0.3	20	"	3.0
21	0.1	20	"	2.9[**]
21	0.43	20[*]	"	3.3
21	0.43	5	"	1.2
21[*]	0.43	20	"	3.3
14	0.43	20	"	7.7
14	0.43	20	"	11.6[***]

[*]Parameters being compared are inside the rectangle.
[**]Colony morphology suggests damaged colony.
[***]Medium supplemented with rat erythrocytes (Courtney-Mills modification).

+ The 20% O_2 condition actually consisted of a mixture of 8% CO_2 and 92% air. The 5% O_2 condition actually consisted of a mixture of 6% CO_2, 5% O_2, 89% N_2.

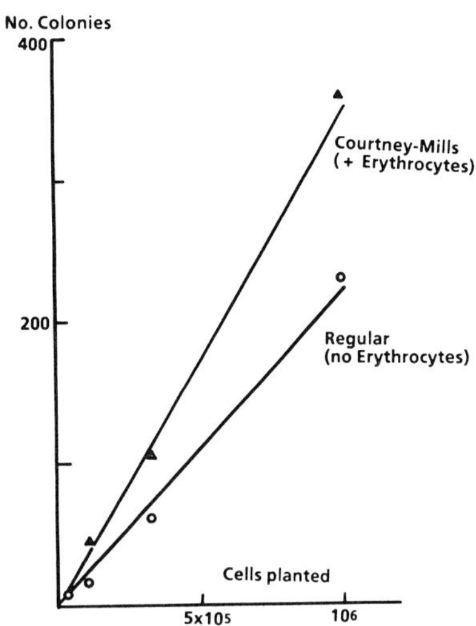

Figure 3. Linear relationship between number of colon 38 cells planted and colonies formed. Cells were planted in the presence of rat erythrocytes (Courtney-Mills modification) or in its absence.

is about 5-fold more cytotoxic to colon 38 than L1210. In contrast, piercidin C_1 is greater than 100-fold more toxic to colon 38. Adriamycin and U-73975 are more cytotoxic to L1210 than colon 38. However, in contrast to the disk-plate assay, the cell-survival assay clearly shows that U-73975 is about 100-fold more cytotoxic to L1210 than colon 38.

In Vivo Activity of Piercidin C_1

Since piercidin C_1 was significantly cytotoxic _in vitro_ to colon 38 cells (LD_{90} <1 ng/ml) and was less cytotoxic to L1210 cells we tested its activity _in vivo_ against colon 38 tumors. The results (Table 5) show that piercidin C_1 was inactive _in vivo_ against colon 38, even when injected peritumorally.

PIERCIDIN

ACIVICIN

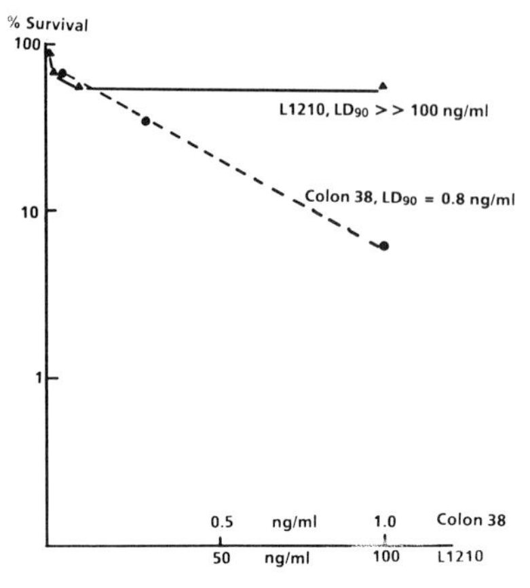

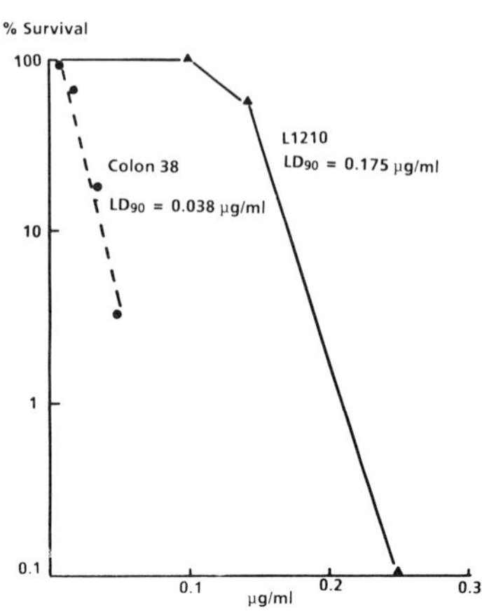

U-73975

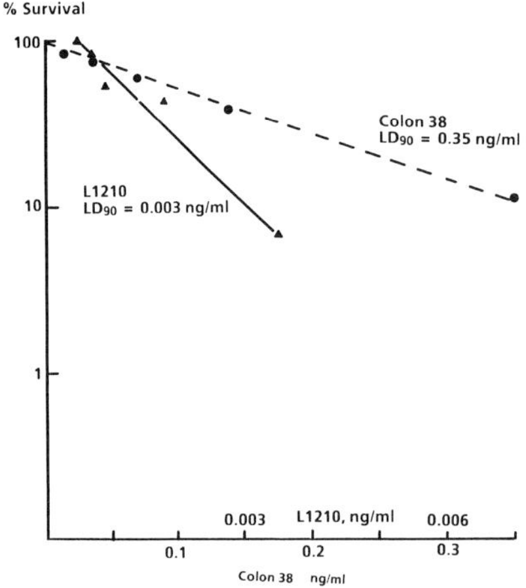

Figure 4. Survival of colon 38 and L1210 cells after continuous exposure to various drugs.

We entertained two possibilities for this discrepancy: (i) the drug requires long time of contact to exert cytotoxicity but the plasma level is not maintained at a high enough level for that period or (ii) Piercidin C_1 is cytotoxic to tumor cells in suspension but may be inactive against a tumor mass. Of course, other possibilities may also exist.

373

Table 4

Cytotoxicity of Drugs After Continuous Exposure
of Colon 38 and L1210 in a Cell Survival Assay

| Drug | LD$_{90}$ (ng/ml) | | LD$_{90}$ L1210 | | Sensitivity |
	L1210	Colon 38	LD$_{90}$ Colon 38		
Acivicin	175	38	4.6		Colon 38 >L1210
Piercidin C$_1$	>>100	0.8	>>100		Colon 38 >L1210
Adriamycin	30	120	0.25		L1210 >Colon 38
U-73975	0.003	0.35	0.008		L1210 >Colon 38

Table 5

Evaluation of Antitumor Effect of Piercidin C$_1$
Against Mouse Colon 38 Carcinoma In Vivo[a]

Route	Dose[b] (mg/kg/day)	Toxic Death/ Total	Animal Weight[c] Change (g)	Mean Tumor[d] Weight (mg)	TGI[e] (%)	Comments[f]
I.P.	1.75	8/8			Toxic	
	0.88	5/8			Toxic	
	0.44	0/8	5.2	714	35	Inactive
S.C.	1.0	8/8			Toxic	
(peri-	0.5	6/8			Toxic	
tumor)	0.25	0/8	5.6	768	30	Inactive
	0.125	0.8	6.0	963	12	Inactive

[a] Tumor fragments (2 mm^3) were implanted s.c. by trocar in the axilla (8 mice/group) on Day 0.

[b] Administered on Days 2 to 10 for a total of 9 injections.

[c] Mean animal weights were obtained on Days 2 and 20.

[d] The tumor weight was estimated from Day 22 tumor volume (mm^3) calculated as length x width^2/2.

[e] Percent tumor growth inhibition = [1-(mean tumor weight of drug-treated group/mean tumor weight of vehicle-treated control group)] x 100%. The mean tumor weight of the untreated control on Day 22 was 1088 mg.

[f] Activity (NCI criteria): Active, $\geq$58% TGI; highly active, $\geq$90% TGI.

Table 6

LD$_{90}$ After 1 hr vs. Continuous Drug Exposure

	Colon 38 (LD$_{90}$ ng/ml)			L1210 (LD$_{90}$ ng/ml)		
	1 hr[*]	Cont.[+]	Ratio[++]	1 hr	Cont.	Ratio
Acivicin	>1000	50	>20	41×10^3	175	234
Piercidin C$_1$	30	0.5	60		>>100	
Adriamycin	500	120	4.2	150	28	5
U-73975	3.5	0.35	10	0.026	0.0035	7

[*]1 hr exposure.
[+]Continuous exposure.

[++]Ratio = LD$_{90}$ 1 hr/LD$_{90}$ continuous

Table 6 compares the doses needed to cause 90% lethality after a short (1-2 hr) or a long exposure to drug. The ratio of LD$_{90}$ for 1 hr and continuous exposure is low for Adriamycin and U-73975 and is highest for piercidin. Although other possibilities exist, this high ratio for piercidin suggests that the drug requires a long time of contact to exert its cytotoxicity. This increases the possibility that the plasma level may not be maintained at a cytotoxic level for a sufficient period of time to demonstrate efficacy.

The lethality of 1 hr exposure to piercidin C$_1$ for cells in suspension and for tumor slices are compared in Figure 5. The LD$_{90}$ of piercidin C$_1$ after 1 hr exposure of cells in suspension was 30 ng/ml compared to >>100 ng/ml when tumor fragments were exposed to the drug. It is quite clear that piercidin C$_1$ is much less cytotoxic to tumor slices which might explain the lack of activity of this drug against colon 38 _in_ _vivo_.

DISCUSSION

We have used the disk-plate assay to confirm Corbett's (4) observation that several compounds are more cytotoxic to solid tumor (colon 38) cells than to rapidly growing leukemia (L1210) cells. Further quantitation of this assay was undertaken by substituting

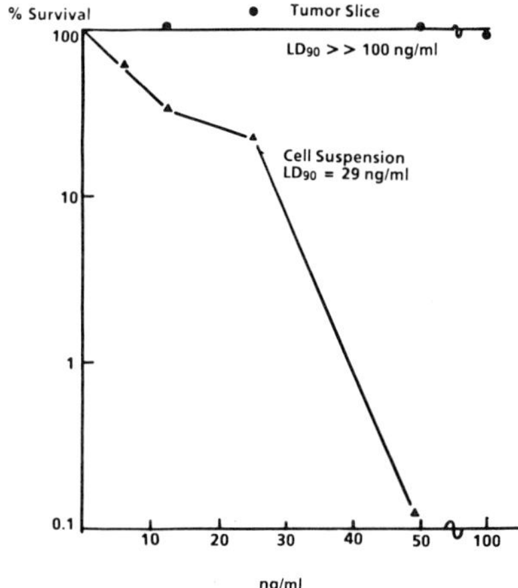

Figure 5. Survival of colon 38 cells, after 1 hr exposure to drug, either as a single cell suspension or as tumor slice.

cell-survival as an end point instead of measurement of zone of inhibition. Differences between the results of the 2 assays (Tables 1 and 4) was observed. For example, U-73975 was 125-fold more cytotoxic to L1210 than colon 38 in the survival assay as compared to 7-fold difference in the disk-plate assay.

The survival assay also allowed us to attempt to correlate the cytotoxic effect of the drug (expressed as LD_{90}) in vitro to the antitumor effect expected in vivo. For example, piercidin C_1, which was highly cytotoxic to colon 38 cells in vitro (LD_{90} <1 ng/ml) could be expected to be effective against colon 38 tumors in vivo. However, the drug was inactive in vivo.

In the absence of any information about drug concentration in the plasma and in the tumor, it was not possible to completely explain the lack of activity of piercidin C_1 in vivo. However, piercidin C_1 was clearly much less cytotoxic to a multicellular tumor mass (i.e. tumor slices) than to single cells. Similar results, namely lower cytotoxicity of drugs for a multicellular mass as compared to single cells, have also been reported for spheroids (11,12). Spheroids, by virtue of their multicellularity and the presence of hypoxic and drug resistant cells in their interior, are considered to be a representative model for solid tumors. Therefore, the use of tumor slices in this assay may result in a better correlation between _in vitro_ and _in vivo_ results.

Our experience indicated that preparation of tumor slices of uniform size was slow and not reproducible. Krumdieck et al. (13) have described a tissue slicer microtome (which is commercially available) that rapidly prepares slices of uniform thickness in a sterile environment.

Our results clearly show large quantitative differences in the sensitivity of L1210 or colon 38 to certain drugs. For example, piercidin C_1 is more than 100-fold more cytotoxic to colon 38 than L1210. It would be interesting to know if this difference will hold true for other solid tumors and leukemias.

Our studies raise an important question which still needs to be answered: What causes the difference in sensitivity to certain durgs between L1210 and colon 38 at the cellular level? For example, acivicin and piercidin C_1 are respectively 4-fold and 100-fold more cytotoxic to colon 38 than to L1210. In contrast, Adriamycin and U-73975 are 4-fold and 100-fold more cytotoxic to L1210 than colon 38. Could this difference be accounted for by differences in drug uptake by the 2 cell lines? Adriamycin and U-73975 both interact with DNA and cause DNA damage. Therefore, differences in the rate of DNA repair between the 2 cell lines could cause differential drug sensitivity. Since piercidin causes mitochondrial damage, the obvious question would be whether the drug causes more mitochondrial damage to colon 38 than L1210 cells (14).

The Upjohn Company Cancer Research Unit, (Drs. D.G. Martin and L.J. Hanka) collaborated with Dr. T. Corbett (Wayne State University) to screen fermentation broths and pure compounds (using the disk plate assay) from 1983 to 1988. This process did not yield any novel compounds with high antitumor activity _in vivo_. About 10,000 fermentation broths (mostly from streptomycetes fermentation) were screened of which 100 broths were differentially active _in vitro_. From these 100 broths, 13 compounds were isolated which can be classified as follows: (i) 8 known antitumor com-

pounds (ii) 3 known compounds with no activity _in vivo_ (e.g., piercidin C_1) (iii) 2 novel compounds with marginal or no activity
in vivo.

Six thousand synthetics were also screened of which 200 were
tested _in vivo_. Only 2 compounds, which were unrelated to previously identified antitumor agents, were found to have modest _in
vivo_ activity. (This analysis of our efforts with this screen was
obtained from Drs. J.P. McGovren and P.A. Aristoff.)

Overall, the yield of novel _in vivo_ active compounds from
this screening process was disappointingly low. The following modifications to the screen could improve its output: (a) Changing
the source of raw materials to be screened (marine or plant or
fastidious micro-organisms instead of steptomycetes) would increase the probability of discovering novel compounds. (b) Cells
from drug-insensitive human tumor xenografts could be used in
screening for new antitumor agents. (c) Finally, tumor slices used
as a secondary screen could improve the correlation between _in
vitro_ and _in vivo_ activity.

ACKNOWLEDGMENTS

We acknowledge the help of Dr. C. Hall in studying the
histology of colon 38 tumors and Mrs. C.A. Kiewiet in preparing
the manuscript.

REFERENCES

1. Corbett TH, Valeriote FA, Baker LH: Is the P388 murine tumor
    no longer adequate as a drug discovery model. Invest. New
    Drugs 5:3-20, 1987.
2. Staquet MJ, Byar DP, Green SB, Rozencweig M: Clinical pre-
    dictivity of transplantable tumor systems in the selection of
    new drugs for solid tumors. Rationale for a three-stage stra-
    tegy. Cancer Treat. Rep. 67:753-765, 1983.
3. Corbett TH, Valeriote FA: Rodent models in cancer chemo-
    therapy. In: Rodent Tumor Models in Experimental Cancer
    Chemotherapy. RE Kallman (ed), Pergamon Press.
4. Corbett TH: A selective soft-agar assay for drug discovery.
    Proc. AACR 25:325, 1984.
5. Smith KS, Badiner GJ, Li LH et al: Modified _in vitro_ two
    tumor assay for solid tumor selective drugs. Proc. AACR
    30:613, 1989.

6. Courtney VC, Mills J: An _in vitro_ colony assay for human tumors grown in immune-suppressed mice and treated _in vivo_ with cytotoxic agents. Brit. J. Cancer 37:261-268, 1978.
7. Adams EG, Crampton SL, Bhuyan BK: Effect of 7-con-O-methyl-nogarol on DNA synthesis, survival, and cell cycle progression of Chinese hamster ovary cells. Cancer Res. 42:4981-4987, 1981.
8. Kelly RC, Gebhard I, Wicnienski N et al: Coupling of cyclopropapyrroloindole (CPI) derivatives. The preparation of CC-1065, ent-CC-1065, and analogs. J. Am. Chem. Soc. 109:6837-6838, 1987.
9. Martin DG, Duchamp DJ, Chidester CC: The isolation, structure and absolute configuration of U-42126, a novel antibiotic. Tetrahedron Let. 27:2549-2552, 1973.
10. Yoshida S, Takahasi N: Piercidins: Naturally occurring inhibitors against mitochondrial respiration. Heterocycles 10:425-467, 1978.
11. Li LH, Bhuyan BK, Wallace TL: Comparison of cytotoxicity of a monolayer and spheroid system. Proc. AACR 30:612, 1989.
12. Durand RE: Chemosensitivity testing in V79 spheroids: Drug delivery and cellular microenvironment. JNCI 77:247, 1986.
13. Krumdieck CL, DosSantos JE, Ho K: A new instrument for the rapid preparation of tissue slices. Anal. Biochem. 104:118-123, 1988.
14. Horgan DJ, Ohno H, Singer TP: Studies on the respiratory chain-linked reduced nicotinamide adenine dinucleotide dehydrogenase. J. Biol Chem. 104:118-123, 1968.

22

5-FLUOROURACIL: SCHEDULE OPTIMIZATION IN METASTATIC COLORECTAL CANCER

Norwood R. Anderson and Jacob J. Lokich

INTRODUCTION

Initially synthesized as a pyrimidine antagonist over three decades ago, the fluorinated pyrimidine, 5-fluorouracil (FUra), has historically formed the foundation of virtually all chemotherapy combinations in the treatment of advanced digestive cancers. With the development of newer chemotherapeutic agents such as VP-16, cisplatin and its analogues, and to a lesser extent the anthracycline doxorubicin, FUra has been partially supplanted in the treatment of cancers of the upper digestive tract. It remains, however, the sole chemotherapeutic agent with reproducible clinical efficacy in the treatment of cancers of the lower digestive system, i.e. colon and rectum.

Recent technological advances in drug delivery systems have allowed an increasingly safe administration of this agent with resultant improved rates of tumor response seen in advanced colorectal cancer. These drug delivery improvements have permitted the development of new schedules of administration of FUra that have optimized its clinical effect in a variety of human tumors and in advanced colorectal cancer in particular. A brief review of the history of FUra administration followed by a discussion of the use of prolonged venous infusion (PVI) of FUra in colorectal cancer is, therefore, indicated to understand these technological advances and to translate them into more clinically effective treatment programs. Based on such understanding, it is possible to envision future innovations in the use of FUra administration that may further optimize the clinical efficacy of this agent in these common cancers.

Clinical Efficacy of FUra: Historic Review

The major cytotoxic effects of FUra are produced both through the incorporation of its cytotoxically active metabolites into the cancer cell ribonucleic acid and through inhibition of thymidine synthesis by the inactivation of the signally important enzyme thymidylate synthetase achieved by the FUra metabolite fluoro-deoxyuridine-5′-monophosphate (FdUMP). FUra incorporation directly into cellular deoxyribonucleic acid via other active metabolites may also play an important role in the observed anti-tumor effect of FUra. Recent clinical trials showing increased responsiveness with the addition of folinic acid (at a variety of dose levels) to FUra have stressed the major importance of the inhibition of thymidylate synthetase as the possible primary mode of action of FUra.

Soon after its synthesis by Heidelberger, et. al. in 1957 (1), FUra became the "standard" drug treatment for advanced colorectal cancer. Original dosing schedules involved high-dose, rapid intravenous administration of FUra either on a weekly basis or on a daily "loading schedule" titrated for toxicity. Because of lack of unanimity on the preferred schedule of delivery, Ansfield, et. al. studied 492 patients with advanced colo-rectal or breast cancers with four schedules of FUra in 1976 to determine the optimal use of FUra clinically (2). This randomized trial compared an intensive loading schedule (12 mg/Kg/day for five consecutive days followed by weekly maintenance) with two weekly schedules without initial intensive therapy and a weekly oral schedule. Analysis of response data in the 198 patients with colo-rectal cancer revealed a 33% response rate with the loading dose schedule and almost identical response rates of 13%, 14% and 13% for the other schedules, indicating a clear superiority for the loading schedule in terms of clinical response. Toxicity was primarily hematologic in all arms with neutropenia being dose limiting and significantly more common in the loading schedule than in the other study arms.

381

The Ansfield report became the basis of clinical practice and guideline for the clinical use of FUra with subsequent reports in the 1970's and 1980's indicating clinical response in the range of 15-20% for colo-rectal cancer (3-5). Recently, however, trials utilizing more rigorous definitions of response have suggested that 10% may be a more realistic response rate for single-agent bolus FUra. Erlichman, et. al. found a 7% response rate (4/61 patients) for a bolus loading schedule of FUra at a dose of 425 mg/M^2/day for five days monthly in a randomized trial of FUra and folinic acid versus FUra alone in advanced colo-rectal cancer (6). Similarly, the Nordic Gastrointestinal Tumor Adjuvant Therapy Group recently reported their evaluation of a randomized trial of sequential methotrexate plus FUra and leucovorin compared to singe-agent bolus FUra at a dose of 600 mg/M^2/day for two consecutive days every two weeks (7). An objectively measured response of 3% (3/91 patients) was observed for the bolus FUra group. The results of these two recent studies are summarized in table form along with five other recently reported trials comparing bolus FUra combined with either leucovorin or methotrexate (TABLE 1). Taken collectively, these well conducted, randomized, multi-institutional trials indicate a response rate of between 3-17% for bolus FUra alone with most of the studies reporting responses considerably under 10% (8-12).

Although there is great variety in the dose of FUra employed in current trials - as seen by an analysis of Table 1 - most contemporary studies utilize an "intensive" schedule of five successive days of treatment repeated monthly instead of schedules utilizing weekly bolus administration. Despite this relatively dose-intensive schedule of FUra administration - recently reviewed by Arbuck (13) - response rates remain discouragingly low when FUra is employed as a single agent and given by bolus delivery. Despite these disappointing results utilizing FUra on a bolus schedule, this schedule of administration remains the mainstay of therapy for advanced colo-rectal cancer today. Newer technologies allowing for improved drug delivery along with new drug development in the 1980's however, have resulted in the introduction of

Table 1

Clinical Efficacy of Bolus FUra in Advanced Colorectal Cancer

INSTITUTION	AUTHOR [REFERENCE]	FUra DOSE	NO. PTS.	RESPONSE CR	PR	%	MEDIAN SURVIVAL (MOS.)	% ALIVE: 1 YR[c]	2 YR[c]
PRINCESS MARGARET HOSPITAL	ERLICHMAN [5]	370 mg/M^2/DAY x EVERY 28 DAYS	61	0	4	7	9.6	25	15
NORDIC G.I. ADJUVANT TUMOR TREATMENT GROUP	[6]	600 mg/M^2/DAY x 2 EVERY 14 DAYS	91	0	3	3	6.0[b]	20	5
MAYO CLINIC; NORTH CENTRAL CANCER TREATMENT GROUP	O'CONNELL [8]	500 mg/M^2/DAY x 5 EVERY 28 DAYS	39	0	4	10	8.0	35	10
ROSWELL PARK	PETRELLI [9]	450 mg/M^2/DAY x THEN 200 mg/M^2/DAY EVERY 2 DAYS x 6 EVERY 28 DAYS	22	0	2	9	11.0[b]	40	15
ROSWELL PARK	PETRELLI [14]	500 mg/M^2/DAY x 5 EVERY 28 DAYS	107	0	13	12	11.5[b]	45	15
NORTHERN CALIFORNIA ONCOLOGY GROUP	VALONE [11]	12 mg/Kg/DAY x 5 THEN 15 mg/Kg/WEEK	52	4	5	17	11.5	45	15
CITY OF HOPE	DOROSHOW [12]	370 mg/M^2/DAY x EVERY	0	5	13	13.0	55	10	

[a]ACTUARIAL SURVIVAL
[b]ESTIMATED PROBABILITY OF SURVIVAL
[c]CALCULATED FROM SURVIVAL CURVES

more innovative therapeutic modalities with the possibility of greater clinical effect.

Technology of Prolonged Venous Infusion (PVI)

Spurred by the development of hyperalimentation technology, continuous ambulatory infusion of chemotherapeutic agents became logistically feasible in the latter half of the 1970's. The two major advances permitting the clinical investigation of PVI were the development and production of reliable venous access options and ambulatory infusion pumps. A detailed discussion of the various devices and infusion pumps now available is outside the scope of this review. It is sufficient, however, to state that virtually any style of ambulatory infusion pump (i.e. high flow rate, low flow rate, high volume reserve, low volume reserve, multivariate programmable, chronoprogrammable, etc.) is commercially available to be utilized with an effective venous access system, thereby, making PVI a logistical and clinical possibility.

With advances in the technology of venous access devices along with increased surgical experience, initial concerns regarding the risks of infection and venous thrombosis of the surgically implanted devices have diminished considerably. In a relative early report reviewing the complications of implanted venous access catheters appearing in 1985, Lokich and Bothe, et. al., reported a 9% (8/92 catheters) incidence of infection with only 2/8 patients developing septicemia from the implanted devices (14). A recent review of The Cancer Center experience has revealed seventeen cases of access-related infection in 600 patients with only seven cases (1.2%) of documented sepsis (15). While venous thrombosis incited by the presence of the venous access device remains the major potential morbidity of the surgically implanted ports, occurring in 16-30% of patients, Bern, et. al., recently reported a statistically significant decrease in the incidence of local thrombosis with the prophylactic use of very low dose warfarin at 1 mg/day (16). Such studies clearly indicate that with increasing use and experience, the implanted access ports are becoming more reliable and safer indicating that they can be recommended for routine use in clinical practice. Such safety and reliability, therefore, permit a more detailed evaluation of the clinical utility and efficacy of PVI for the treatment of advanced colo-rectal carcinoma.

Pharmacologic Rationale for Infusional FUra

The theory underlying the clinical use of PVI for chemotherapeutic agents is founded primarily on three scientific principles: (1) the <u>pharmacokinetics</u> of antineoplastic agents; (2) the <u>cytokinetic</u> profile of any individual agent in any given malignancy; and (3) the demonstration of <u>schedule dependency</u> for drug delivery. In contrast, conventional bolus chemotherapy, although taking pharmacokinetics, cytokinetics and schedule dependency profile of chemotherapeutic agents into account, is primarily based on the demonstration of <u>dose-related response</u> as seen in many clinical and pre-clinical trials.

In general, most antineoplastic agents effect only that portion of the malignant cell pool of any given tumor that is actively "in cycle" and dividing at the time of drug exposure. In most situations a cytokinetic analysis of the majority of cells in a given tumor at any one instance shows these cells to be in the "quiescent" portion of their cell cycles (G_0) making them at least relatively immune to the cytotoxic effect of even the highest concentration of chemotherapeutic agent. PVI, at least theoretically, provides a potential mechanism of overcoming this resistance by providing prolonged, continuous, relatively low-dose exposure of drug, thereby, allowing exposure of a greater percentage of actively dividing (and thereby potentially "chemo-sensitive") cancer cells to the cytotoxic potential of any individual agent.

The second major rationale for PVI is based on the recognition of the pharmacokinetic profile of individual chemotherapeutic agents. Most of the commonly employed antineoplastic agents have relatively short plasma half-lives varying from a few minutes to a few hours depending on individual drug variations such as liver extraction, physiological excretion and protein binding. At best, however, only a small portion of administering bolus chemotherapy

is actually delivered to the cancer cell with only a fraction of
the total cell mass of any individual tumor being susceptible to
the effect of that drug during its exposure. PVI provides a theoretic basis for overcoming this metabolic obstacle by providing
continuous drug exposure resulting in prolonged measurable concentrations of active antineoplastic agents in the plasma, thereby
providing continual drug exposure for hours, days or even weeks at
a time.

Similarly, the more schedule-dependent and cycle-specific any
given chemotherapeutic agent, the more the theoretic rationale for
the use of that agent in an infusional schedule. Providing more
prolonged drug exposure of a cell-specific agent will theoretically result in the exposure of more malignant cells to the cytotoxic potential of the administered agent as progressively more
cells "cycle" into the phase during which the drug is specifically
active.

In many respects, the antimetabolites in general and FUra in
particular, represent the prototypical chemotherapeutic agents to
include in an infusional schedule. The major cytotoxic effect of
FUra occurs during S-phase of the cell cycle with a demonstrated
mean plasma half-life of approximately eleven minutes after bolus
administration (17). Therefore, only a small percentage of tumor
cells are theoretically susceptible to the antimetabolite effect
of a single bolus of FUra. In addition to this cell-cycle specificity, FUra exhibits considerable schedule dependency as seen by
data indicating that longer duration of exposure to FUra results
in significantly increased cellular toxicity as measured in total
cell kill (18,19). By utilizing PVI of FUra, more tumor cells
are, therefore, exposed to its toxic metabolites as they pass
through S-phase in their individual cell cycles.

<u>Infusional FUra: Clinical Experience</u>

Seifert and Baker, et. al. (20), were the first investigators
to test the efficacy of a continuously administered infusion of
FUra. They randomized 68 patients with advanced carcinoma of the
colon or the rectum to receive either bolus FUra at a dose of 12

mg/Kg/day for five successive days (36 patients) or a 120-hour infusion of FUra at a dose of 30 mg/Kg/day (32 patients). The results of this seminal study were reported in 1975 and are tabula-
ted in Table 2. The patients were age and sex matched in each

Table 2

Bolus Versus Prolonged Infusion of
Fluorouracil for Colo-Rectal Carcinoma

Treatment	No. Pts.	Response			Median Survival[a] (Mos.)	% Alive[b]	
		CR	PR	%		1 Yr.	2 Yr.
Bolus-12 mg/Kg/day x 5 every 28 days	36	0	8	22	2	15	N/A
Infusion-30 mg/Kg/day x 5 every 28 days	34	1	14	44	8	20	N/A

[a]Actuarial survival
[b]Calculated from survival curves

N/A = Not Available

Seifert, P., et al. Cancer 36:123-128, 1975.

group and had similar distribution and extent of tumor for response measurements. Twenty-two percent of bolus-treated patients
(8/36) evidenced objective regression of tumor while 44% of (15/
34) of the PVI-treated patients showed demonstrable response. Despite this difference in response rates, the over-all survival for
both groups was similar at 5.5-6 months, although a more detailed
analysis revealed that more of the PVI-treated patients survived
longer when compared to the bolus-treated patients.

The more important discovery of Seifert's study, however, was
the uncovering of very different patterns of toxicity for the bolus and the PVI-treatment arms. Similar to previous reports, they
found that hematologic toxicity in the form of neutropenia was the
dose-limiting toxicity for the bolus schedule with two toxic

387

deaths (6%) attributed to neutropenia and related sepsis. In the
PVI-group, however, myelotoxicity was uncommon and never associated with leukopenia <2000 cells/mm^3. Mucocutaneous toxicity with
stomatitis and cutaneous eruption was dose-limiting in the PVI-
treated group. Seifert concluded that the use of FUra as a PVI
over five days resulted in greater response rates with increased
clinical safety as compared to bolus FUra, resulting in the elimination of the major toxic effect of bolus administration - namely
neutropenia and the risk of related sepsis.

Since the original Seifert report describing the Wayne State
experience, there have been many contemporary Phase I and Phase II
trials of various infusional schedules of FUra as a single-agent.
There have also been two randomized Phase III prospective trials
of PVI-FUra reported within the last two years. Before detailing
recent results utilizing prolonged venous infusion (duration of
infusion greater than five days), we will briefly summarize some
of the reports dealing with shorter infusional schedules and then
comment on the concept of dose intensity as it relates to FUra
administration by infusional schedule.

Shorter Duration (24-48 hours) and Intermediate Duration (5 days)
Infusions

Basing their study on a previous Phase I report of Hill, Ansfield, et. al. (21), indicating that a 48-hour infusion of FUra at
fourteen day intervals was technically feasible and associated
with acceptable toxicity, Shah, et. al. (22), treated 94 patients
in a non-randomized fashion with three different dose schedules of
short-term infusional FUra: 72-hour infusion (30/mg/Kg/day) every
21 days; 72-hour infusion (30/mg/Kg/day) every 14 days; 48-hour
infusion (30 mg/Kg/day) every seven days. The optimal treatment
for response and survival was the 48-hour infusion at weekly intervals with a response rate of 30% and median survival of 14
months compared to response rates of 9% and 16% and median survival of 9 and 9.5 months for the other dose schedules. As in
Seifert's trial, the major toxicity for these infusional schedules
was mucocutaneous with no hematologic toxicity observed.

388

Hum and Bateman (23) and Hartman, et. al (24), extended the
duration of infusion to 120 hours for patients previously treated
with bolus FUra. Hum reported no effectiveness for the PVI route
in these bolus-refractory patients while Hartman reported a 10%
response rate in this difficult group of patients. Hartman recommended the consideration of the use of PVI in these bolus-refractory patients because of its lack of toxicity and clinical efficacy approaching bolus FUra in chemotherapy-naive patients.

<u>Intermediate Duration Infusion (5 days) with Cisplatin</u>

Based on her initial Phase II trial of the combination of
5-day infusion of FUra plus weekly bolus cisplatin (CP) in patients with advanced, measurable colo-rectal cancer (25), Kemeny,
et. al. performed a randomized Phase III prospective trial of
infusional FUra (1000 mg/M^2/day for five days every four weeks)
with or without CP (20 mg/M^2/day for five days every four weeks)
(26) (Table 3). One hundred twenty-two previously untreated patients were randomized with 63 receiving FUra plus CP and 61 re-

Table 3

Randomized Study of Continuous Infusion Fluorouracil (FUra)
Versus Fluorouracil Plus Cisplatin (CP) in Patients
with Metastatic Colorectal Cancer

Treatment	No. Pts.	CR	Response PR	%	Median Survival (Mos.)	% Alive 1 Yr. 2 Yr.
FUra-1000 mg/M^2/day x every 28 days CP -20 mg/M^2/day x every 28 days	61	0	15	25	10	Not Stated
FUra-1000 mg/M^2/day x every 28 days	59	0	2	3	12	Not Stated

Kemeny, N., et al. J. Clin. Onc. 8:313-318, 1990.

ceiving FUra alone. Age, sex and site of disease distribution were equally matched in each treatment group. Toxicity was significantly greater in the FUra + CP group with considerably more nausea and vomiting as well as twelve instances of World Health Organization grade 3/4 hematologic toxicity (neutropenia) as compared to no instances of hematologic toxicity in the FUra only group. Fifteen of sixty-one (25%) evaluable patients treated with FUra plus CP demonstrated partial response as compared to 2/59 (3%) for the FUra only treatment group. Despite these benefits in response, the FUra plus CP group did not show any increase in either duration of response (median 6 months and 4.7 months for the FUra plus CP and FUra only groups respectively) or in total survival (median, 10 months and 12 months respectively).

<u>Prolonged Duration Infusion (more than 5 days)</u>

With the development of safe venous access devices and the availability of ambulatory drug delivery pumps, Lokich, et al., performed the first Phase I study of PVI-FUra administration in 1981 (27). Seventeen patients with various advanced stage cancers received 19 courses of FUra at doses ranging from 200 mg/M^2/day to 600 mg/M^2/day with interruption of the infusion dictated by the development of stomatitis. At dose rates of 300 mg/M^2/day, the length of the PVI was reduced to less than ten days. As previously observed by Seifert, this study found no myelosuppression with any of the doses employed. Lokich concluded that a safe starting dose for further PVI investigation of FUra was 300 mg/M^2/day recommending further trials to determine the clinical efficacy of infusional FUra.

Combining Lokich's Phase I results with the 1975 report of Seifert indicating the potential of improved response rates and greater therapeutic index of PVI-FUra, various Phase II trials utilizing PVI-FUra have been reported in the last five years. These six clinical studies, reported in primarily abstract form (28-33), are summarized in Table 4. Collectively, they represent treatment results on 284 previously untreated patients with advanced measurable colo-rectal cancer. While many criticisms of

Table 4

Single-Arm Phase II Trials of Constant Infusion
5-Fluorouracil in Metastatic Colorectal Cancer:
A Compendium of Results

Author (Reference)	Patients Treated	Patients Responding	Toxicity
Leichman (28)	16	5 (31%)	Mucocutaneous
Belt (29)	26	10 (39%)	Stomatitis Hand-Foot
Molina (30)	25	11 (44%)	Hand-Foot
Wade (31)	100	53 (53%)	Mucocutaneous Hand-Foot
Hansen (32)	91	30 (33%)	Hand-Foot Mucocutaneous
Kuo (33)	26	11 (42%)	Mucocutaneous Hand-Foot
TOTALS	284	120 (42%)	

these trials may be raised - they were all single-institution,
non-randomized, non-controlled studies employing varying response
criteria - taken together they certainly give additional insight
into the PVI use of FUra. Clinical response rates reported in
these trials between 31%-53% are considerably greater than for any
reported bolus FUra treatment and toxicity data universally indicate substantially decreased toxicity compared to bolus FUra.
This toxicity advantage is seen most clearly in the total absence
of neutropenia and neutropenia-associated sepsis, thereby producing a therapeutic option with a significantly increased therapeutic index. Despite these major advantages, however, no improvement in survival of PVI-FUra as compared to bolus FUra was noted
in any of these single-institution Phase II studies.

In 1989, the Mid-Atlantic Oncology Program (MAOP) completed
the first prospective Phase III randomized trial in advanced measurable colo-rectal cancer comparing the efficacy of bolus FUra
versus PVI-FUra. In this study, 174 patients were randomly assign-

ed to receive either a bolus loading schedule of FUra at 500 mg/M^2/day times five every five weeks versus a PVI dose of 300 mg/M^2/day for 70 consecutive days. The bolus dose of 500 mg/M^2/day was chosen to maximize the possibility of response to the bolus administration schedule while the 300 mg/M^2/day dose for the PVI was selected based on Lokich's original Phase I study. No patient had received prior chemotherapy and all had measurable disease. Utilizing stringent response criteria requiring indepen-dent confirmation by x-ray or scan documented response, the tumor response for the bolus group was 7% (6/87 patients) and for the PVI group 30% (26/87 patients) - a statistically significant dif-ference (Table 5).

Table 5

A Prospective Randomized Comparison of Continuous
Infusional 5-Fluorouracil with a Conventional
Bolus Schedule in Metastatic Colorectal Cancer

	TREATMENT ARM	
	Infusional FUra	Bolus FUra
Total No. Patients:	87	87
Median Patient Age:	54.6	61.1
Sex (Male/Female):	44/43	44/43
Site of Indicator Lesion:		
Liver	55 (63%)	57 (66%)
Peritoneum	9 (10%)	8 (9%)
Lung	15 (17%)	18 (21%)
Other	8 (9%)	4 (5%)
No Previous Chemotherapy	87	87
Performance Status 0/1:	78 (90%)	81 (93%)
Response:		
Partial Response	22 (25%)	6 (7%)
Complete Response	4 (5%)	0
Total Response	26 (30%)	6 (7%)
Drug Related Deaths:	0	4 (5%)
Median Survival (Months):	10	11

Lokich, J., et al. J. Clin. Onc. 7:425-432, 1989.

In addition to showing a marked difference in response rate for the two groups, the study further demonstrated a significant difference in toxicity in the two groups, (Table 6). In the bolus treatment group, 14% developed severe neutropenia (white blood

Table 6

A Prospective Randomized Comparison of Continuous
Infusional 5-Fluorouracil with a Conventional
Bolus Schedule in Metastatic Colorectal Cancer
Comparative Pattern of Toxicity for
Infusional FUra Versus Bolus FUra

Toxicity	Grade	Infusional FUra	Bolus FUra
Leukopenia	2 ($<3,000/MM^3$)	0	16 (21%)
	3 ($<2,000/MM^3$)	1 (1%)	11 (14%)
	4 ($<1,000/MM^3$)	0	6 (8%)
Thrombocytopenia	2 ($<90,000/MM^3$)	3 (4%)	4 (5%)
	3 ($<50,000/MM^3$)	1 (1%)	2 (3%)
	4 ($<25,000/MM^3$)	0	1 (1%)
Stomatitis	2 (Treatment Needed)	17 (20%)	15 (19%)
	3 (Unable to Eat)	3 (4%)	9 (12%)
	4 (Hospitalization)	0	1 (1%)
Dermatitis		0	3 (4%)
Hand-Foot Syndrome		20 (24%)	0
Drug-Related Death		0	4 (5%)

Lokich, J., et al. J. Clin. Onc. 7:425-432, 1989.

count between 1000-2000/mm^3) with 8% developing life-threatening neutropenia (white blood count less than 1000/mm^3). Four pat- ients (5%) in the bolus arm died from sepsis during the neutro- penic phase of their treatment. Only one patient in the PVI arm developed severe neutropenia and no life-threatening toxicity was observed. Thrombocytopenia was considerably less common than neu- tropenia in both groups, although more likely to occur in the bo- lus arm than the PVI arm.

A second common toxicity of FUra, stomatitis, occurred infrequently in both groups and dermatitis was an insignificant problem in either group. The most common toxicity seen in the PVI arm was the development of palmar-plantar erythro-dysesthesia ("hand-foot syndrome"), previously described by Lokich and Moore (35) and frequently cited in many of the previously reported Phase II trials. This reversible syndrome, characterized by painful swelling and erythroderma of the soles of the feet, palms of the hands and distal fingers, occurred in 24% (20/87) of the PVI-treated patients and was never life-threatening although it did cause dose attenuation or a period of withdrawal of therapy to allow spontaneous resolution of symptoms. Despite these impressive differences in toxicity and response highly favoring the PVI group, survival was similar in the two groups with a median survival of 10 months for the PVI-group and 11 months for the bolus group. There was, however, a non-statistically significant trend toward an advantage in the "tail" of the survival curve for the PVI group.

Based on this study the MAOP subsequently undertook a second randomized trial in advanced measurable colorectal cancer, this time prospectively comparing treatment with PVI-FUra (300 mg/M^2/ day for 70 days) versus the same dose of FUra plus weekly bolus cisplatin (20 mg/M^2/week) (36). One hundred eighty-four patients were randomized for treatment with 90 receiving PVI-FUra alone and 94 receiving PVI-FUra plus cisplatin therapy. All patients had measurable advanced metastatic disease and none had received prior chemotherapy. A total of 179 patients were eligible for analysis for survival and toxicity and 168 were evaluable for tumor response. The two groups were matched equally for age, sex, and site of disease, extent of disease and performance status. Response rates were similar in the two groups with 33% (28/85) responders in the cisplatin/FUra arm and 35% (29/83) in the FUra-only arm. Median survival for the cisplatin/FUra group was 11.8 months and an identical 11.2 months for the FUra-only group. Toxicity was similar to that reported in the previous MAOP trial with the exception of the anticipated increased gastrointestinal toxicity in the cisplatin-treated patients.

When combined with the results of the initial MAOP trial, this study provides considerable information relative to PVI-FUra versus bolus FUra in the treatment of metastatic colorectal cancer (Table 7). Two hundred fifty-five patients are evaluable for re-

Table 7

Compendium of Results of Two Randomized Infusional Versus Bolus 5-Fluorouracil Trials in Metastatic Colorectal Cancer

Treatment	No. Pts.	Response CR	PR	%	Median Survival (Mos.)	% Alive 1 Yr.	2 Yr.
FUra-500 mg/M^2/day x 5 then every 28 days	85	0	6	7	11	44	11
FUra-300 mg/M^2/day Infusion x 70 days	87	4	22	30	10	44	17
FUra-300 mg/M^2/day Infusion x 70 days PLUS Cisplatin-20 mg/M^2/wk	85	2	26	33	11.8	48	13
FUra-300 mg/M^2/day Infusion	83	2	27	35	11.2	52	16

sponse and survival in the PVI-FUra arms of these two prospectively randomized trials with a combined total of 83/255 (32.5%) patients responding compared to the 7% (6/85) seen in the bolus group. In addition, complete responses were observed in all three PVI-FUra arms with a combined total of 8/255 (3%) complete responders. Neither study, however, revealed survival advantage for PVI over bolus FUra although toxicity was markedly reduced and no drug-related deaths were seen in any of the 255 PVI-treated patients.

At least three randomized clinical trials are currently on-going to test the MAOP conclusions about PVI-FUra and to attempt biochemical modulation of FUra. MAOP itself is currently enrolling patients in a randomized trial of PVI-FUra alone versus PVI-FUra plus weekly bolus N-phosphonoacetyl-L-aspartate (PALA) with approximately 70 patients having been enrolled thus far. A preliminary data analysis will be forthcoming when accrual reaches 80 patients. The Eastern Co-Operative Oncology Group (ECOG) likewise is currently randomizing patients to a four arm study comparing bolus FUra to bolus FUra plus cisplatin, PVI-FUra and PVI-FUra plus cisplatin. Caudry and Maire in Bordeaux have entered 54 patients thus far in a randomized trial comparing bolus FUra plus folinic acid to PVI-FUra alone to PVI-FUra plus mitomycin-C plus cyclophosphamide (37). Preliminary analysis of their data does not indicate any clear superiority of one of the programs over another. Collectively, these trials, which should be published within the next two years, should further clarify the role of PVI-FUra in treatment of metastatic colorectal cancer.

Dose Intensity and Response Analysis for FUra

Recently, Hryniuk, et. al. (38), and Young (39) have stressed the importance of dose-intensity of administered chemotherapy as a potential major determinant of the cytotoxicity of any chemotherapeutic agent or combination of agents. An analysis of Erlichman's trial utilizing the commonly employed "intensive" bolus administration of 425 mg/M^2/day FUra for five successive days repeated every 28 days (6), the Nordic Gastrointestinal Tumor Adjuvant Treatment Group bolus regimen of 600 mg/M^2/day times two days twice monthly (7), and the Memorial Sloan-Kettering Cancer Center study of 1000 mg/M^2/day PVI-FUra for five days every four weeks (25), compared to the original MAOP trial of 300 mg/M^2/day PVI-FUra for 70 consecutive days (34) with respect to dose intensity reveals considerable differences in the actual dose intensity of the four trials. Such differences may, in fact, have significant bearing on the disparate responses seen in these well conducted prospectively randomized trials (Table 8). All four studies

Table 8

Dose-Intensity Analysis of 5-Fluorouracil
Administration in Relation to Response

| | Author (Reference) | | | |
| | Erlichman (6) | Nordic (7) | Kemeny (26) | Lokich (34) |
Schedule:	Bolus	Bolus	Infusion	Infusion
FUra Dose:	425 Mg/M^2/dx5	600 MG/M^2/dx2	1 GM/M^2/dx5	300 MG/M^2/dx70
Cycle:	Every 28/d	Every 14/d	Every 28/d	Daily x 70/d
Dose Intensity: (Gg. FUra/Week)	0.53	0.60	1.25	2.1
Number Patients:	61	91	59	89
Primary Metastatic Site:				
Liver	46 (75%)	54 (59%)	37 (66%)	59 (68%)
Lung	6	31	10	18
Other	9	6	12	12
Response Rates				
Complete	0	0	0	4
Partial	4	3	2	22
Total	4 (7%)	3 (3%)	2 (3%)	26 (30%)
Median Survival: (Months)	9.6	6	12	10.3
Drug-Related Death:	0	0	1	0

evidenced similar demographic data but there is a considerably
higher response rate in the PVI-FUra group of the MAOP trial with
26/89 (30%) responders compared to 7% (4/61), 3% (3/91), and 3%
(2/59) in the Erlichman, Nordic, and Memorial trials respectively. Analyzed for dose-intensity, the MAOP trial provides a dose
intensity of 2.1 gm/M^2/week of FUra compared to 1.25 gm/M^2/week
in the 120-hour infusion reported by Kemeny, and 0.53 gm/M^2/week
in Erlichman's bolus group and 0.6 gm/M^2/week in the Nordic
trial. This translates into 68% greater dose intensity exposure
utilizing PVI-FUra compared to the five-day infusion, 290% greater

compared to Erlichman's bolus data, and 250% greater compared to the Nordic group bolus schedule. Such a significant dose intensity difference may partially explain the higher response observed in the MAOP trial. These data, finally, indicate the clinical importance of both an optimal dose and optimal duration of treatment with PVI-FUra in order to obtain the dose intensity of treatment which is the pre-requisite for tumor cell kill.

Summary of PVI Trials

These data indicate that PVI-FUra is currently technologically feasible utilizing available venous access devices and ambulatory infusion pumps. Results of Phase II and randomized Phase III trials indicate a clear superiority of PVI-FUra over bolus FUra both in terms of percent responders and in therapeutic index with considerably enhanced safety of administered PVI-FUra. A total of 539 patients have been analyzed in these six Phase II and two Phase III trials, thereby minimizing any statistical bias and lending considerable statistical credibility to the observed results. This increased response rate - achieved at significantly reduced toxicity - argues forcefully for the continuation of clinical trials comparing infusional and bolus FUra plus biochemical modulators (i.e. leucovorin) to assess the clinical efficacy of infusional drug delivery. Quality of life analyses and expense analyses comparing infusional to bolus FUra should also be conducted to assess over-all feasibility and practicality of the infusional schedule.

Despite this definite improvement in response rates, however, there is still no study of PVI-FUra that indicates a clear-cut survival advantage for the infusional schedule. This should not be surprising since response rates have consistently been significantly less than 50% in this setting, making such a survival advantage unlikely. Further advances and new directions are, therefore, indicated utilizing both bolus and infusional FUra as comparative treatment foundations in efforts to improve clinical responsiveness until it impacts significantly on survival in colorectal cancer.

<u>New Directions in FUra Therapy</u>

Recently many reports dealing with the biochemical modulation and immunological modulation of FUra have appeared in the literature utilizing a wide variety of modulating agents. While these reports have generally used bolus FUra as the schedule against which response is measured, some trials have utilized a PVI schedule for FUra. The awareness of the importance of daily circadian rhythms and their influence on the biologic behavior of cancer cells as well as non-cancerous cells, has likewise led to heightened interest in the use of chronobiologically programmed infusion systems of FUra. Such innovative additions to single-agent bolus or infusional FUra are required to improve further its clinical spectrum of activity while striving to maintain the improved therapeutic index realized with the infusional schedule of administration.

Current trials utilizing both schedules of FUra in combination with known biochemical modulators [folinic acid, N-phosphono-acetyl-L-aspartic acid (PALA), hydroxyurea, and methylmercapto-purine riboside (MMPR)] or immunologic modulators (interferon or tumor necrosis factor) as well as the use of innovative circadian-rhythm-driven infusion systems and double biochemical modulation are currently on-going in this regard. Such studies should strive to maintain the maximum dose intensity of FUra since the FUra represents the active cytotoxic agent in these combinations and its dose should not be reduced below an optimal level in order to maximize the clinical effectiveness seen with this classical chemotherapeutic agent.

REFERENCES

1. Heidelberger C, Chaudhari NK, Danneberg P et al: The fluorinated pyrimidines: A new class of tumor-inhibitory compounds. Nature 179:663-666, 1957.
2. Ansfield F, Koltz J, Nealon T et al: A phase III study comparing the clinical utility of four regimens of 5-fluorouracil. Cancer 39:34-40, 1977.
3. Douglass HOJ, Lavin PT, Woll J et al: Chemotherapy of advanced measurable colon and rectal carcinoma with oral 5-fluorouracil, alone or in combination with cyclophosphamide

or 6-thioguanine, with intravenous 5-fluorouracil or beta-2'
-deoxythioguanosine or with oral 3(4-methyl-cyclohexyl)-1-
(2-chloroethyl)-1-nitrosourea: A Phase 2-3 study of the
Eastern Co-operative Oncology Group. Cancer 42:2538-2545,
1978.

4. Presant CA, Denes AE, Liu C, Bartolucci AA: Prospective
randomized reappraisal of 5-fluorouracil in metastatic
colorectal carcinoma. A comparative trial with 6-thiogua-
nine. Cancer 53:2610-2614, 1984.

5. Windshitl H, Scott M, Schutt A et al: Randomized Phase 2
studies in advanced colorectal carcinoma: A North Central
Cancer Treatment Group Study. Cancer Treat. Rep. 67:1001-
1008, 1983.

6. Ehrlichman C, Fine S, Wong A, Elhakim T: Randomized trial of
fluorouracil and folinic acid in patients with metastatic
colorectal carcinoma. J. Clin. Onc. 6:469-475, 1988.

7. Nordic Gastrointestinal Tumor Adjuvant Treatment Group.
Superiority of sequential methotrexate, fluorouracil and
leucovorin to fluorouracil alone in advanced symptomatic
colorectal carcinoma: A randomized trial. J. Clin. Onc.
7:1437-1446, 1989.

8. O'Connell MJ: A phase III trial of 5-fluorouracil and leucovorin in the treatment of advanced colorectal cancer.
Cancer 63:1026-1030, 1989.

9. Petrelli N, Herrera L, Rustum Y et al: A prospective randomized trial of 5-fluorouracil versus 5-fluorouracil and
high-dose leucovorin versus 5-fluorouracil and methotrexate
in previously untreated patients with advanced colorectal
carcinoma. J. Clin. Onc. 5:1559-1565, 1987.

10. Petrelli N, Douglass HOJ, Herrera L et al: The modulation of
5-fluorouracil with leucovorin in metastatic colorectal carcinoma: A prospective randomized trial. J. Clin. Onc.
7:1419-1426, 1988.

11. Valone FH, Friedman MA, Wittinger PS et al: Treatment of
patients with advanced colorectal carcinoma with fluorouracil
alone, high-dose leucovorin plus fluorouracil, or sequential
methotrexate, fluorouracil, and leucovorin: A randomized
trial of the Northern California Oncology Group. J. Clin.
Onc. 7:1427-1436, 1989.

12. Doroshow JH, Multhauf P, Leong L et al: Prospective randomized comparison of fluorouracil versus fluorouracil plus
high-dose continuous infusion leucovorin calcium for the
treatment of advanced measurable colorectal cancer in patients previously unexposed to chemotherapy. J. Clin. Onc.
8:491-501, 1990.

13. Arbuck SG: Overview of clinical trials using 5-fluorouracil
and leucovorin for treatment of colorectal cancer. Cancer
63:1036-1044, 1989.

14. Lokich J, Bothe A, Benotti P, Moore C: Complications and
management of implanted venous access catheters. J. Clin.
Onc. 3:710-717, 1985.

15. Moore C. Personal communication.

16. Bern M, Lokich J, Wallach S et al: Very low doses of warfarin can prevent thrombosis in central venous catheters. Ann. Int. Med. 112:423-428, 1990.

17. MacMillan WE, Wolberg WH, Welling PG: Pharmacokinetics of 5-fluorouracil in humans. Cancer Res. 38:3479-3482, 1978.

18. Calabro-Jones PM, Byfield JE, Ward JF, Sharp TR: Time-dose relationships for 5-fluorouracil cytotoxicity against human epithelial cancer cells in vitro. Cancer Res. 42:4413-4420, 1982.

19. Drewinko B, Yang LY: Cellular basis for the inefficacy of 5-fluorouracil in human colon carcinoma. Cancer Treat. Rep. 69:1391-1398, 1985.

20. Seifert P, Baker LH, Reed ML, Vaitkevicius VK: Comparison of continuously infused 5-fluorouracil with bolus injection in treatment of patients with colorectal adenocarcinoma. Cancer 36:123-128, 1975.

21. Hill JG II, Grage TB, Wilson W, Ansfield FJ: 5-Fluorouracil intravenous infusion for 48 hours repeated every two weeks. J. Surg. Onc. 23:60-70, 1972.

22. Shah A, MacDonald W, Goldie J et al: A comparison of three dose schedules. Cancer Treat. Rep. 69:739-742, 1985.

23. Hum GJ, Bateman JR: Five-day infusion with 5-fluorouracil (5-FU; NSC-19893) for gastroenteric carcinoma after failure on weekly 5-FU therapy. Cancer Chemo. Rep. 59:1177-1179, 1975.

24. Hartman HA, Kessinger A, Lemon HM, Foley JF: Five-day continuous infusion of 5-fluorouracil for advanced colorectal, gastric, and pancreatic adenocarcinoma. J. Surg. Onc. 1:227-238, 1979.

25. Kemeny N, Niedzwiecki D, Reichman B et al: Cisplatin and 5-fluorouracil infusion for metastatic colorectal carcinoma. Cancer 63:1065-1069, 1989.

26. Kemeny N, Israel K, Niedzwiecki D: Randomized study of continuous infusion fluorouracil versus fluorouracil plus cisplatin in patients with metastatic colorectal cancer. J. Clin. Onc. 8:313-318, 1990.

27. Lokich J, Bothe A, Fine N, Perri J: Phase I study of protracted venous infusion of 5-fluorouracil. Cancer 48:2565-2568, 1981.

28. Leichman L, Leichman CG, Kinzie J et al: Long term low dose 5-fluorouracil in advanced measurable colon cancer: No correlation between toxicity and efficacy. Proc. Am. Soc. Clin. Onc. 4:86, 1985 (abstract).

29. Belt RJ, Davidven ML, Myron MC, Barrett S: Continuous low-dose 5-fluorouracil for adenocarcinoma: Confirmation of activity. Proc. Am. Soc. Clin. Onc. 4:90, 1985 (abstract).

30. Molina R, Fabian C, Slavik M, Dahlberg S: Reversal of palmar-plantar erythrodysesthesia by B6 without loss of response in colon cancer patients receiving 200 mg/M^2/day continuous infusion 5-FU. Proc. Am. Soc. Clin. Onc. 6:74, 1987 (abstract).

31. Wade JL, Herbst S, Greenberg A: Prolonged venous infusion of 5-fluorouracil for metastatic colon cancer: A Follow-up Report. Proc. Am. Soc. Clin. Onc. 7:94, 1988 (abstract).

32. Hansen R, Quebbeman D, Ausman R et al: Continuous systemic
    5-fluorouracil infusion in advanced colorectal cancer:
    Results in 91 patients. J. Surg. Onc. 40:177-181, 1989.
33. Kuo S, Finck S, Cho J et al: Continuous ambulatory infus-
    ional 5-fluorouracil chemotherapy in advanced colorectal
    cancer: A single institutional retrospective study. Proc.
    Am. Soc. Clin. Onc. 8:126, 1989 (abstract).
34. Lokich J, Ahlgren J, Gullo J et al: A prospective randomized
    comparison of continuous infusion fluorouracil with a conven-
    tional bolus schedule in metastatic colorectal carcinoma: A
    Mid-Atlantic Oncology Program Study. J. Clin. Onc. 7:425-
    432, 1989.
35. Lokich J, Moore C: Chemotherapy-associated palmar-plantar
    erythrdysesthesia syndrome. Ann. Int. Med. 101:798-800,
    1984.
36. Lokich J, Ahlgren J, Gullo J et al: A prospective randomized
    study of continuous infusion 5-fluorouracil with or without
    weekly bolus cisplatin in metastatic colorectal carcinoma.
    In press.
37. Caudry M, Maire JP: Personal communication.
38. Hryniuk WM, Figueredo A, Goodyear M: Application of dose
    intensity to problems in chemotherapy of breast and colo-
    rectal cancer. Sem. Onc. 14:(Suppl. 4) 3-11, 1987.
39. Young RC: Mechanisms to improve chemotherapy effectiveness.
    Cancer 65:815-822, 1990.

23

PRECLINICAL ANTITUMOR EFFICACY OF TAXOTERE (RP56976, NSC 628503),
A TAXOL ANALOG AND OF RP60475 (NSC645008), A NEW BENZOPYRIDOINDOLE

Marie-Christine Bissery, Ph.D. and Francois Lavelle, Ph.D.

INTRODUCTION

Two compounds are currently being developed at Rhone-Poulenc Rorer. The first one, Taxotere, is a semisynthetic compound obtained using a precursor of natural origin. The second one, RP60475, is a synthetic compound representing a new family of antitumor agents.

In this short review, we present the preclinical activity of both compounds which are now undergoing clinical evaluation.

TAXOTERE

Taxotere [RP56976; NSC628503; N-debenzoyl-N-(tert-butoxycarbonyl)-10-deacetyltaxol, Figure 1] is a new semisynthetic taxol

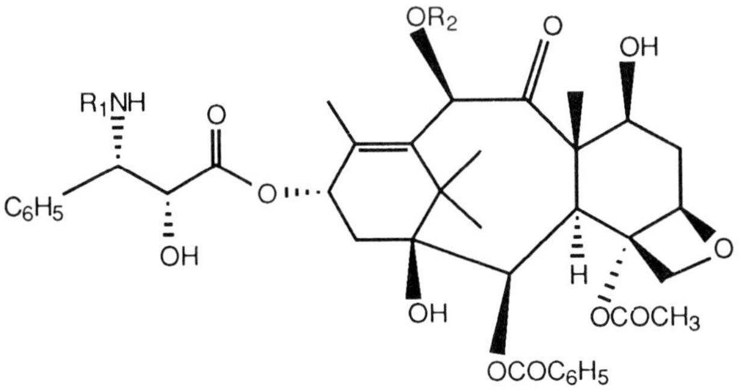

Taxotere : R_1 = -COOC(CH_3)_3 ; R_2 = H

Taxol : R_1 = -COC_6H_5 ; R_2 = -COCH_3

Figure 1. Structure of Taxotere

analog prepared at the Institut de Chimie des Substances Natur-
elles of the Centre National de la Recherche Scientifique (Gif sur
Yvette, France). It was obtained through partial synthesis using
a precursor 10-deacetylbaccatin III, which can be extracted from
needles of the European Yew, Taxus baccata (1,2,3). It was first
selected using a tubulin test (4). Taxotere was found to be the
most potent analog in inhibiting microtubule disassembly with an
ID_{50} of 0.2 μM (concentration of drug leading to 50% inhibition
of the rate of microtubule disassembly) (5). It was also found
the most cytotoxic analog _in vitro_ against P388 leukemic cells
with an IC_{50} of 0.13 μg/ml (concentration inhibiting 50% of the
cell proliferation) (5). In addition, Taxotere was found to be
more soluble than Taxol in the polysorbate 80/ethanol (V/V) solvent system (5). Therefore Taxotere was selected for preclinical
evaluation as a potential anticancer agent.

Taxotere was tested against transplantable tumors of mice
representing a variety of tissue types and behavior patterns
(6,7,8). The antitumor activity at optimal dosages is summarized
in Table 1 (9,10,11). Taxotere has a good spectrum of efficacy
in vivo against murine transplantable tumors. Eleven tumor models
were evaluated and 9 of them responded to intravenously administered Taxotere. The agent cured early stage SC colon 38 adenocarcinoma and pancreatic ductal adenocarcinoma 03. It was also found
very active by NCI standards against B16 melanoma, and colon adenocarcinoma 51. It was found active to a lesser extent against
Lewis lung carcinoma, Glasgow Osteogenic Sarcoma, IP P388 and
L1210 leukemias. Modest activity was found against colon carcinoma 26 with a treatment starting day 1, but colon 26 treated on
day 3 did not respond to Taxotere in separate experiments. The
agent was found inactive against M5076 sarcoma and MA 16/C adenocarcinoma. Finally, Taxotere was found schedule-independent
(10,11).

Because of its good preclinical activity, its unique mechanism of action, and the development of an efficient semisynthetic
process using a renewable source of natural chemical precursor,

TABLE 1

Summary of _In Vivo_ Antitumor Effects of Taxotere
in Mouse Transplantable Tumors at Optimal Dose

Tumor[a]	Schedule (days)	Optimal Total Dose mg/kg	T/C X 100	Score[b]	Log_{10} Cell Kill	Score[c] SRI
B16 (s.c./i.v.)	4,6,8,10	53.6	0	++	3.0	++++
C38 (s.c./i.v.)	3,5,7	70.5	0	++	TFS[d]	NA[e]
C51 (s.c./i.v.)	3,5,7	38.1	2	++	2.3	+++
C26 (s.c./i.v.)	1-4	20.0	33	+	-	-
PO3 (s.c./i.v.)	3,5,7,9	82.0	0	++	TFS	NA
3LL (s.c./i.v.)	3-7	116.0	6	++	1.2	++
MA 16/C (s.c./i.v.)	3,5,7	43.2	48	-	-	-
GOS (s.c./i.v.)	3-7	93.0	27	+	1.2	+
M5076 (s.c./i.v.)	3-7	43.0	51	-	-	-
P388 (i.p./i.v.)	1-4	92.8	155[f]	+	3.6	++
L1210 (i.p./i.v.)	1-4	86.8	170	++	4.2	++

[a] Tumor implantation site/Taxotere injection site
[b] NCI: National Cancer Institute score criteria
[c] SRI: Southern Research Institute score criteria

	NCI[b]		SRI[c]	
high activity			Solid Tumors	Leukemias
	++ < 10% T/C for s.c. tumors		++++ >2.8	6.0 - 7.5
	>150% T/C for L1210		+++ 2.0 - 2.8	4.5 - 5.4
	>175% T/C for P388		++ 1.3 - 1.9	3.0 - 4.4
active				
	+ 11.42% T/C for s.c. tumors		+ 0.7 - 1.2	1.5 - 2.9
	125-140% T/C for L1210			
	120-174% T/C for P388			
inactive				
	- > 42% T/C for s.c. tumors		- <0.7	<1.5
	<125% T/C for L1210			
	<120% T/C for P388			

[d] TFS: Tumor Free Survivors
[e] NA: Not Applicable
[f] T/C = 100 + ILS

Taxotere has entered Phase I clinical trials in both Europe and
the U.S.

RP60475

A series of substituted 5H-benzo[e]pyrido[4,3-b]indoles were
synthesized at the Institut Curie (Orsay, France) as candidate
antineoplastic agents (12,13). The compounds were evaluated both
in vitro and _in vivo_. One of the most active compounds in the

series was RP60475, 11-(3-dimethylaminopropyl-amino)-3-hydroxy-8-methyl-7H-benzo[e] pyrido[4,3-b] indole, dimethanesulfonate (NSC 645008) (Figure 2).

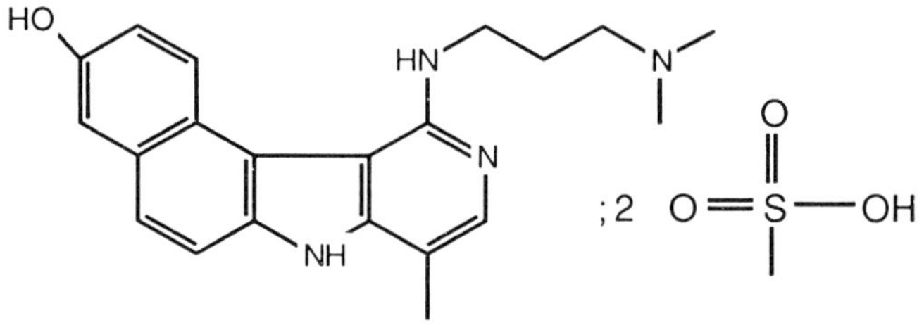

HO
HN
N
N
NH
;2   O = S — OH
O

Figure 2.   Structure of RP60475

This compound was found solid tumor selective _in vitro_ in the soft-agar-colony-formation disk-diffusion-assay (method described in Chapter 3) (12,13).   RP60475 was selectively cytotoxic for the two solid tumors tested, colon adenocarcinoma 38 and pancreatic ductal adenocarcinoma 03, as compared to L1210 leukemia (15 μg/disk:L1210 = 375 zu; C38 = 750 zu PO3 = 850 zu, 1 zu = 32.5 μm) (12).   It was also found to inhibit Topoisomerase II (13).

In vivo, RP60475 was tested against 11 transplantable tumors of mice characterized by different sensitivities to chemotherapeutic agents (6,7,8).   The results are summarized in Table 2 (14).   Clearly, RP60475, administered intravenously, has a broad spectrum of antitumor activity.   All the tumors evaluated responded to RP60475, nine of them being responsive at the Decision Network-2 level (T/C <10%), which is the level used by the NCI to justify further development.

Of interest, RP60475 meets most of the criteria listed by Corbett et al. for the advancement of a solid tumor active agent toward clinical development (Chapter 3).   RP60475 is solid tumor selective (Criteria #1).   It produces greater than a 2 log cell kill in two tumor systems from a single course of treatment, colon adenocarcinoma 38 and pancreatic ductal adenocarcinoma 03, the two _in vitro_ responsive tumors, and also in Mammary adenocarcinoma 16/C and in Glasgow Osteogenic sarcoma (Criteria #3).   It is

TABLE 2

Summary of In Vivo Antitumor Effects of Taxotere
in Mouse Transplantable Tumors at Optimal Dose

Tumor[a]	Schedule (days)	Optimal Total Dose mg/kg	Score[b] (NCI)
C38 (s.c./i.v.)	3-7,9	36.0	++
C51 (s.c./i.v.)	3-7	55.5	++
C26 (s.c./i.v.)	3-7	57.5	++
PO3 (s.c./i.v.)	3-7	93.0	++
MA16/C (s.c./i.v.)	3-7	53.4	++
MA14 (s.c./i.v.)	4-8	57.5	++
MA44 (s.c./i.v.)	3-7	43.2	+
GOS (s.c./i.v.)	6-11	72.0	++
3LL (s.c./i.v.)	3,5,7	65.1	+
P388 (i.p./i.v.)	1-4	92.4	++
L1210 (i.p./i.v.)	1-4	96.8	++

[a] Tumor Implantation site/RP 60475 injection site
[b] NCI: National Cancer Institute score criteria

high activity
++ < 10% T/C for s.c. tumors
>150% T/C for L1210
>175% T/C for P388

active
+ 11-42% T/C for s.c. tumors
125-149% T/C for L1210
120-174% T/C for P388

inactive
- > 42% T/C for s.c. tumors
<125% T/C for L1210
<120% T/C for P388

active at 2 non-toxic dosage levels in at least 3 tumor models,
with the drug administered at a different site than the tumor implantation site (Criteria #4). No long delayed lethality was
observed 150 days post tumor implantation. (Criteria # 5). In
addition, RP60475 is water soluble, it is stable in solution at
room temperature for more than 3 months, and the dosage levels
required for activity are well below the 1100 mg/kg rule (Table
2).

Criteria #2 (efficacy on human tumor xenografts) and Criteria
#6 (activity against a tumor with the multidrug resistant pheno-
type, are presently under evaluation.

RP60475 is entering Phase I clinical evaluation based on its broad spectrum of antitumor activity.

CONCLUSION

This brief account on the discovery of Taxotere and RP60475 is representative of some of the strategies used at Rhone-Poulenc Rorer for drug screening and preclinical evaluation, that will hopefully lead to clinically active anticancer agents.

ACKNOWLEDGEMENTS

The authors gratefully acknowledge the technical assistance of the staff of the Experimental Therapeutic Laboratory of the Oncology Department and Loretta Lisow for secretarial assistance.

REFERENCES

1. Colon M, Guenard D, Gueritte-Voegelein F, Potier P: Process for preparing derivatives of baccatin III and of 10-deacetyl baccatin III. US Patent N° 4924012, granted 5/8/1990.
2. Denis JN, Greene AE, Guenard D et al: A highly efficient, practical approach to natural taxol. J. Am. Chem. Soc. 110:5917-5919, 1988.
3. Mangatal L, Adeline MT, Guenard D et al: Application of the vicinal oxyamination reaction with asymmetric induction to the hemisynthesis of taxol and analogues. Tetrahedron 45:4177-4190, 1989.
4. Shelanski ML, Gaskin F, Cantor CR: Microtubule assembly in the absence of added nucleotides. Proc. Nat. Acad. Sci. 70:765-768, 1973.
5. Gueritte-Voegelein F, Guenard D, Lavelle F et al: Relationships between the structure of taxol analogues and their antimitotic activity. J. Med. Chem. 34:992-998, 1991.
6. Corbett TH, Leopold WR, Dykes DJ et al: Toxicity and anticancer activity of a new triazine antifolate (NSC 127755). Cancer Res. 42:1701-1715, 1982.
7. Corbett TH, Roberts BJ, Leopold WR et al: Induction and chemotherapeutic response of two transplantable ductal adenocarcinomas of the pancreas in C5781/6mice. Cancer Res. 44:717-726, 1984.
8. Geran RI, Greenberg NH, MacDonald MM et al: Protocols for screening chemical agents and natural products against animal tumors and other biological systems (third edition). Cancer Chemother. Rep. Part. 3:1-103, 1972.
9. Lavelle F, Fizames C, Gueritte-Voegelein F et al: Experimental properties of RP 56976, a Taxol derivative. Proc. AACR 30:2254, 1989.

10. Bissery MC, Bayssas M, Lavelle F. Preclinical evaluation of
    intravenous Taxotere (RP 56976, NSC 628503), a Taxol analog.
    Proc. AACR 31:417, 1990.
11. Bissery MC, Guenard D, Gueritte-Voegelein F, Lavelle F.
    Experimental antitumor activity of Taxotere (RP 56976, NSC
    628503), a Taxol Analog. Cancer Res. In Press, 1991.
12. Nguyen CH, Lhoste JM, Lavelle F et al: Synthesis and anti-
    tumor activity of 1-[(dialkylamino)alkyl] amino]-4-methyl-5H-
    pyrido [4,3-b]benzo-[e]- and -benzo[g])indoles. A new class
    of antineoplastic agents. J. Med. Chem. 33:1519-1528, 1990.
13. Lavelle F, Nguyen CH, Bissery MC et al: Structure-activity
    relationships in the pyrido-benzo-indole series, a new class
    of antitumor agents. Proc. AACR 31:417, 1990.
14. Bissery MC, Nguyen CH, Bisagni E, Lavelle F. Preclinical
    evaluation of RP 60475, a pyrido-benzo-indole antitumor
    agent. Proc. AACR 31:417, 1990.